Access Videos, Fitness Programs, and More!

Self-Study Companion Website resources included with any new book.

Access to MyFitnessLab, including assignments and eText, sold separately. To purchase access, visit www.mypearsonstore.com.

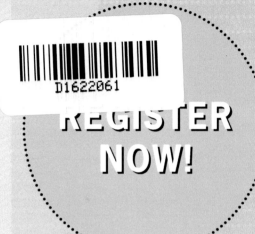

REGISTER NOW!

Registration will let you:

- **See It!** with exercise videos, lab demos, and *ABC News* videos.
- **Hear It!** with audio case studies and audio tutor sessions.
- **Do It!** with interactive labs.
- **Live It!** with customizable fitness programs.

Registration also gives you access to multiple practice quizzes, mobile apps, web links, and more.

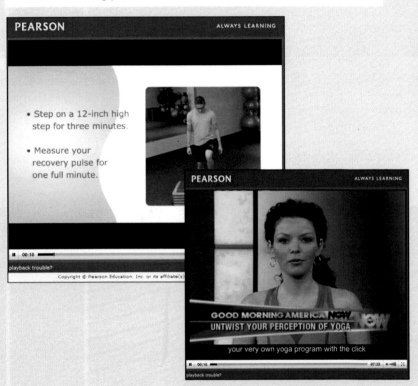

www.pearsonhighered.com/powers

TO REGISTER

1. Go to www.pearsonhighered.com/powers
2. Click on your book cover.
3. Select any chapter from the drop-down menu and click "Go."
4. Click "See It" and then click one of the video options.
5. Click "Register."
6. Follow the on-screen instructions to create your login name and password.

Your Access Code is:

USWPTW-SETUP-GOPAK-XYLAN-SOTUN-DALES *

Note: If there is no silver foil covering the access code, it may already have been redeemed, and therefore may no longer be valid. In that case, you can purchase access online using a major credit card or PayPal account. To do so, go to www.pearsonhighered.com/powers, follow steps 1–4 above, and click "Buy Access."

TO LOG IN

1. Go to www.pearsonhighered.com/powers
2. Click on your book cover.
3. Select any chapter from the drop-down menu and click "Go."
4. Click "See It" and then click one of the video options.
5. Enter your login name and password.

Hint:
Remember to bookmark the site after you log in.

Technical Support:
http://247pearsoned.custhelp.com

Stop!

Did you register? Don't miss out!

Turn back one page to register and get help preparing for exams... whenever and wherever you need it.

www.pearsonhighered.com/powers

PRE-COURSE/POST-COURSE ASSESSMENT

Name _____   Date(s): _____

As you complete the key fitness/wellness lab assessments in this course, record your results in the "Pre-Course Assessment" column. At the end of the course, re-do the labs, record your results in the "Post-Course Assessment" column, and see the progress you have made!

LAB	PRE-COURSE ASSESSMENT	POST-COURSE ASSESSMENT
Lab 2.3: Using a Pedometer to Count Your Steps	Average steps taken per day: _____	Average steps taken per day: _____
Lab 2.4: Identifying Barriers to Physical Activity	Barrier 1. Lack of time: _____ Barrier 2. Social and environmental influences: _____ Barrier 3. Lack of resources: _____ Barrier 4. Lack of motivation: _____	Barrier 1. Lack of time: _____ Barrier 2. Social and environmental influences: _____ Barrier 3. Lack of resources: _____ Barrier 4. Lack of motivation: _____
Lab 3.1: Measuring Cardiorespiratory Fitness	**1.5-mile run test** Finish time: _____ Fitness category: _____ **1-mile walk test** Finish time: _____ Fitness category: _____ **Submaximal cycle test** Heart rate: _____ Fitness category: _____ **3-minute step test** 1 minute recovery HR: _____ (bpm) Fitness category: _____	**1.5-mile run test** Finish time: _____ Fitness category: _____ **1-mile walk test** Finish time: _____ Fitness category: _____ **Submaximal cycle test** Heart rate: _____ Fitness category: _____ **3-minute step test** 1 minute recovery HR: _____ (bpm) Fitness category: _____
Lab 4.1: Evaluating Muscular Strength	**Chest press** 1 RM/BW ratio: _____ Fitness category: _____ **Leg press** 1 RM/BW ratio: _____ Fitness category: _____	**Chest press** 1 RM/BW ratio: _____ Fitness category: _____ **Leg press** 1 RM/BW ratio: _____ Fitness category: _____
Lab 4.4: Measuring Muscular Endurance	**Push-up assessment** Repetitions: _____ Category: _____ **Curl-up assessment** Repetitions: _____ Category: _____	**Push-up assessment** Repetitions: _____ Category: _____ **Curl-up assessment** Repetitions: _____ Category: _____
Lab 5.2: Assessing Flexibility	**Sit-and-reach test** Reach distance (centimeters): _____ Fitness category: _____ **Shoulder flexibility test** Left side reach distance (inches): _____ Fitness category: _____ Right side reach distance (inches): _____ Fitness category: _____	**Sit-and-reach test** Reach distance (centimeters): _____ Fitness category: _____ **Shoulder flexibility test** Left side reach distance (inches): _____ Fitness category: _____ Right side reach distance (inches): _____ Fitness category: _____
Lab 6.1: Assessing Body Composition	**Skinfold test** Sum of 3 skinfolds: _____ Percent body fat estimate: _____ Classification: _____ **Waist-to-hip ratio** Waist: _____ Hip: _____ Waist-to-hip ratio: _____ Disease risk classification: _____ **BMI** BMI: _____ kg/m^2 Weight classification: _____	**Skinfold test** Sum of 3 skinfolds: _____ Percent body fat estimate: _____ Classification: _____ **Waist-to-hip ratio** Waist: _____ Hip: _____ Waist-to-hip ratio: _____ Disease risk classification: _____ **BMI** BMI: _____ kg/m^2 Weight classification: _____
Lab 8.1: Analyzing Your Diet (Three-day nutrient summary from SuperTracker on ChooseMyPlate.gov)	Average total calories: _____ kcal Average calories from fat: _____ kcal Average protein intake: _____ gm Average carbohydrate intake: _____ gm Average fiber intake: _____ gm Average fat intake: _____ gm Average cholesterol intake: _____ mg Average sodium intake: _____ mg	Average total calories: _____ kcal Average calories from fat: _____ kcal Average protein intake: _____ gm Average carbohydrate intake: _____ gm Average fiber intake: _____ gm Average fat intake: _____ gm Average cholesterol intake: _____ mg Average sodium intake: _____ mg
Lab 9.1: Determining Ideal Body Weight	% body fat: _____ Weight: _____ lb BMI: _____ kg/m^2 Ideal weight: _____ kg	% body fat: _____ Weight: _____ lb BMI: _____ kg/m^2 Ideal weight: _____ kg
Lab 9.2: Estimating Daily Caloric Expenditure	Estimated calorie intake: _____ Estimated daily caloric expenditure: _____	Estimated calorie intake: _____ Estimated daily caloric expenditure: _____
Lab 10.2: Understanding Your Risk for Cardiovascular Disease	Family risk for CVD, total points: _____ Lifestyle risk for CVD, total points: _____ Additional risks for CVD, total points: _____	Family risk for CVD, total points: _____ Lifestyle risk for CVD, total points: _____ Additional risks for CVD, total points: _____
Lab 11.1: Stress Index Questionnaire	Number of Yes answers: _____ Stress category: _____	Number of Yes answers: _____ Stress category: _____
Lab 14.1: Determining Your Cancer Risk	Number of Yes answers: _____	Number of Yes answers: _____
Lab 15.1: Inventory of Attitudes and Behaviors toward Sexually Transmitted Infections	Number of True answers: _____ Number of False answers: _____ Risk level: _____	Number of True answers: _____ Number of False answers: _____ Risk level: _____
Lab 16.1: Alcohol Abuse Inventory	Number of Yes answers: _____ How risky is your alcohol use? _____	Number of Yes answers: _____ How risky is your alcohol use? _____

BEHAVIOR CHANGE CONTRACT

Choose a health behavior that you would like to change, starting this quarter or semester. Sign the contract at the bottom to affirm your commitment to making a healthy change and ask a friend to witness it.

My behavior change will be:

_____

My long-term goal for this behavior change is:

_____

Barriers that I must overcome to make this behavior change are (things that I am currently doing or situations that contribute to this behavior or make it hard to change):

1. _____

2. _____

3. _____

The strategies I will use to overcome these barriers are:

1. _____

2. _____

3. _____

Resources I will use to help me change this behavior include:

A friend/partner/relative _____

A school-based resource _____

A community-based resource _____

A book or reputable website _____

In order to make my goal more attainable, I have devised these short-term goals:

Short-term goal _____ Target date _____ Reward _____

Short-term goal _____ Target date _____ Reward _____

Short-term goal _____ Target date _____ Reward _____

When I make the long-term behavior change described above, my reward will be:

_____ Target date _____

I intend to make the behavior change described above. I will use the strategies and rewards to achieve the goals that will contribute to a healthy behavior change.

Signed _____ Date _____

Witness _____ Date _____

Coach Your Students Toward
Total Fitness & Wellness

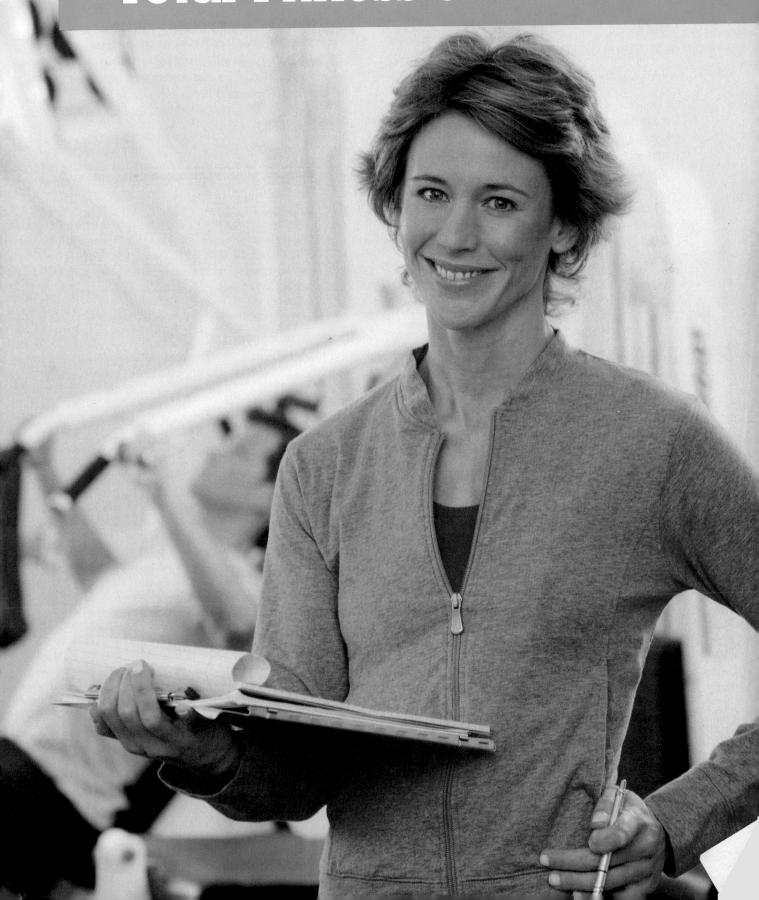

NEW!
Sample Fitness and Wellness Programs

These new and redesigned programs, appearing in chapters 1, 3–5, 7–8, and 11–12, offer easy-to-follow schedules to successfully reach fitness and wellness goals.

Customizable "pre-fab" programs and related tracking features on the book's website make it easy to jump into a fitness or wellness program and stick with it, with mobile phone access for training on the go.

New wellness programs set weekly wellness plans into motion for increasing general physical activity, improving nutrition, and managing stress. Gradual adjustments and built-in rewards and breaks make wellness goals realistic and attainable.

	Activity Time	Monday	Tuesday	Wednesday	Thursday	Friday	Saturday	Sunday
Week 1	Lunch Break		10 min walk		10 min walk		10 min walk	10 min walk
	Study Break	1 set of 25 crunches, 1 set of 15 push-ups, 1 set of 15 dips		1 set of 25 crunches, 1 set of 15 push-ups, 1 set of 15 dips		1 set of 25 crunches, 1 set of 15 push-ups, 1 set of 15 dips	10 min walk	10 min walk
Week 2	Lunch Break		15 min walk		15 min walk		15 min walk	15 min walk
	Study Break	1 set of 25 crunches, 1 set of 20 push-ups, 2 sets of 10 dips	15 min yoga DVD	1 set of 25 crunches, 1 set of 20 push-ups, 2 sets of 10 dips	15 min yoga DVD	1 set of 25 crunches, 1 set of 20 push-ups, 2 sets of 10 dips	15 min walk	15 min walk (morning) 15 min yoga DVD (afternoon)
Week 3	Lunch Break		15 min walk		15 min walk		20 min walk	20 min walk
	Study Break	2 sets of 25 crunches, 2 sets of 15 push-ups, 2 sets of 15 dips	20 min yoga DVD	2 sets of 25 crunches, 2 sets of 15 push-ups, 2 sets of 15 dips	20 min yoga DVD	2 sets of 25 crunches, 2 sets of 15 push-ups, 2 sets of 15 dips	20 min walk	20 min walk (morning) 20 min yoga DVD (afternoon)

Redesigned fitness programs are organized by week, with color coding and other textual features to distinguish intensity levels and activity days.

DENSE AND HARD-TO-READ
*Total Fitness & Wellness, **5th Edition***
▼

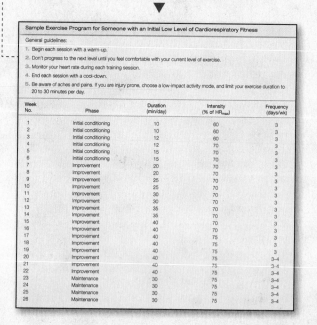

Sample Exercise Program for Someone with an Initial Low Level of Cardiorespiratory Fitness

General guidelines:
1. Begin each session with a warm-up.
2. Don't progress to the next level until you feel comfortable with your current level of exercise.
3. Monitor your heart rate during each training session.
4. End each session with a cool-down.
5. Be aware of aches and pains. If you are injury prone, choose a low-impact activity mode, and limit your exercise duration to 20 to 30 minutes per day.

Week No.	Phase	Duration (min/day)	Intensity (% of HRmax)	Frequency (days/wk)
1	Initial conditioning	10	60	3
2	Initial conditioning	10	60	3
3	Initial conditioning	12	60	3
4	Initial conditioning	12	70	3
5	Initial conditioning	15	70	3
6	Initial conditioning	15	70	3
7	Improvement	20	70	3
8	Improvement	20	70	3
9	Improvement	25	70	3
10	Improvement	25	70	3
11	Improvement	30	70	3
12	Improvement	30	70	3
13	Improvement	35	70	3
14	Improvement	35	70	3
15	Improvement	40	70	3
16	Improvement	40	70	3
17	Improvement	40	75	3
18	Improvement	40	75	3
19	Improvement	40	75	3
20	Improvement	40	75	3–4
21	Improvement	40	75	3–4
22	Improvement	40	75	3–4
23	Maintenance	30	75	3–4
24	Maintenance	30	75	3–4
25	Maintenance	30	75	3–4
26	Maintenance	30	75	3–4

CLEAR AND EASY-TO-FOLLOW
*Total Fitness & Wellness, **6th Edition***
▼

Beginner Cardiorespiratory Training Program

	Monday	Tuesday	Wednesday	Thursday	Friday	Saturday	Sunday
Initial Conditioning							
Week 1	10 min		10 min		10 min		
Week 2	10 min		10 min		10 min		
Week 3	12 min		12 min		12 min		
Week 4	12 min		12 min		12 min		
Week 5	15 min		15 min		15 min		
Week 6	15 min		15 min		15 min		
Improvement							
Week 7	20 min		20 min		20 min		
Week 8	20 min		20 min		20 min		
Week 9	25 min		25 min		25 min		
Week 10	25 min		25 min		25 min		
Week 11	30 min		30 min		30 min		
Week 12	30 min		30 min		30 min		
Week 13	35 min		35 min		35 min		
Week 14	35 min		35 min		35 min		
Week 15	40 min		40 min		40 min		
Week 16	40 min		40 min		40 min		
Week 17	40 min		40 min		40 min		
Week 18	40 min		40 min		40 min		
Maintenance							
Week 19	40 min		40 min		40 min		
Week 20	40 min		40 min		40 min		40 min	
Week 21	40 min		40 min		40 min		40 min	
Week 22	30 min		30 min		30 min		30 min	
Week 23	30 min		30 min		30 min		30 min	
Week 24	30 min		30 min		30 min		30 min	
Week 25	30 min		30 min		30 min		30 min	
Week 26	30 min		30 min		30 min		30 min	

Intensity Key
60% of HRmax
70% of HRmax
75% of HRmax

Chapter 7: Creating Your Total Fitness & Wellness Plan

The new chapter teaches students the fundamentals of putting together fitness and wellness programs. Students learn to successfully set goals, plan weekly routines, develop strategies to combat backsliding, and target behavior to modify for improved fitness and wellness.

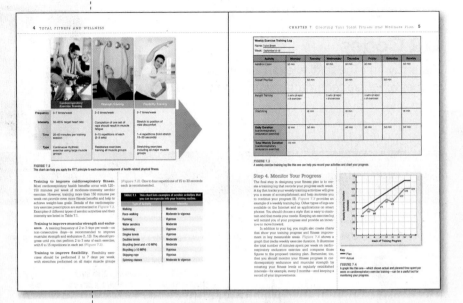

Coaching Corner

This feature box, appearing twice in every chapter, represents the "teacher's voice" in the text—giving students practical advice and tips on helpful strategies to put into action and giving hints or feedback on how to overcome fitness and wellness obstacles.

COACHING corner

Every step is necessary in the journey toward reaching your fitness and wellness goals. Sometimes, however, you may find yourself drifting from your original intentions. Consider the following questions as you continue to cement your commitment to a fitness and wellness program. You can discuss your answers with someone who might help hold you accountable for following your plan.

- What are the three most important reasons you have decided to commit to this plan?

- How do you know when your life is in or out of balance?

- On days you do not "feel" like following your plan, what are other options you can use that are "better than nothing at all"?

- Explain your plan and your goals to a close friend. Discuss how that person can best help you when you do not feel like following your plan.

3 reasons for my wellness plan . . .

COACHING YOUR STUDENTS
ON TODAY'S TECHNOLOGY

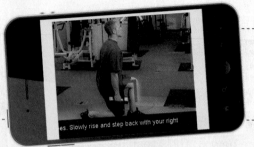

QR Codes

Instantly link the text to exercise videos demonstrating proper exercise techniques with new QR codes.

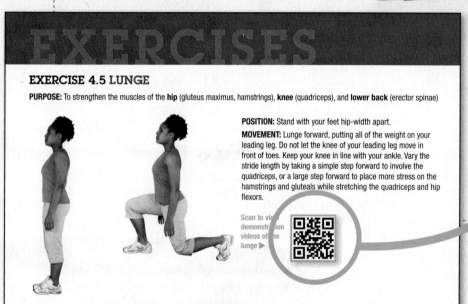

EXERCISES

EXERCISE 4.5 LUNGE

PURPOSE: To strengthen the muscles of the **hip** (gluteus maximus, hamstrings), **knee** (quadriceps), and **lower back** (erector spinae)

POSITION: Stand with your feet hip-width apart.

MOVEMENT: Lunge forward, putting all of the weight on your leading leg. Do not let the knee of your leading leg move in front of toes. Keep your knee in line with your ankle. Vary the stride length by taking a simple step forward to involve the quadriceps, or a large step forward to place more stress on the hamstrings and gluteals while stretching the quadriceps and hip flexors.

Scan to view demonstration videos of the lunge ▶

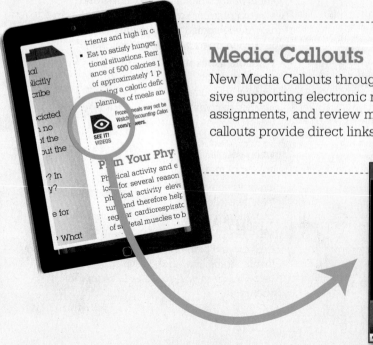

Media Callouts

New Media Callouts throughout the text direct students to extensive supporting electronic media, including videos, audio files, assignments, and review materials. In the eText version, media callouts provide direct links to the media resources.

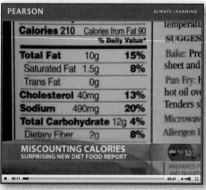

New timelines in the **Steps for Behavior Change** feature boxes present students with practical steps they can take to make immediate and lasting behavior change.

STEPS FOR BEHAVIOR CHANGE

Are you reluctant to strength train?

Answer the following questions to assess the barriers that prevent you from starting a strength-training program.

Y N

☐ ☐ I feel intimidated by other people in the strength-training facility.
☐ ☐ I cannot find time in my schedule to exercise.
☐ ☐ I do not know how to use the various machines or free weights.
☐ ☐ I do not know how to begin a strength-training program.

If you answered yes to more than one question, check out the following tips to help you break through the barriers.

TIPS TO EASE YOURSELF INTO A STRENGTH-TRAINING ROUTINE

Tomorrow, you will:

☑ Research the fitness facilities in your area. Fitness facilities cater to a wide range of clients, from beginners to professional body builders. Try to find one that is convenient, affordable, and contains enough of the basic equipment to meet your strength-training goals.

Within the next 2 weeks, you will:

☑ Join a fitness facility. After doing your research for a facility, join the one that meets the criteria above and also makes you feel welcome and comfortable.

☑ Take an orientation tour through the fitness facility to familiarize yourself with the machines and equipment.

☑ Consider hiring a personal trainer at the facility if you feel you need more individualized instruction. Most facilities have fitness professionals who will assess your overall strength and suggest a starting program.

By the end of the semester, you will:

☑ Make a commitment to set aside 30–60 minutes a day for training, and do not allow others to interfere with your personal time. Personal fitness does require a time commitment, but you are worth the investment.

A CLOSER LOOK

How Many "Friends" Do You Have?

Having a strong or large support network is typically associated with better stress management and mental health. But what is the effect if the social network is an online network? As more social networking websites have been developed, more and more adolescents and young adults are developing large online and text social networks. Does having a network of 500 or more "friends" really mean one has a stronger support network? Texting and the use of social networks are not necessarily problematic, but they can be for some. People use sites differently and for different reasons. How and why you choose to use these sites can affect the impact that use has on social relationships and health. It appears that extraverts use social network sites to enhance their social relationships and interactions, whereas introverts use them for social compensation. Studies also have shown that more time spent using social network sites is associated with depression, psychological distress, and lower self-esteem. Furthermore, some might experience increases in anxiety when the use of social networking sites is limited or stopped. So how do you know whether your texting or use of social network sites is problematic? If you have multiple "yes" answers to the following questions, you might want to re-evaluate your use of online social networking and texting.

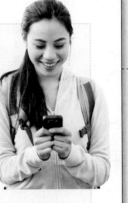

- Do you spend less time in face-to-face interactions than you do in online interactions? Or have your online "friends" replaced people in your life?
- Do you experience symptoms of stress or anxiety when you are unable to text, update your status, or interact using a social network site?
- Do you frequently text or use social network sites at times that are considered inappropriate (e.g., class, work, church, or on a date)?

- Do you compare your life to the lives of those in your network? Do you feel bad or inadequate when you make comparisons?
- Have your texting and social network habits had a negative impact on your relationships, grades, work performance, or any other aspect of your life?
- Does the time spent texting and using social network sites impact your time management?

Sources: Chou, H. T., and N. Edge. "They are happier and having better lives than I am": The impact of using Facebook on perceptions of others' lives. *Cyberpsychology, Behavior and Social Networking* 15(2):117–121, 2012; Durocher, J. J., Lufkin, K. M., M. E. King, and J. R. Carter. Social technology restriction alters state-anxiety but not autonomic activity in humans. *American Journal of Physiology: Regulatory, Integrative and Comparative Physiology* 301(6):R1773–1778, 2011; Kujath, C. L. Facebook and MySpace: Complement or substitute for face-to-face interaction? *Cyberpsychology, Behavior and Social Networking* 14(1–2):75–78, 2011; Kuss, D. J., and M. D. Griffiths. Online social networking and addiction: A review of the psychological literature. *International Journal of Environmental Research and Public Health* 8(9):3528–3552, 2011; Mango, A. M., T. Taylor, and P. M. Greenfield. Me and my 400 friends: The anatomy of college students' Facebook networks, their communication patterns, and well-being. *Developmental Psychology* 48(2):369–390, 2012; O'Dea, B., and A. Campbell. Online social networking amongst teens: Friend or foe? *Studies in Health Technology and Informatics* 167:133–138, 2011; Wilson, K., S. Fornasier, and K. M. White. Psychological predictors of young adults' use of social networking site. *Cyberpsychology, Behavior and Social Networking* 13(2):173–177, 2010.

A Closer Look feature boxes present relevant topics to address real-world issues and experiences.

A vibrant **redesign** makes the book look modern and approachable.

ADD AN ASSISTANT COACH TO YOUR LINEUP
WITH MyFitnessLab

MyFitnessLab
www.myfitnesslab.com

The new MyFitnessLab from Pearson has been designed and refined with a single purpose in mind: to help educators create that moment of understanding for their students. The MyFitnessLab system helps instructors maximize class time with customizable, easy-to-assign, and automatically graded assignments that motivate students to learn outside of class and arrive prepared for the lecture. By complementing your teaching with our engaging technology and content, you can be confident your students will arrive at that moment—the moment of true understanding.

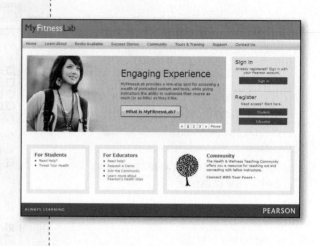

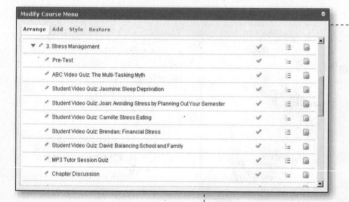

NEW!
Over 150 Pre-built Assignments

Instructors can lessen their prep time and simplify their lives with preloaded quiz and test questions (specific to the textbook) that they can assign and/or edit, a gradebook that automatically records student results from assigned tests, and the ability to customize the course as much (or as little) as desired.

Exercise Videos

More than 100 videos of exercises are available—allowing students access to additional instruction on their own time, and giving them the ability to exercise in the comfort of their own homes. Selected videos with assignable, gradable quiz questions make assigning homework on proper form, technique, and safety easy to do.

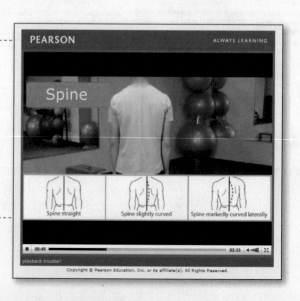

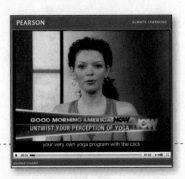

NEW! ABC News Videos

These videos bring fitness and wellness topics to life and are available on the Instructor Resource DVD, MyFitnessLab, and the Companion Website.

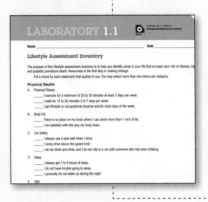

NEW!
Labs in Electronic Format

All labs are available online in interactive PDF format and are assignable through MyFitnessLab.

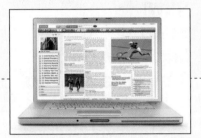

NEW!
Pearson eText

Students can access the text whenever and wherever they have access to the Internet. The powerful functionality of the eText includes the ability to create notes, highlight text in different colors, create bookmarks, zoom, click on hyperlinked words to view definitions, and view in single-page or two-page view.

Media callouts throughout the text provide direct links to the extensive supporting electronic media, including videos, audio files, assignments, and review materials.

Dedicated instructor and student support via Internet chat at http://247pearsoned.custhelp.com or the dedicated customer service line, 800-677-6337.

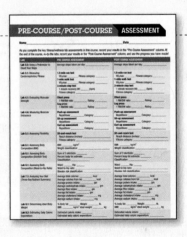

NEW!
Pre- and Post-Evaluations

You can now easily measure before and after results for both Student Learning Outcomes and Fitness Evaluations. A 50-question exam can be assigned at the start of the course, and again at the end, to effectively measure Student Learning Outcomes. Additionally, an editable version of the pre-/post-fitness assessment from the beginning of the book is available so students can track before and after results.

TOOLS TO HELP YOU
COACH BETTER

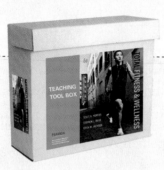

Teaching Tool Box

978-0-321-88424-4 • 0-321-88424-8

Save hours of valuable planning
time with one comprehensive
course planning kit. In one handy
box, adjuncts, part-time, and full-time faculty will find a wealth
of supplements and resources that reinforce key learning from
the text and suit virtually any teaching style.

The Teaching Tool Box includes:

- Instructor Resource DVD
- Instructor Resource and Support Manual and Test Bank
- *User's Quick Start Guide* reference guide
- Access to MyFitnessLab course management website
- *Great Ideas: Active Ways to Teach Health and Wellness*
- *Behavior Change Log Book and Wellness Journal*
- *Eat Right! Healthy Eating in College and Beyond*
- *Take Charge of Your Health!* Worksheets
- *Teaching with Student Learning Outcomes*
- *Teaching with Web 2.0*
- *Food Composition Table*

Student Supplements

MyFitnessLab
www.myfitnesslab.com

Behavior Change Log Book and Wellness Journal
978-0-321-80317-7 • 0-321-80317-5

Live Right! Beating Stress in College and Beyond
978-0-321-49149-7 • 0-321-49149-1

*Eat Right! Healthy Eating
in College and Beyond*
978-0-805-38288-4 • 0-805-38288-7

Take Charge of Your Health! Worksheets
978-0-321-49942-4 • 0-321-49942-5

Food Composition Table
978-0-321-66793-9 • 0-321-66793-X

Companion Website
www.pearsonhighered.com/powers

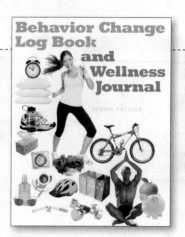

NEW!
Behavior Change Logbook and Wellness Journal

The Behavior Change Logbook
and Wellness Journal helps
students achieve a healthy
behavior change. This edition
has been revised to appear more
student-friendly, with more
intuitive navigation to match
the steps of the behavior change
project. Get started on making a
healthy behavior change today!

New to This Edition:

- New behavior change topics
- New evaluation section to
  assist with end-of-semester
  reports
- Expanded nutrition, weight
  management, and fitness
  sections
- Updated worksheets and journal prompts

TOTAL
Fitness &
Wellness

BRIEF EDITION

TOTAL
Fitness &
Wellness

FOURTH EDITION

Scott K. Powers
University of Florida

Stephen L. Dodd
University of Florida

Erica M. Jackson
Delaware State University

PEARSON

Boston   Columbus   Indianapolis   New York   San Francisco   Upper Saddle River
Amsterdam   Cape Town   Dubai   London   Madrid   Milan   Munich   Paris   Montréal   Toronto
Delhi   Mexico City   São Paulo   Sydney   Hong Kong   Seoul   Singapore   Taipei   Tokyo

Executive Editor: Sandra Lindelof
Associate Editor: Erin Schnair
Editorial Manager: Susan Malloy
Director of Development: Barbara Yien
Developmental Editor: Brent Goff
Editorial Assistant: Briana Verdugo
Assistant Media Producer: Sade McDougal
Senior Managing Editor: Deborah Cogan
Production Project Manager: Dorothy Cox
Production Management and Compositor:
   PreMediaGlobal

Cover and Interior Designer: Yvo Riezebos
Illustrator: Precision Graphics
Senior Photo Editor: Donna Kalal
Photo Researcher: Marta Johnson
Senior Manufacturing Buyer: Stacey Weinberger
Executive Marketing Manager: Neena Bali
Cover Photo Credit: Artiga Photo/Corbis (front);
   bloomua/Fotolia (back)

Credits and acknowledgments borrowed from other sources and reproduced, with permission, in this textbook appear on the appropriate page within the text and on page CR-1.

Website links are subject to change. Please visit this book's website at www.pearsonhighered.com/powers for updated links.

Library of Congress Cataloging-in-Publication Data

Powers, Scott K. (Scott Kline), 1950-
   Total fitness & wellness / Scott K. Powers, University of Florida, Stephen L. Dodd, University of Florida, Erica M. Jackson, Delaware State University.—Sixth edition.
     pages cm
   Includes bibliographical references and index.
   ISBN-13: 978-0-321-84052-3
   ISBN-10: 0-321-84052-6
   1. Physical fitness—Textbooks.   2. Health—Textbooks.   I. Dodd, Stephen L.   II. Jackson, Erica M.   III. Title.
   IV. Title: Total fitness and wellness.
   RA781.P66 2014
   613—dc23

                                        2012034980

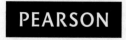

www.pearsonhighered.com

ISBN 10: 0-321-84052-6; ISBN 13: 978-0-321-84052-3 (Student Edition)
ISBN 10: 0-321-88366-7; ISBN 13: 978-0-321-88366-7 (Brief Edition)
ISBN 10: 0-321-86218-X; ISBN 13: 978-0-321-86218-1 (Exam Copy)
ISBN 10: 0-321-88480-9; ISBN 13: 978-0-321-88480-0 (à la Carte Edition)

To Jen, Haney, and Will. Your love and encouragement have always meant more than you will ever know.

—Stephen L. Dodd

To my mother, who encouraged me to pursue academic endeavors.

—Scott K. Powers

Brief Contents

Contents

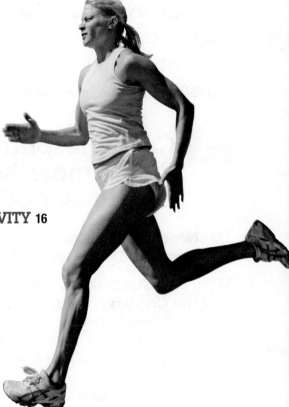

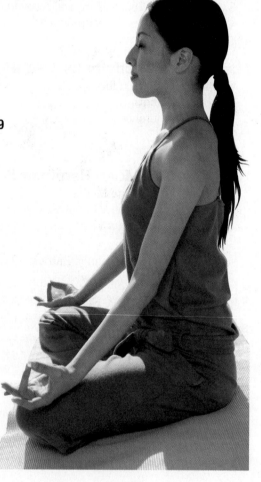

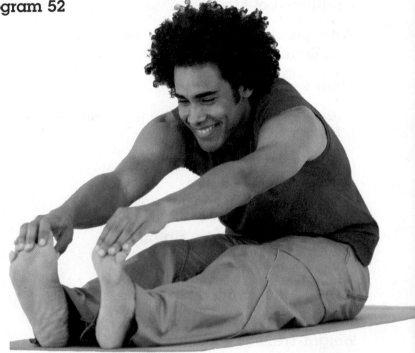

4 Improving Muscular Strength and Endurance 75

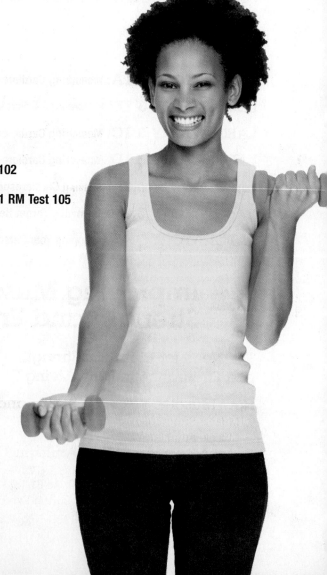

5 Improving Flexibility 113

6 Body Composition 143

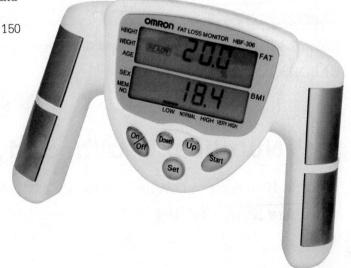

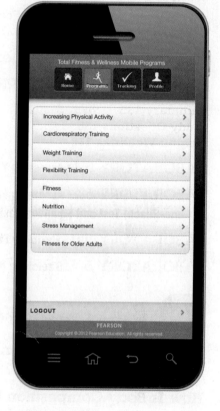

8 Nutrition, Health, and Fitness 191

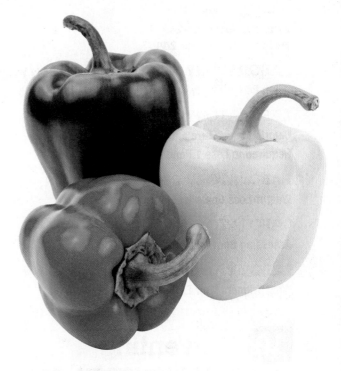

9 Exercise, Diet, and Weight Control 227

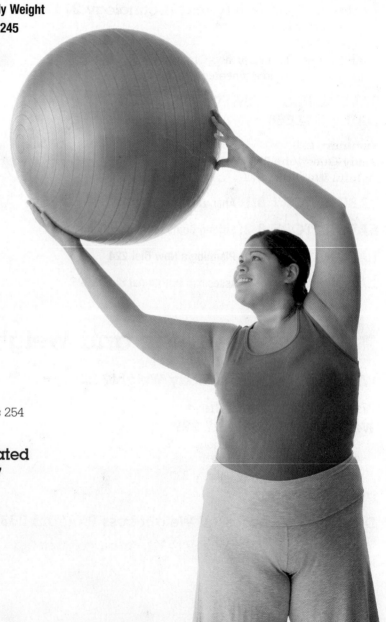

11 Stress Management 273

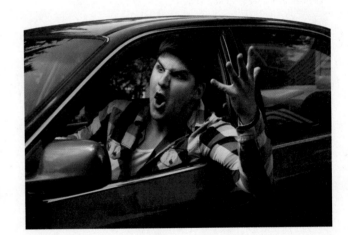

Feature Boxes

Labs and Programs

Videos with QR Codes

Preface

Good health is our most precious possession. Although we tend to appreciate it only in times of illness or injury, more and more of us are realizing that good health is not simply the absence of disease. Indeed, there are degrees of health, or wellness, and lifestyle can have a major impact on many of its components.

Intended for an introductory college course, *Total Fitness and Wellness, Brief Edition* focuses on helping students effect positive changes in their lifestyles, most notably in exercise and diet. The interaction of exercise and diet and the essential role of regular exercise and good nutrition in achieving total fitness and wellness are major themes of the text.

Total Fitness and Wellness, Brief Edition, Fourth Edition, was built on a strong foundation of both exercise physiology and nutrition. The text provides clear, objective, research-based information to college students during their first course in physical fitness and wellness. By offering a research-based text, we hope to dispel many myths associated with exercise, nutrition, weight loss, and wellness. In particular, we show students how to evaluate their own wellness level with respect to various wellness components, such as fitness level and nutritional status. Indeed, the title of the book reflects our goals.

Numerous physical fitness and wellness texts are available today. Our motivation in writing *Total Fitness and Wellness, Brief Edition,* Fourth Edition, was to create a unique, well-balanced physical fitness and wellness text that covers primary concepts of physical fitness and wellness and also addresses other important issues such as behavior change, stress management, and prevention of cardiovascular disease.

New to This Edition

- **Chapter 7, Creating Your Total Fitness and Wellness Plan,** provides students with practical, step-by-step instructions on developing both fitness and wellness plans.
- **Sample fitness and wellness programs** have been added throughout the text, offering easy-to-follow instructions for implementing successful fitness and wellness programs. Sample programs appear in Chapters 1, 3–5, 7–8, and 11. The programs are also available in a mobile format for training on the go.

- **New Coaching Corner feature boxes** give practical advice, tips, and strategies to put into action and offer hints on how to overcome fitness and wellness obstacles.
- **New QR codes** instantly link exercise photos in the text to videos demonstrating proper exercise techniques. Simply scan the QR codes in the book with your smartphone or tablet by following these easy instructions:
  1. Download a QR code reader from your app store, or use a built-in code reader if your device has one.
  2. Scan the code using the QR code reader.
  3. View content online. You will automatically be redirected to exclusive online extras. (*Note:* Data usage charges may apply.)
- **New media icons** direct students to the extensive supporting material available on the companion website, including assessments, online labs, and additional web content. In the eText versions, these callouts provide direct links to the media assets.
- **Steps for Behavior Change boxes** include new **specific timelines and goals** for completion.
- **A vibrant redesign** brands the book as both **contemporary** and **user friendly.** Chapter-opening photos have also been updated, graphs have been improved, and exercise photos have been silhouetted.
- **Content changes cover the latest research and statistics,** including objectives from *Healthy People 2020* and myplate.gov. **Updated coverage** includes current topics of student interest such as eating disorders, stress-management strategies, barefoot running, Pilates, diabetes and pre-diabetes, ergogenic dietary supplements, at-home fitness equipment, antioxidants, and emotional health.
- **MyFitnessLab** has been expanded to include more assignable, gradable content for every chapter. Instructors can now assign as many as six assignments per chapter—all with just a click of a button. Assigning and grading homework has never been easier!
- **Online labs have been improved** with clearer organization on the companion website and easier-to-use interactive PDFs that can be saved, printed, or e-mailed to an instructor.

Chapter-by-Chapter Revisions

Chapter 1 Understanding Fitness and Wellness

- Added a new Sample Program on increasing general physical activity.
- Revised and updated objectives for *Healthy People 2020*.
- Introduced SMART goals in behavior modification and in Lab 1.1.
- Included Lab 1.5 on evaluating fitness products (previously found elswhere in the book).
- Enhanced Figures 1.1, 1.2, 1.3, and 1.4, and added new photos.

Chapter 2 General Principles of Exercise for Health and Fitness

- Updated the Consumer Corner on how to choose the best exercise shoe.
- Added a new section on removing barriers to physical activity and Lab 2.4 on identifying barriers to physical activity.
- Added a new figure representing the FIT principle (Figure 2.5).
- Updated and enhanced Figures 2.2, 2.3, and 2.6, and added new photos.

Chapter 3 Cardiorespiratory Endurance: Assessment and Prescription

- Revised and improved the Sample Programs for cardiorespiratory training.
- Updated content on calculating target heart rate and heart rate classifications (Table 3.1).
- Added a new table on exercises and activities to improve cardiorespiratory fitness and the number of calories expended per 30-minute workout (Table 3.2).
- Added a new Closer Look on barefoot running.
- Reorganized Lab 3.4 to match the new Sample Program design and added a behavior modification assessment.
- Enhanced Figures 3.3, 3.5, 3.7, 3.8, and 3.9, and added new photos.

Chapter 4 Improving Muscular Strength and Endurance

- Revised the Sample Programs for muscular strength.
- Created a new figure with guidelines and precautions prior to beginning a strength-training program (Figure 4.9).
- Enhanced Figures 4.5, 4.7, and 4.8, and added new photos.

Chapter 5 Improving Flexibility

- Revised the Sample Programs for flexibility.
- Added a new section on preventing poor posture and Lab 5.1 on evaluating posture.
- Updated Table 5.1 on the top potential contributors to lower back pain along with sample stretches to maintain a healthy back.
- Created a new figure on avoiding hazardous exercises (Figure 5.5).

Chapter 6 Body Composition

- Revised and updated content on overweight and obesity in the United States, including updated statistics.
- Updated the description of bioelectrical impedance analysis.
- Revised the section on using body composition to determine your ideal body weight.
- Added a new body mass index figure (Figure 6.5).
- Updated and enhanced Figures 6.2, 6.3, and 6.6, and added new photos.

Chapter 7 Creating Your Total Fitness and Wellness Plan

- New! Chapter includes new content, figures, labs, and Sample Programs for planning fitness and wellness programs.
- Closer Look features on choosing a health-care provider and a glossary of medical specialists, previously found elsewhere in the book, are now integrated into the chapter.

Chapter 8 Nutrition, Health, and Fitness

- Added a Sample Program for nutritional planning.
- Revised and updated content on MyPlate to replace MyPyramid.

- Updated the section on the 2010 *Dietary Guidelines for Americans*.
- Added a new section on vegetarian diets.
- Integrated material on dietary reference intakes into the text.
- Added Table 8.5 with examples of low or nonfat alternatives to commonly eaten foods.
- Revised Table 8.6 to include the latest recommended dietary allowances of micronutrients.
- Enhanced Table 8.7 with improved diet suggestions for a college-aged female weighing 132 pounds.
- Revised Table 8.8 to reflect the latest classifications for nutritional supplements.
- Updated Lab 8.1 with recommendations for using the SuperTracker feature on ChooseMyPlate.gov.
- Updated Lab 8.3 with recommendations for using MyPlan SuperTracker.
- Added a new MyPlate graphic.
- Created a new figure on the influence of exercise intensity on fuel use (Figure 8.8).
- Updated and improved Figures 8.1, 8.2, 8.3, 8.5, and 8.7, and added new photos.

Chapter 9 Exercise, Diet, and Weight Control

- Updated obesity statistics throughout the chapter.
- Added new content on the genetic factors that contribute to obesity.
- Added a new Closer Look on facts and myths about popular diet plans.
- Added a new Closer Look on fructose and supplements.
- Revised Table 9.3 with updated myths and facts about weight loss.
- Added a new figure to visually compare energy expenditure and energy intake (Figure 9.1).
- Added a new figure with the social or environmental influences that result in overeating (Figure 9.3).
- Enhanced Figure 9.2, and added new photos.

Chapter 10 Preventing Cardiovascular Disease

- Included the latest data for the prevalence of cardiovascular disease in the United States.
- Revised the sections on cardiovascular disease risk factors.
- Added Figure 9.1 with projections of the increase in health-care cost of cardiovascular disease from 2010 to 2030.

- Enhanced Figures 10.5 and 10.6, and added new photos.

Chapter 11 Stress Management

- Added a new Sample Program for stress management.
- Updated the section on managing stressors.
- Created a new Closer Look on social networking.
- Enhanced Figures 11.2 and 11.3.

Text Features and Learning Aids

- **Thought-provoking chapter-opening quizzes** address common myths and misconceptions about fitness.
- **A fresh new design** throughout makes the text more accessible, engaging, and visually appealing than ever before.
- **Lab exercises** allow students to apply textual information to practical issues, encouraging the immediate development of healthy lifestyle choices and a core fitness plan.
- **New! Coaching Corner** boxes represent the "teacher's voice" throughout the text, offering helpful hints and strategies to overcome fitness and wellness obstacles.
- **A Closer Look** boxes give the reader insight into special topics such as low carb diets, road rage, muscle cramps, and anabolic steroids.
- **Consumer Corner** boxes teach students to be informed and discerning health and fitness consumers, guiding them to make the best fitness and wellness decisions in a market full of fads, gimmicks, and gadgets.
- **Appreciating Diversity** boxes present current health research, covering issues such as how the risk of cardiovascular disease varies across the United States and the search for obesity-related genes.
- **Steps for Behavior Change** boxes focus students on evaluating their own behaviors (e.g., Are you a fast food junkie? Are you reluctant to strength train?). New timelines present students with practical steps they can take to make meaningful behavior change.
- **Consider This!** grabs students' attention with surprising statistics and information, prompting them to pause and consider the long-term consequences of specific health behaviors.
- **End-of-chapter material** includes Chapter Summaries, Study Questions, and Weblinks. Suggested Readings and updated References appear in their own section at the end of the book.

Supplemental Materials

Available with *Total Fitness and Wellness, Brief Edition,* Fourth Edition, is a comprehensive set of ancillary materials designed to facilitate teaching and to enhance learning.

Instructor Supplements

MyFitnessLab

www.myfitnesslab.com

The new MyFitnessLab from Pearson has been designed and refined with a single purpose in mind: to help educators create that moment of understanding with their students. The MyFitnessLab system helps instructors maximize class time with customizable, easy-to-assign, and automatically graded assignments that motivate students to learn outside of class and arrive prepared for the lecture. By complementing your teaching with our engaging technology and content, you can be confident your students will arrive at that moment—the moment of true understanding.

In the Live It area:

- **New Sample Fitness and Wellness Programs** from the text help students commit to a new fitness or wellness routine. Links to exercise demonstrations and technique videos provide further guidance for students just getting started on a fitness or wellness program.
- **Behavior Change Logbook and Wellness Journal** is provided in interactive PDF format for easy assigning and submitting.
- *Take Charge of Your Health!* **worksheets** in interactive PDF format offer more options for self-assessment and developing behavior change plans.

In the Read It area:

- **New Pearson eText** gives students access to the text whenever and wherever they have access to the Internet. Pearson eText pages look exactly like the printed text and offer powerful new functionality for students and instructors. Users can create notes, highlight text in different colors, create bookmarks, zoom, click on hyperlinked words and phrases to view definitions, and view in single-page or two-page view.
- **New RSS feeds,** provided by various news sources, give students easy online access to hot health topics such as Zumba, multivitamins, carb diets, etc., which are updated daily.
- Within the eText, **new media icons** (See It! Do It!, etc.) link directly to supporting material in MyFitnessLab, including videos, assessments, online labs, and additional web content.

In the See It area:

- **More than 100 exercise videos** demonstrate strength training and flexibility exercises with resistance bands, stability balls, free weights, and gym machines. The exercise videos are also available for download onto iPods or media players.
- **Over 30 ABC News video clips** bring fitness and wellness topics to life. Related quizzing is available for assigning and automatic grading.

In the Hear It area:

- **New Audio/Visual Student Reviews** pertaining to each chapter's content support classroom lectures and enhance self-study options. Short quizzes are available for assigning and automatic grading.
- **Audio case studies** challenge students to make conclusions about what they have just heard, helping students see the relevance to their own lives.

In the Do It area:

- **Pre-course/post-course assessment** lets students evaluate their own fitness and wellness status both before and after taking the course.
- **New interactive labs** are available online to students, allowing them to assess their levels of fitness and wellness, learn core skills, and develop behavior change plans to track their progress. Students can easily complete the labs and e-mail them to you directly—eliminating the need for paper entirely.

In the Review It area:

- **Multiple-choice and true/false Practice Quizzes** for every chapter are automatically graded, so students can get feedback on their work and check their understanding of the material.
- **Online glossary** is a quick and easy resource for students to locate definitions for the terms they don't know.
- **Interactive flashcards** allow students to build a deck of flashcards from the key terms in every chapter, review them online, print them out to review, or even export them to their mobile phone.

Teaching Toolbox

Save hours of valuable planning time with one comprehensive course planning kit. In one handy box, adjuncts, part-time, and full-time faculty will find a wealth of supplements and resources that reinforce key learning from the text and suit virtually any teaching style. The Teaching Tool Box includes:

- **Instructor Resource DVD** with all art, photos, and tables from the text; PowerPoint lecture slides; a computerized Test Bank; ABC News videos; exercise demonstration videos; Active Lecture (clicker) Questions; Quiz Show Game PowerPoint slides; PDF transparency masters; and Test Bank Word files.

- **Instructor Resource and Support Manual and Test Bank** with detailed chapter outlines incorporating IRDVD assets, in-class discussion questions, and activities, additional resources, first-time teaching tips, sample syllabi, and tips for using MyFitnessLab. The Test Bank includes over 1000 questions in multiple-choice, true/false, and short-essay formats.

- **User's Quick Start Guide** for getting up and running using the materials in the Teaching Tool Box.

- **MyFitnessLab Access Kit** with more than 150 separate assignments, a gradebook, and an annotatable eText.

- **Great Ideas: Active Ways to Teach Health and Wellness,** a manual of ideas for classroom activities that can be adapted to various topics and class sizes.

- **Teaching with Student Learning Outcomes** publication containing useful suggestions and examples for successfully incorporating outcomes into a fitness and wellness course.

- **New Teaching with Web 2.0** handbook introducing popular new online tools and offering ideas for incorporating them into a fitness and wellness course.

- **Behavior Change Logbook with Wellness Journal,** newly revised to include updated worksheets, nutrition information, journals, and fitness logs.

- **New Food Composition Table** containing detailed nutrition information about thousands of foods.

- **Live Right! Beating Stress in College and Beyond** booklet on handling life's challenges including sleep, finances, time management, academic pressure, and relationships.

- **Eat Right! Healthy Eating in College and Beyond** booklet of guidelines, tips, and recipes for healthy eating.

- **Take Charge of Your Health!** self-assessment worksheets.

Student Supplements

MyFitnessLab

www.myfitnesslab.com

This online course management system has been redesigned for greater usability and is loaded with valuable resources, including preloaded content for online or hybrid courses. See the full descripion of assets under the Instructor Supplements above.

Companion Website

www.pearsonhighered.com/powers

The *Total Fitness and Wellness* companion website has been extensively updated and reorganized in the same manner as MyFitnessLab to help make learning fun. Students can access a Behavior Change Planner that guides them from assessment through behavior change evaluation (Live It); view ABC News video clips and more than 80 new demonstration exercise videos (See It); listen to MP3s (Hear It); check out RSS feeds of fitness- and health-related news stories (Read It); fill in electronic versions of labs, self-assessments, and pre- and post-course fitness assessments (Do It); and take practice quizzes as well as download flashcards to their mobile phone (Review It).

Behavior Change Log Book and Wellness Journal

978-0-8053-7844-3 / 0-8053-7844-8

This booklet helps students track their daily exercise and nutritional intake and create a personalized long-term nutrition and fitness program. It has been newly revised to include updated worksheets, nutrition information, and fitness logs.

Live Right! Beating Stress in College and Beyond

978-0-321-49149-7 / 0-321-49149-1

This full-color booklet offers useful tips and practical suggestions for coping with a variety of life's challenges or preventing stress. Topics include improving sleep, managing finances, coping with academic pressure, and developing healthy relationships.

Eat Right! Healthy Eating in College and Beyond

978-0-8053-8288-4 / 0-8053-8288-7

This handy, full-color booklet provides practical guidelines, tips, shopper's guides, and recipes for putting healthy eating principles into action. Topics include healthy eating in the cafeteria, dorm room, and fast food restaurants; eating on a budget; weight management tips; vegetarian alternatives; and guidelines on alcohol and health.

Take Charge of Your Health! Worksheets

978-0-321-49942-4 / 0-321-49942-5

Twelve new worksheets have been added to this edition's collection of self-assessment actvities, providing a total of 50 self-assessment exercises in a pad that can be packaged with the text.

New Lifestyles Pedometer

978-0-321-51803-3 / 0-321-51803-9

Take strides to better health with this pedometer, a first step toward overall health and wellness. This pedometer measures steps, distance (miles), activity time, and calories, and provides a time clock.

MyDietAnalysis

MyDietAnalysis, developed by the nutrition database experts at ESHA Research, Inc., offers an accurate, reliable, and easy-to-use program with nearly 20,000 foods and multiple reports. The program allows students to track their diet and activity for up to three profiles and to assess the nutritional value of their food composition.

Food Composition Table

978-0-321-66793-9 / 0-321-66793-X

This comprehensive booklet provides detailed nutritional information on thousads of foods and is correlated with MyDietAnalysis.

Acknowledgments

First and foremost, this edition of *Total Fitness and Wellness, Brief Edition* reflects the valuable feedback provided by many people throughout the country. As always, this edition could not have been completed without the work of an enormous number of people at Pearson. From the campus sales representatives to the president of the company, they are truly first rate, and our interaction with them is always delightful.

There were several key people in the process. Our Acquisitions Editor, Sandra Lindelof, has been the primary force behind assembling the team and directing the process, and her input has been invaluable. Several new additions to the team have been important in both the revisions of the text and the production process. In particular, the authors would like to thank Erin Schnair for significant contributions to this fourth edition. Moreover, special thanks go to Susan Malloy, who offered valuable input during the revision process, and to Brent Goff, who served as a development editor for the addition of a new chapter. Dorothy Cox served as Production Supervisor and has expertly guided the manuscript through each stage of production. Other specific duties were expertly handled by the following professionals; we offer them our utmost appreciation for their efforts: Neena Bali, Executive Marketing Manager; Sade McDougal, Assistant Media Producer; Briana Verdugo, Editorial Assistant; Deborah Cogan, Senior Managing Editor; Tracy Duff of PreMediaGlobal, Senior Project Manager; Marta Johnson, Photo Researcher; and Yvo Riezebos, Cover and Text Designer.

Claire Alexander, Molly Ward, Cathy Nolan (Moraine Valley Community College), Mary Winfrey-Kovell (Ball State University), and John Kowalczyk (Walden University) have made major contributions to the ancillaries, and Kurt Sollanek has made major contributions to the book content. Also, thanks go to Amanda Salyer-Funk for her contribution to the new Coaching Corner feature boxes.

Finally, there is a long list of professionals whose reviews of the text's content and style or participation in a fitness and wellness forum have helped to shape this book. We owe these individuals a tremendous debt of gratitude:

Ezzeldin Aly, *Graceland University*
Kym Atwood, *University of West Florida*
Stephen Ball, *University of Missouri*
Angela Cress, *Southwestern Illinois College*
Mandi Dupain, *Millersville University*
Michael Dupper, *University of Mississippi*
Robert Femat, *El Paso Community College*
Megan Franks, *Lone Star College*
Jennifer Gordon, *Springfield Technical Community College*
Ken Grace, *Chabot College*
Kirkland Hall, *University of Maryland Eastern Shore*
Tim Hilliard, *Fitchburg State University*
Elizabeth Howley, *James Madison University*
Josiah Johnson, *San Antonio College*
Mary Kemp, *Carroll Community College*
Gary Ladd, *Southwestern Illinois College*
Angela Baldwin, *Lanier Berry College*
Rosemary Lindle, *University of Maryland*
Mike Manning, *Indiana Wesleyan University*
Kathleen Meyer, *Clemson University*
Kris Moline, *Lourdes University*
Miguel Narvaez, *Saint Bonaventure University*
Lori Patten, *St. Cloud State University*
Charles J. Pelitera, *Canisius College*
Mary Jo Saunders, *James Madison University*
Robin Siara, *Rio Hondo Community College*
Jennifer Spry-Knutson, *Des Moines Area Community College*
Susan M. Tendy, *United States Military Academy*
Mary Winfrey-Kovell, *Ball State University*

Many thanks to all!

Scott K. Powers
University of Florida

Stephen L. Dodd
University of Florida

Erica M. Jackson
Delaware State University

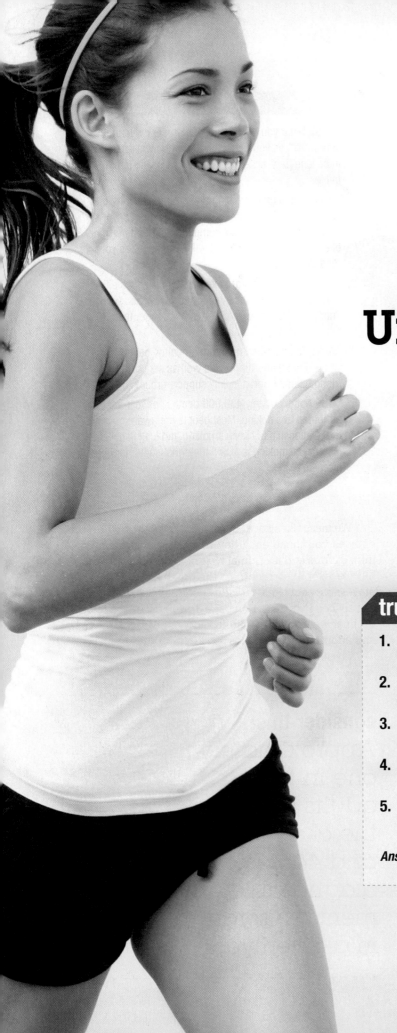

Understanding Fitness and Wellness

true or false?

1. Your **physical activity** as a college student has no effect on your health later in life.
2. You definitely have a high level of **wellness** if you exercise and eat a healthy diet.
3. As little as 30 minutes of **brisk walking** most days of the week can improve your health.
4. Most people do not need help to make a health **behavior change**.
5. **Smoking** is the leading cause of preventable death in the United States.

Answers appear on the next page.

Maria is a college freshman who is away from home for the first time and starting to gain a little weight. In high school, Maria had been active with after-school sports, and her mother kept healthy food around the house and cooked meals for the family. After soccer or softball practice, Maria would go home, have dinner with her family, and study. Since coming to college, Maria has not been involved in sports and rarely finds time to go to the gym. Her eating habits are erratic, and she's spending more time partying with her friends, forgoing much study and sleep time in the process. Like many college students, Maria is excited to be away from home and "on her own," but she is a little overwhelmed by all of the choices she now has to make about what to eat and how to spend her time.

Do you relate to Maria? Are you less physically active now than when you were in high school? Has your diet changed for the worse since you've assumed control of what you eat? Do you think your level of wellness is better or worse than when you left home?

In this book, you will learn about behaviors that can put you on the path to optimal wellness. In this first chapter, we present the concept of wellness, discuss the health benefits of exercise, and outline the major components of physical fitness. Understanding the role that exercise plays in your own health and wellness can help motivate you to sustain a lifetime of physical fitness.

What Is Wellness?

Not so long ago, *good health* was defined as the absence of disease. But then, in the 1970s and 1980s, many exercise scientists and health educators became dissatisfied with this limited definition. These visionary health professionals believed that health includes physical fitness and emotional and spiritual health as well. Their revised concept of good health is called **wellness** (1). You can achieve a state of wellness by practicing a healthy lifestyle that includes regular physical activity, proper nutrition, eliminating unhealthy behaviors (that is, avoiding high-risk activities such as reckless driving, smoking, and drug use), and maintaining good emotional and spiritual health (1). Let's discuss the components of wellness, and what it means to enjoy a healthy lifestyle, in more depth now.

Six Components of Wellness

To enjoy an optimal state of wellness, you need to achieve physical, emotional, intellectual, spiritual, social, and environmental health. Do you get regular physical and dental exams? Do you stay close to and communicate with friends and family? Do you recycle? These choices and habits can all contribute to a healthy lifestyle, and they all fall under the components of wellness.

answers

1. **FALSE** What you do as a college student will affect your health as you get older. Students who are active in college have lower risk for heart disease later in life.
2. **FALSE** Although exercising and eating a healthy diet are very positive wellness habits, they don't cover everything. There are six components that determine overall wellness, which you will learn about as you read this chapter.
3. **TRUE** Regular moderate exercise can produce a lot of health benefits. However, for certain goals, such as improving fitness, you will have to do more than 30 minutes of moderate activity.
4. **FALSE** To adopt and maintain a healthy behavior, you will need information, as well as support from friends, family, and possibly support groups.
5. **TRUE** Approximately 430,000 deaths per year are attributed to smoking. Most people are aware of the relationship between smoking and lung cancer. Moreover, smoking is also a major risk factor for heart disease.

Wellness is also a dynamic concept in that the choices you make each day move you along a continuum. At one end is optimal well-being associated with a high level of functioning. At the other end is a low level of wellness that likely includes poor physical and mental health (see **Figure 1.1** on page 3). You can move toward optimal well-being by eliminating unhealthy behaviors and adopting healthy ones.

consider this!

Approximately one in four adults between the ages of 18 and 44 has a diagnosable mental disorder in a given year.

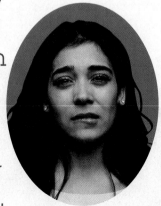

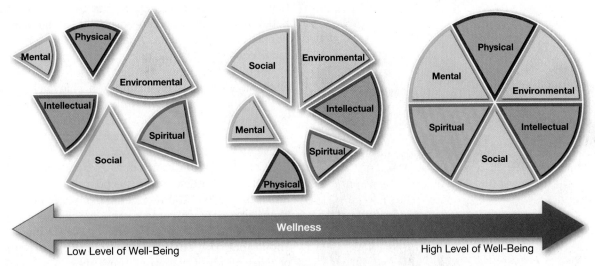

FIGURE 1.1
When the wellness components are well integrated and working together, you can enjoy the benefit of optimal well-being.

Physical Health   Physical health refers to all the behaviors that keep your body healthy. One of the key aspects of maintaining a healthy body is physical fitness. Physical fitness can have a positive effect on your health by reducing your risk of disease and improving your quality of life. Getting proper nutrition, performing self-exams, and practicing personal safety are other important physical health behaviors.

Emotional Health   Emotions play an important role in how you feel about yourself and others. Emotional health (also called mental health) includes your social skills and interpersonal relationships. Your level of self-esteem and your ability to cope with the routine stress of daily living also are aspects of emotional health.

   The cornerstone of emotional health is emotional stability, which describes how well you deal with the day-to-day stresses of personal interactions and the physical environment. Most people are well equipped to handle life's ups and downs, but inability to handle everyday situations can lead to poor emotional health or mental health disorders, such as depression and anxiety disorders, in many people. In fact, mental disorders are the leading cause of disability for people aged 15–44 years (2). Emotional wellness means being able to respond to life situations in an appropriate manner and not remaining in extreme high or low emotional states.

Intellectual Health   You can maintain intellectual health by keeping your mind active through life-long learning. College is the ideal place to develop this wellness component, partly because it exposes you to new ideas and ways of thinking about life. Attending lectures, engaging in thoughtful discussions with friends

or teachers, and reading are excellent ways to promote intellectual health. Maintaining good intellectual health can also increase your ability to define and solve problems, and continuous learning and thinking can provide you with a sense of fulfillment. Take advantage of opportunities to broaden your mind. Listen to audio books in the car, keep up with current events by watching the news or reading it online, and do not shy away from friendly debate.

Spiritual Health   The term *spiritual* means different things to different people. Most definitions of spiritual health include having a sense of meaning and purpose. Many people define spiritual health according to their religious beliefs, but it is not limited to religion. People may also find meaning in helping others and being altruistic, through prayer, or enjoying the beauty of nature. Whether you define spiritual health as religious beliefs or the establishment of personal values, it is an important aspect of wellness, is closely linked to emotional health, and also influences physical health (3).

   Optimal spiritual health includes the ability to understand your basic purpose in life; to experience love, joy, pain, peace, and sorrow; and to care for and respect all living things. Anyone who has experienced a

wellness The state of healthy living achieved by the practice of a healthy lifestyle, which includes regular physical activity, proper nutrition, eliminating unhealthy behaviors, and maintaining good emotional and spiritual health.

(e.g., asthma). Drinking water that has been contaminated with harmful bacteria can lead to infection, and drinking water that contains carcinogens (cancer-producing agents) increases the risk of certain types of cancers.

Your environment can also have a positive influence on wellness. For example, a safe environment evokes feelings of comfort and security, which impact your emotional health. Moreover, if your environment is safe, you are more likely to spend time outside being active and improving your physical health.

Our relationship with our environment is a two-way street. We discussed the positive and negative impacts the environment can have on our health. Now, let's discuss some examples of how people's behaviors might influence the environment. Think about your own behaviors: Do you recycle regularly, or does much of your trash end up in a landfill? Do you carpool or take public transportation when you can, or are you leaving a large carbon footprint? Achieving total wellness requires learning about the environment and protecting yourself against environmental hazards that threaten your health and well-being, as well as being aware of your impact on the environment.

HEAR IT!
CASE STUDY
How can Omar connect his physical, mental, and spiritual health? Listen to the online case study at www.pearsonhighered.com/powers.

Interaction of Wellness Components

None of the components of wellness works in isolation; in fact, all six work closely together. For example, people with an anxiety or depressive disorder who also have a chronic physical illness report more physical symptoms than those who do not have a mental health disorder (4). Also, strong spirituality is associated with lower rates of mental disorders, better immune function, and greater participation in health-promoting behaviors (3, 5). Although the wellness components are interrelated, practicing healthy behaviors related to one aspect of wellness is not a guarantee of a high level of total wellness. Rather, total wellness is achieved through a balance of physical, intellectual, social, emotional, spiritual, and environmental health.

LIVE IT!
ASSESS YOURSELF
Assess your behavior with the *Health Behavior Self-Assessment* Take Charge Of Your Health! Worksheet online at **www.pearsonhighered.com/powers**.

MAKE SURE YOU KNOW...

- *Wellness* is defined as a state of optimal health achieved by living a healthy lifestyle.

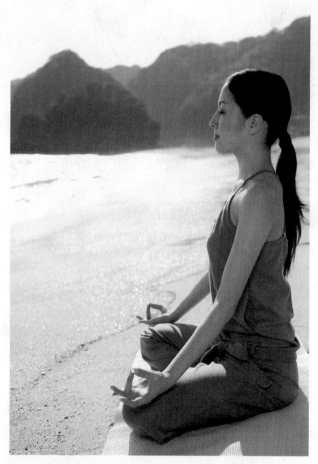

Meditating or spending time outdoors can help you improve spiritual health.

beautiful sunset or smelled the first scents of spring can appreciate the pleasure of maintaining optimal spiritual health.

Social Health Social health is the development and maintenance of meaningful interpersonal relationships. The result is the creation of a support network of friends and family. Good social health helps you feel confident in social interactions and provides you with emotional security. It is not necessarily the number of people in your support network, but the quality of those relationships that is important. Developing strong communication skills is one behavior that is crucial for maintaining a strong social network.

Environmental Health Environmental health includes the influence of the environment on your health, as well as your behaviors that affect the condition of the environment. Our environment can have a positive or negative impact on our total wellness. For example, air pollution and water contamination are two important environmental factors that can harm physical health. Breathing polluted air can lead to a variety of respiratory disorders

Wellness Issues across the Population

Your behaviors have a significant impact on your level of health and wellness. However, there are factors beyond your control that contribute to your wellness and your risk for certain chronic diseases and conditions. Ethnicity, sex, age, family history, and socioeconomic status affect your risk of developing diabetes, cancer, cardiovascular disease, obesity, and other conditions.

For example, black Americans have a higher risk of developing hypertension (high blood pressure) compared to the U.S. population as a whole. Similarly, diabetes is more common in Native Americans and Latinos than in people from other ethnic backgrounds. Further, men and women differ in their risk for heart disease, osteoporosis, and certain types of cancer.

Aging also can affect the ability to achieve wellness. For instance, the risk of chronic diseases (e.g., heart disease and cancer) increases with age. Finally, people of low socioeconomic status often have less access to quality health care and experience higher rates of obesity, heart disease, and drug abuse. The goal for everyone is to achieve optimal wellness, but individual and demographic differences can present special challenges in achieving wellness. This important issue will be discussed throughout this book.

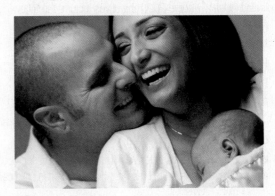

- There are six interacting components of wellness: physical health, emotional health, intellectual health, spiritual health, social health, and environmental health.

Wellness Goals for the Nation

All countries, including the United States, have a vested interest in having a healthy population. A nation of unhealthy people drains national resources by reducing worker productivity and increasing the amount of money the government has to spend on health care. To improve the overall well-being of Americans, the U.S. government has established a set of wellness goals known as *Healthy People*.

The *Healthy People* initiative seeks to prevent unnecessary disease and improve the quality of life for all Americans. The wellness goals were first presented in *Healthy People* reports published in 1980 and have since been revised every 10 years based on the progress toward meeting the objectives. Each report includes a broad range of health and wellness objectives based on 10-year agendas. *Healthy People 2020* is the current set of goals for the nation. The overarching goals are to attain high-quality, longer lives free of preventable disease, injury, and premature death; to achieve health equity, eliminate disparities, and improve the health of all groups (see the Appreciating Diversity box above); to create social and physical environments that promote good health for all; and to promote quality of life, healthy development, and healthy behaviors across all life stages. For more details on the current goals and objectives of *Healthy People 2020,* see the Closer Look box on page 6, or visit www.healthypeople.gov.

MAKE SURE YOU **KNOW...**

- *Healthy People* is a set of wellness goals set by the U.S. government for the American people.
- The main goals of *Healthy People 2020* are to attain high-quality, longer lives free of preventable disease, injury, and premature death; to achieve health equity, eliminate disparities, and improve the health of all groups; to create social and physical environments that promote good health for all; and to promote quality of life, healthy development, and healthy behaviors across all life stages.

Assess your health with the *Multidimensional Health Locus of Control* Take Charge Of Your Health! Worksheet online at **www.pearsonhighered.com/powers.**

LIVE IT!
ASSESS
YOURSELF

What Is Exercise, and Why Should I Do It?

When you hear the word *exercise,* do you picture someone in a gym running on a treadmill? Or do you imagine hiking up a scenic mountain with a group of friends? Actually, both activities can be exercise, and both are good for your health. In fact, there are numerous fun and interesting ways to exercise. So if going to the gym is not your thing, there are many other ways you can be active and improve your health. One part of designing your personal fitness program is to find out what works best for *you.*

Understanding *Healthy People 2020*

Government agencies and public health professionals have recently developed the *Healthy People 2020* objectives needed to meet the new overreaching goals for the nation. They will collect data to chart our progress on meeting the new goals. Selected *Healthy People 2020* objectives include the following:

- Reduce the proportion of adults who engage in no leisure-time activity.
- Reduce the female breast cancer death rate.
- Reduce the prostate cancer death rate.
- Reduce the melanoma death rate.
- Increase the proportion of physician office visits that include counseling or education related to nutrition or weight.
- Increase the number of states with nutrition standards for foods and beverages provided to preschool-aged children in child care.

- Increase the proportion of adolescents who are connected to a parent or other positive adult caregiver.
- Reduce the proportion of adolescents who engage in disordered eating behaviors in an attempt to control their weight.
- Reduce the proportion of persons engaging in binge drinking of alcoholic beverages.
- Increase the proportion of older adults who are up to date on a core set of clinical preventive services.
- Increase the proportion of adults who get sufficient sleep.

Source: U.S. Department of Health and Human Services, Office of Disease Prevention and Health Promotion, www.healthypeople.gov.

Exercise Is One Type of Physical Activity

Although the terms *physical activity* and *exercise* are often used interchangeably, they do not mean the same thing. **Physical activity** includes all physical movement, regardless of the level of energy expenditure or the reason you do it (6). Physical activity can be occupational, lifestyle, or leisure time. Occupational activity is the activity that you carry out in the course of your job as, for example, a restaurant server or construction worker. Lifestyle activity includes housework, walking to class, or climbing the stairs to get to your apartment or dorm room. Leisure-time physical activity is any activity you choose to do in your free time.

Exercise is a type of leisure-time physical activity (6). Virtually all conditioning activities and sports are considered exercise because they are planned and help maintain or improve physical fitness. The main thing that distinguishes exercise from other types of physical activity is that exercise is done specifically for health and fitness.

When we use the term *physical activity,* it encompasses exercise, but exercise does not include all types of physical activity. For example, riding your bike to work for transportation is lifestyle physical activity, and lifting heavy boxes at work is occupational physical activity. Both of these activities will improve health and are examples of how an active lifestyle or job can affect health even when a person does not participate in a regular structured exercise program. Typically, exercise produces the greatest health benefits, but you still can receive a lot of health benefits with regular physical activity. (You'll learn more about this in Chapter 2.)

There Are Numerous Health Benefits of Physical Activity

If you ask people whether they exercise regularly, the answer often is no. People have many reasons for not exercising. However, most of us are aware that there are many health benefits of regular physical activity and exercise. In addition to making us look better by improving muscle tone and levels of body fat, regular exercise helps improve our energy levels and our ability to perform everyday tasks. Perhaps even more important, it can help you achieve total wellness (2, 7–15).

The importance of regular physical activity in promoting good health and wellness is emphasized in the 1996 Surgeon General's report on physical activity and health (16). This report concludes that lack of physical activity is a major public health problem in the United States and that all Americans can improve their health by engaging in as little as 30 minutes of light- to moderate-intensity physical activity most days of the week. The Surgeon General's report recognizes numerous health benefits of physical activity and exercise (Figure 1.2), which we will discuss next. Keep in mind that different levels of physical activity or exercise are needed for different health benefits. You will learn more about the recommended amounts of activity needed for health and fitness throughout the book.

Reduced Risk of Heart Disease **Cardiovascular disease (CVD)** (i.e., any ailment of the heart and blood vessels) is a major cause of death in the United States. In fact, one of every three Americans dies of CVD (17). Regular physical activity and exercise can significantly

COACHING **corner**

Take some time to notice how your levels of wellness change from day to day. Revisit this activity often throughout the semester to gain a more robust understanding of how your well-being changes.

- One a scale of 1 to 10 (10 being completely well), how do you rank your wellness in each of the dimensions in this chapter?
- Identify people, tasks, obligations, or desires that affect your wellness.

- Create a list of all of the things that tend to add to your stress level and another list of all the things that give you strength or energy. Are there relationships between those items?
- Identify specific actions you take each day that are intended to affect your well-being.

What is my wellness level?

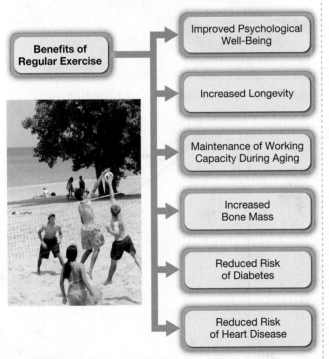

Benefits of Regular Exercise
→ Improved Psychological Well-Being
→ Increased Longevity
→ Maintenance of Working Capacity During Aging
→ Increased Bone Mass
→ Reduced Risk of Diabetes
→ Reduced Risk of Heart Disease

FIGURE 1.2
Regular exercise can yield several long-term benefits for your health.

reduce your risk of developing CVD (1, 7, 8, 10, 11, 17–21). Further, strong evidence suggests that regular physical activity reduces the risk of dying during a heart attack (see **Figure 1.3** on page 8) (22–25). Note from Figure 1.3 that exercise training can reduce the magnitude of cardiac injury during a heart attack by more than 60% (23, 24). Many preventive medicine specialists argue that these facts alone are reason enough

for engaging in regular physical activity and exercise (7, 18, 26). (Chapter 10 provides a detailed discussion of exercise and CVD.)

Reduced Risk of Diabetes **Diabetes** is a disease characterized by high blood sugar (glucose) levels. Untreated diabetes can result in numerous health problems, including blindness and kidney dysfunction. Regular physical activity and exercise can reduce the risk of a specific type of diabetes, called type 2, by improving the regulation of blood glucose (9, 27, 28). (We will discuss diabetes in more detail in Chapter 6.)

Increased Bone Mass The bones of the skeleton provide a mechanical lever system to permit movement and protect internal organs. Clearly, then, it is important to maintain strong and healthy bones. Loss of

physical activity Any movement of the body produced by a skeletal muscle that results in energy expenditure, especially through movement of large muscle groups.

exercise Planned, structured, and repetitive bodily movement done to improve or maintain one or more components of fitness.

cardiovascular disease (CVD) Any disease of the heart and blood vessels.

diabetes A metabolic disorder characterized by high blood glucose levels. Chronic elevation of blood glucose is associated with increased incidence of heart disease, kidney disease, nerve dysfunction, and eye damage.

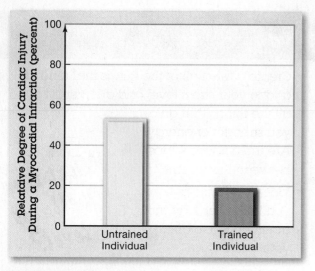

FIGURE 1.3
Regular endurance exercise protects the heart against injury during heart attack. This figure illustrates that during a myocardial infarction (a heart attack), exercise-trained individuals suffer less cardiac injury compared to untrained individuals.

Source: Data from Yamashita, N., et al. Exercise provides direct biphasic cardioprotection via manganese superoxide dismutase activation. *Journal of Experimental Medicine* 189:1699–1706, 1999.

bone mass and strength is called **osteoporosis**, and it increases the risk of bone fractures. Although osteoporosis can occur in men and women of all ages, it is more common in older adults, particularly women.

Exercise can improve bone health by strengthening your bones. Mechanical force applied by muscular activity is a key factor in regulating bone mass and strength. Numerous studies have demonstrated that regular exercise increases bone mass, density, and strength in young adults (29–31). In particular, weight-bearing activities, such as running, walking, and resistance training, are important for bone health. Further, research on osteoporosis suggests that regular exercise can prevent bone loss in older adults and is also useful in treating osteoporosis (29).

Easier Aging As people age, they gradually lose their physical capacity to do work. As we grow older, our ability to perform strenuous activities (e.g., running, cycling, or swimming) progressively declines. Although this decline may begin as early as the 20s, the most dramatic changes occur after about age 60 (32–34). Regular exercise training can reduce the rate of decline in physical working capacity as we age (32, 35, 36). Notice the differences in physical working capacity among highly trained, moderately trained, and inactive individuals in **Figure 1.4**. The key point is that although physical working capacity declines with age, regular exercise can reduce the rate of this decline, increasing your ability to enjoy a lifetime of physical recreation and an improved quality of life that comes with it.

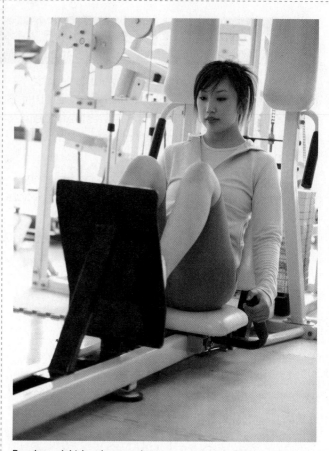

Regular weight-bearing exercise can prevent loss of bone mass.

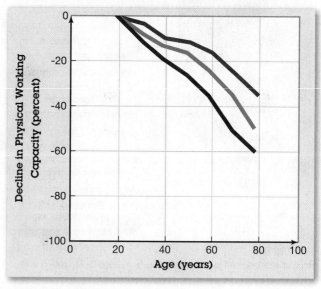

Key

— Highly Trained
(60 min of exercise a day)
— Moderately Trained
(30 min of exercise a day)
— Untrained (sedentary)

FIGURE 1.4
Regular exercise can reduce the natural decline in working capacity that occurs as we age.

Increased Longevity Although controversial, a growing amount of evidence suggests that regular physical activity and exercise (combined with a healthy lifestyle) increase longevity (7, 8, 25, 37–39). For example, a classic study of Harvard alumni over the past 30 years reported that men with a sedentary lifestyle have a 31% greater risk of death from all causes than men who report regular physical activity (8). Studies including women also show that sedentary and low fit women also have a higher risk of death (40, 41). These findings translate into a longer life span for people who exercise and have more active lifestyles. The primary factor for this increased longevity is thought to be their lower risk of both heart attack and cancer (7, 8).

Improved Psychological Well-Being Strong evidence indicates that regular exercise improves psychological well-being in people of all ages. The mental health benefits of regular exercise include reduced risk for anxiety disorders and depression (42). Also, people report feeling less anxious and stressed after an exercise session, even up to 8 hours afterward. These mental benefits lead to an improved sense of well-being in the physically active individual. (We will further discuss the role of exercise as a method of reducing psychological stress in Chapter 11.)

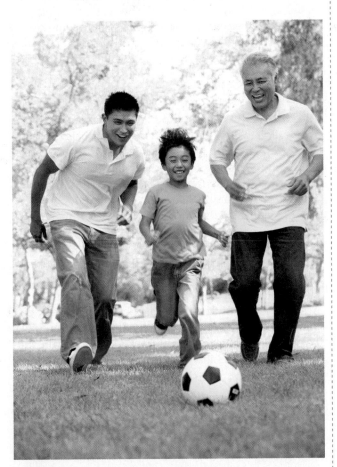

Regular physical activity can help you live longer.

MAKE SURE YOU KNOW...

- Regular physical activity and exercise reduce the risk of both heart disease and diabetes.
- Exercise increases bone mass in young people and strengthens bone in older adults.
- Regular exercise maintains physical working capacity as the person ages.
- Regular physical activity and exercise have been shown to increase longevity and improve quality of life.
- Exercise promotes psychological well-being and reduces risk of depressive and anxiety disorders.

Exercise and Activity for Health-Related Fitness

Exercise conditioning programs can be divided into two broad categories according to their goals: (1) health-related physical fitness and (2) sport- or skill-related physical fitness. This book focuses on health-related fitness. The overall goal of a total health-related physical fitness program is to optimize the quality of life (1, 42). The specific goals of this type of fitness program are to reduce the risk of disease and to improve total physical fitness so that daily tasks can be completed with less effort and fatigue. In contrast, the single goal of sport- and skill-related fitness is to improve physical performance in a specific sport. Note, though, that the "weekend warrior" engaged in a total health-related physical fitness program will likely also improve physical performance in many sports.

Most fitness experts agree that there are five major components of total health-related physical fitness:

1. Cardiorespiratory endurance
2. Muscular strength
3. Muscular endurance
4. Flexibility
5. Body composition

In addition to these, some fitness experts include motor skill performance as a sixth component. Motor skills are movement qualities, such as agility and coordination, that help athletes improve their performance. Although motor skills are important for sport performance, they are not directly linked to improving health in young adults and are therefore not considered a major component of health-related physical fitness. However, these motor skills might increase in importance as people age, because good balance, coordination, and agility may help reduce the risk of falls in older adults.

osteoporosis A condition that results from the loss of bone mass and strength.

Let's examine each of the five components of fitness in more depth.

Cardiorespiratory Endurance

Cardiorespiratory endurance (sometimes called *aerobic fitness* or *cardiorespiratory fitness*) is often considered the key component of health-related physical fitness. Cardiorespiratory endurance is a measure of the heart's ability to pump oxygen-rich blood to the working muscles during exercise and of the muscles' ability to take up and use the oxygen. The oxygen delivered to the muscles is used to produce the energy needed for prolonged exercise.

In practical terms, cardiorespiratory endurance is the ability to perform endurance-type exercises such as distance running, cycling, and swimming. Someone who has achieved a high measure of cardiorespiratory endurance is generally capable of performing 30 to 60 minutes of vigorous exercise without undue fatigue. (Chapter 3 discusses the details of exercise training designed to improve cardiorespiratory fitness.)

Muscular Strength

Muscular strength is evaluated by how much force a muscle (or muscle group) can generate during a single maximal contraction. In practical terms, this means how much weight an individual can lift during one maximal effort.

Muscular strength is important in almost all sports. Sports such as football, basketball, and events in track and field require a high level of muscular strength. Even

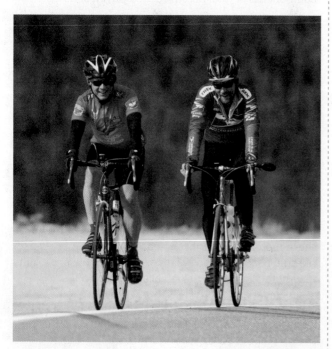

Cyclists who bike for long distances exhibit strong cardiorespiratory endurance.

nonathletes require some degree of muscular strength to function in everyday life. For example, routine tasks around the home, such as lifting bags of groceries and moving furniture, require muscular strength. Even modest amounts of resistance training (commonly performed as weight training) can improve muscular strength and increase ease of everyday tasks. (The principles of developing muscular strength are presented in Chapter 4.)

Muscular Endurance

Muscular endurance is the ability of a muscle to generate a submaximal force over and over again. Although muscular strength and muscular endurance are related, they are not the same. These two terms can be best distinguished by examples. A person lifting a 150-pound barbell during one maximal muscular effort demonstrates high muscular strength. If she lifts a 75-pound barbell a dozen times, she demonstrates muscular endurance. As one develops muscular strength, endurance typically improves. However, strength does not generally improve with muscular endurance training.

Most sports require muscular endurance. For instance, tennis players, who must repeatedly swing their racquets during a match, require a high level of muscular endurance. Many everyday activities (e.g., carrying your backpack across campus all day) also require some level of muscular endurance. (Techniques of developing muscular endurance are discussed in Chapter 4.)

Flexibility

Flexibility is the ability to move joints freely through their full range of motion. Flexible individuals can bend and twist at their joints with ease. Without routine stretching, muscles and tendons shorten and become tight, retarding the range of motion around joints and impairing flexibility.

Individual needs for flexibility vary. Certain athletes (such as gymnasts and divers) require great flexibility to accomplish complex movements. The average individual requires less flexibility than an athlete. However, everyone needs some flexibility for activities of daily living such as reaching for something on the back of the top shelf. Research suggests that flexibility is useful in preventing some types of muscle–tendon injuries and may be useful in reducing low back pain (43, 44). (Techniques for improving flexibility are discussed in Chapter 5.)

Body Composition

The term **body composition** refers to the relative amounts of fat and lean tissue in your body. The rationale for including body composition as a component of health-related physical fitness is that having a high percentage of body fat (a condition known as obesity) is

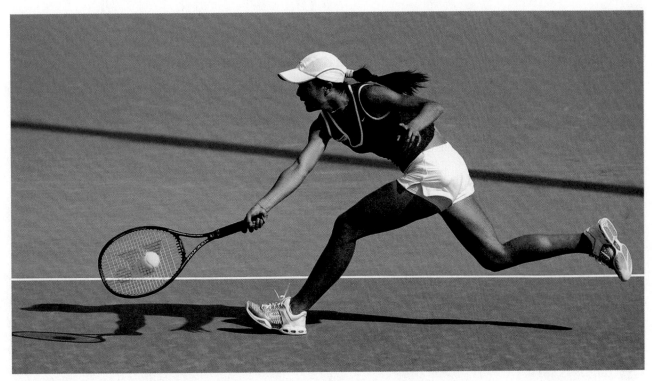

Swinging a tennis racquet repeatedly during a tennis match requires a high level of muscular endurance.

associated with an increased risk of developing CVD, type 2 diabetes, and some cancers. It also contributes to joint stress during movement. In general, being "over-fat" elevates the risk of medical problems.

Lack of physical activity has been shown to play a major role in gaining body fat. Conversely, regular exercise is an important factor in promoting the loss of body fat. (You will learn more about body composition in Chapter 6.)

MAKE SURE YOU KNOW...

- Health-related physical fitness consists of five components: cardiorespiratory endurance, muscular strength, muscular endurance, flexibility, and body composition.

How Can You Make Healthier Behavior Choices?

Remember Maria? She needs to change several behaviors to improve her wellness. Her exercise, eating, sleeping, and time management habits could all be improved. Changing her current behaviors will require some effort on her part, and it will not happen overnight. Unhealthy habits and patterns develop over time, so she cannot expect to change them without time and effort. Fortunately, Maria is committed to improving her health, and she is going to use strategies she learned in her wellness course to make lifestyle behavior changes.

The Stages of Change Model

The **Stages of Change Model** suggests that there is a series of five stages to behavior change:

1. Individuals in the *precontemplation* stage of behavior change do not plan to change their unhealthy behavior. They might not realize the need to change, or they just might not want to change. Because people in this stage are not thinking about changing their behaviors, they might need friends and family to help move to the next stage. The goal

cardiorespiratory endurance A measure of the heart's ability to pump oxygen-rich blood to the working muscles during exercise and of the muscles' ability to take up and use the oxygen.

muscular strength The maximal ability of a muscle to generate force.

muscular endurance The ability of a muscle to generate a submaximal force over and over again.

flexibility The ability to move joints freely through their full range of motion.

body composition The relative amounts of fat and fat-free tissue (muscle, organs, bone) found in the body.

Stages of Change Model A framework for understanding how individuals move toward adopting and maintaining health behavior changes.

STEPS FOR BEHAVIOR CHANGE

Do you have trouble making healthy behavior changes?

Answer the following questions about your typical efforts to change a health behavior.

Y N

☐ ☐ Do you have a specific game plan?

☐ ☐ Do you get help from your friends and family?

☐ ☐ Do you set goals?

☐ ☐ Do you reward yourself for your successes?

If you answered no to most or all of the questions, then you should consider using the behavioral contract in the front of the text.

TIPS FOR USING A BEHAVIORAL CONTRACT AND BEHAVIOR CHANGE STRATEGIES

Tomorrow, you will:

☑ Talk to a friend about signing a behavioral contract with you.

☑ Write out a short- and a long-term SMART goal that you can work to achieve this semester.

☑ Determine your rewards for reaching your goals.

Within the next 2 weeks, you will:

☑ Assess your progress toward reaching your goals and adjust your goals if you realize they are not realistic.

☑ Determine which behavior change strategies will work best for you (i.e., substituting behavior, relapse prevention, stimulus management) and add them to your behavioral contract.

☑ Reward yourself if you reach your short-term goal!

By the end of the semester, you will:

☑ Assess your progress toward your long term goal and reward yourself if you achieve your long-term goal.

☑ Set new goals to achieve.

☑ Continue to use behavioral strategies to help maintain your new healthy behaviors.

---

for people in this first stage is to get good information about healthy behaviors, so they can begin to look at their unhealthy behavior differently.

2. In the *contemplation* stage, a person is aware of the need to change and intends to do so within the next 6 months. People in this stage also need information about healthy behaviors and about the small steps they can make to get closer to changing.

3. During the *preparation* stage, the person is getting ready to make the change within the next 30 days. In some cases, the person might already be making some changes (e.g., increasing lifestyle activity before starting an exercise program). People also begin to take practical steps, such as keeping a detailed schedule in a cell phone or on the computer to list and prioritize daily tasks.

4. In the *action* stage, the behavior change has occurred, but for fewer than 6 months. Using the behavior modification strategies discussed in the next section can help make the new behavior become a habit.

5. After sustaining the behavior change for 6 months, the person enters the *maintenance* stage. During

this stage, the behavior change is more of a habit and requires less conscious effort. As this stage progresses, the temptation to resume old habits steadily decreases. Continuing to use the behavior modification strategies that helped to advance through the earlier stages will help to maintain the change long term.

The length of time that one spends in each stage is highly individual, and progression through the stages is not usually linear. Often, people move back and forth between the stages multiple times before they are able to make the behavior change permanent. Note that a setback does not mean failure. If you experience a lapse to an earlier stage, evaluate why you had the setback, and develop a new plan. Learn from this experience, and do not let it discourage you.

The key element in any behavior change plan is the desire to change. Without a genuine desire to make lifestyle changes, the best behavior change plan is doomed to fail. The rest of this section discusses specific strategies and steps to help you adopt and maintain healthy behaviors.

Behavior Modification

Behavior modification is using the cues that precede a behavior, or the consequences of the behavior, to change that behavior. For example, packing a bag of workout clothes before you go to bed at night and leaving it by your front door is a reminder to take your bag with you the next day so you can stop by the gym after work. If you enjoy the relaxed feeling that results from a good workout, you are likely to keep exercising. Seven commonly used behavior modification strategies are outlined below.

1. *Behavior change contracts* (like the one in the front of this book) include your goals and plans for changing your behavior and are signed by you and a person close to you. Filling out the contract will help you think through your plan, and having another person sign the contract will provide a partner for support and accountability.

2. *Setting realistic short-term and long-term goals* is essential for effective behavior change. (The details of goal setting are outlined at length in Chapter 7.) Briefly, your goals should be what we refer to as SMART goals. SMART is an acronym for Specific, Measureable, Action-oriented, Realistic, and Time-stamped. For example, if you want to lose weight, your SMART goal might be:

   - *Specific and Measurable* – "I want to lose 10 pounds."

   - *Action-oriented* – "I will accomplish this by doing aerobic exercise for at least 45 minutes, 5 days per week, doing resistance training at least 2 days per week, and decreasing my caloric intake by 250 calories per day."

   - *Realistic and Time-stamped* – "I want to reach this goal within 2 months."

3. *Self-monitoring* involves analyzing your behavior to determine what influences your unhealthy behaviors and patterns. Self-monitoring helps you see the things that trigger and reinforce your unhealthy choices so you can make changes. Self-monitoring also can be used to chart your progress as you work toward your goals.

4. *Counter conditioning or substituting behaviors* is replacing an unhealthy behavior choice with a healthier one. Something as simple as keeping fresh fruits and vegetables for snacks instead of potato chips can help you make dietary changes.

5. *Self-reinforcement* is developing a system to reward yourself when you meet your goals. Make sure your reward is meaningful and motivating for reaching your goals.

6. *Decisional balance* involves weighing the positives and negatives of the behavior you want to change. This strategy is usually more helpful for people in the last three stages of change, when they are expecting or experiencing positive outcomes of the new behaviors. In the first two stages, you are more likely to see the negatives of the behavior, so decisional balance might be counterproductive for changing your behavior.

7. *Relapse prevention* is used to keep you from lapsing back to your unhealthy behavior. This strategy involves identifying the "high-risk" situations that are likely to trigger your unhealthy choice and then developing a specific plan of action to avoid or eliminate those situations. If you are trying to drink less alcohol on the weekend and you know that you are likely to drink too much at a campus keg party, you might skip the party and go to a restaurant with your friends instead. Then you might take only enough money for one or two drinks, and rotate the responsibility of being the designated driver. Also, it is important to remember that setbacks are normal and a lapse is not a failure. If you experience a lapse to your old behavior, reevaluate your behaviors and develop a new plan of action.

How can Anita change her behavior in college? Listen to the online case study at **www.pearsonhighered.com/powers.**

HEAR IT! CASE STUDY

What behaviors should you change to live longer? Watch *Months to a Healthier Lifestyle* at **www.pearsonhighered.com/powers.**

SEE IT! VIDEOS

Assessing Your Habits

Before you can change a wellness-related behavior, you must recognize that the behavior is unhealthy and that you can make changes. You also need to identify alternative behaviors for your unhealthy behavior. A good place to begin is a personal assessment of your health risk status. You can use the lifestyle assessment inventory in Laboratory 1.1 to increase your awareness of factors that affect your health. As you complete the lab, develop a list of your less-than-optimal behaviors. Can you identify where you are in the stages of change? Do you need to gather more information before you initiate your behavior change plan? Remember, to be successful in changing the behavior, you must be ready, physically and mentally. Keep in mind that you can control each of these health behaviors but that being aware of them is not enough to bring about change.

After you determine which behaviors you want to change, you can use self-monitoring to study your habits to make the best plan of action. When you assess your patterns, consider why you make the choices you make and why you want to change. Do you have poor dietary habits because you do not know healthy nutrition recommendations, or do you overeat to deal with

COACHING Corner

While in college, students often have strong interactions in the intellectual, social, and physical dimensions. Take a moment to explore your mental, environmental, or spiritual dimension more fully.

- Participate in guided meditation, yoga, or a massage.
- Identify what values are most important to you.

- Practice gratitude by thanking someone publicly.
- Create a piece of art for your own living space.
- Enhance your surroundings so they are more enjoyable to you.

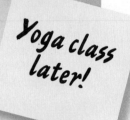
Yoga class later!

stress or emotional problems? Also, you need to assess the things and people in your life that facilitate healthy decisions and that present barriers for healthy decisions.

Finally, when assessing your habits, consider why it is important for you to change. Do you want to change to improve your health and feel better about yourself, or do you want to change to please someone else? Understanding the motivations for your choices will help you develop the best plan to make your changes permanent.

Assess your habits with the *Lifestyle Assessment* Take Charge Of Your Health! Worksheet online at **www.pearsonhighered.com/powers.**
LIVE IT! ASSESS YOURSELF

How can you change your habits and stick with it? Watch *New Year's Resolutions* at **www.pearsonhighered.com/powers.**
SEE IT! VIDEOS

Identifying Behavior Change Barriers

After you have assessed your current behavior patterns, you can focus on the barriers that may prevent you from changing your behavior. For example, you want to start an exercise program, but you have a full load of classes and work part-time in the evening—you may feel that lack of time is a barrier. You want to stop smoking, but all your friends smoke when you hang out together—your barrier would be the social pressure you feel from your friends. Your goal is to reduce or eliminate your barriers, and this is the perfect opportunity to use relapse prevention. (See Chapter 2 for explanation on removing barriers to physical activity.)

Some barriers are easy to work with. Others are complicated, especially when they are influenced by people who are important to you. To go back to our examples, getting up a half-hour earlier might help you overcome the barrier of a perceived lack of time, but to address the social barrier to your quitting smoking you will need

some help from your friends. People who care about you will typically be supportive if they know about your goals, but they cannot help if you do not communicate your desire to change. Telling your friends you want to stop smoking and that you do not want to be with them when they smoke will help them support your decision. Relapse prevention can be very effective in changing behaviors.

Assess your behavior change with the *Weekly Behavior Change Evaluation* Take Charge Of Your Health! Worksheet online at **www.pearsonhighered.com/powers.**
LIVE IT! ASSESS YOURSELF

Changing Unhealthy Behaviors

Now you can begin to develop a game plan for changing your behaviors. After you complete Laboratory 1.1, you might see multiple behaviors you could change to improve your wellness. Do not let your results overwhelm you. Recognize that you do not need to change all of your unhealthy behaviors at the same time. Trying to make too many changes at once is usually very difficult and reduces your chances for success. Setbacks can reduce your motivation to change, but keep in mind that a setback does not mean failure.

Before you can develop your plan of action, you need to have accurate information about the behaviors. You will get a lot of information from this book and from your instructor. However, you might also need to seek out additional resources, such as a counselor at the student health center, a fitness specialist, or a support group. Make sure any outside resources are reputable groups or individuals who are qualified to give you the information and guidance you need (see the Consumer Corner box on the next page for how to identify credible sources of health information).

When deciding which changes you want to make first, consider the number of behaviors you want to change and the effort it will take to change them. Some

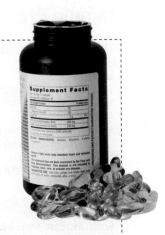

CONSUMER CORNER

Finding Credible Health Information

With all of the health information out there, how do you know what to believe? "Experts" endorse products and plans on infomercials and in magazines, but some of the claims seem too good to be true. To avoid becoming overwhelmed—or worse, being scammed—you have to develop a "healthy skepticism." The next time you visit a website, read a supplement label, or watch an infomercial, ask yourself the following questions:

- Do the claims made about this product seem too good to be true?
- Has all of the supporting research been conducted or funded by the company that makes the product or offers the service?
- Are the claims made about the product supported by quality scientific research?
- Is there information available about short- and long-term effects?
- Does the information fit with the information I am learning in class?

- Are there potential risks and side effects of products and services mentioned?
- Are the experts endorsing the product or service really experts in that field? (For example, a doctor who is a podiatrist might not be the best source for a weight-loss pill.)
- Is there any opposing information available?

Answering yes to the first two questions should always raise a red flag. If you can answer yes to the remaining questions, the product or service might be worth considering. Get the opinion of a trusted professional, such as your instructor or a health care worker at your student health center for further evaluation. Also see Laboratory 1.5 at the end of this chapter for evaluating fitness products.

---

behaviors, such as flossing your teeth regularly or performing monthly self-exams, are simple and do not require as much effort. However, starting a new exercise program, quitting smoking, or changing your diet require more effort. Most people can successfully make more than one simple change at a time. However, for the more complex behaviors, making them one at a time is recommended. Also, breaking them into smaller steps, or **shaping**, is recommended to make the change seem less intimidating. Your success with the simple behaviors and the small steps on the way to the complex behavior will increase your confidence and motivate you to work toward total wellness.

Finally, you need to set goals and develop your specific plan for changing the behavior. Something as simple as putting a monthly reminder on your cell phone to do a self-exam or hanging a plastic tag on your shower head might do the trick. Using counter conditioning by trading a sedentary choice for an active one will increase lifestyle physical activity. However, for many behaviors

you will need a more detailed plan of action. For example, changing your eating habits might include meeting with a dietitian, making grocery lists, planning meals ahead of time, and having an accountability partner. Also, these changes will likely be made in stages. Using shaping will make the change seem more manageable.

MAKE SURE YOU KNOW...

- Knowing your stage of change will help you develop the best plan of action for changing your behavior.
- Behavior modification strategies are very helpful in successfully changing your behavior.
- Assessing your current habits and addressing your barriers are essential before developing your plan for behavior change.

shaping Breaking a behavior or task into small steps to accomplish the larger goal.

Sample Program for Increasing Physical Activity

Scan to plan your individualized program for increasing physical activity. ▶

If you have a busy schedule and find it difficult to fit exercise into your day, there are still ways you can increase your level of physical activity. You might not get the same increase in your fitness level as someone who participates in regular exercise, but you can still improve your health. Getting a pedometer and working to walk 10,000 steps per day,

increasing your lifestyle physical activity, and getting small bouts of moderate activity throughout the day are a few of the things you can do to become more active.

To increase your number of steps per day, try using stairs rather than the elevator, walking to all classes rather than driving, walking to complete errands, and walking up and down extra aisles when grocery shopping. Incorporate physical activity between other commitments by performing exercises in your apartment or living room. Consider trying a fitness DVD or online fitness video, and invite a friend or roommate to join you for a fun social experience.

Goals: Increase steps by 250 per day to reach the target goal of 10,000 steps per day, and increase general physical activity. The number of weeks to reach the goal of at least 10,000 steps per day will vary depending on your starting point.

	Activity Time	Monday	Tuesday	Wednesday	Thursday	Friday	Saturday	Sunday
Week 1	Lunch Break		10 min walk		10 min walk		10 min walk	10 min walk
	Study Break	1 set of 25 crunches, 1 set of 15 push-ups, 1 set of 15 dips		1 set of 25 crunches, 1 set of 15 push-ups, 1 set of 15 dips		1 set of 25 crunches, 1 set of 15 push-ups, 1 set of 15 dips	10 min walk	10 min walk
Week 2	Lunch Break		15 min walk		15 min walk		15 min walk	15 min walk
	Study Break	1 set of 25 crunches, 1 set of 20 push-ups, 2 sets of 10 dips	15 min yoga DVD	1 set of 25 crunches, 1 set of 20 push-ups, 2 sets of 10 dips	15 min yoga DVD	1 set of 25 crunches, 1 set of 20 push-ups, 2 sets of 10 dips	15 min walk	15 min walk (morning) 15 min yoga DVD (afternoon)
Week 3	Lunch Break		15 min walk		15 min walk		20 min walk	20 min walk
	Study Break	2 sets of 25 crunches, 2 sets of 15 push-ups, 2 sets of 15 dips	20 min yoga DVD	2 sets of 25 crunches, 2 sets of 15 push-ups, 2 sets of 15 dips	20 min yoga DVD	2 sets of 25 crunches, 2 sets of 15 push-ups, 2 sets of 15 dips	20 min walk	20 min walk (morning) 20 min yoga DVD (afternoon)

SUMMARY

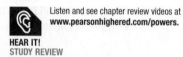

Listen and see chapter review videos at www.pearsonhighered.com/powers.

HEAR IT!
STUDY REVIEW

1. The term *wellness* means "healthy living." Wellness is achieved by practicing a healthy lifestyle, which includes regular physical activity, proper nutrition, eliminating unhealthy behaviors (avoiding high-risk activities such as smoking and drug use), and maintaining emotional and spiritual health.

2. Total wellness can be achieved only by a balance of physical, emotional, intellectual, spiritual, social, and environmental health. The components of wellness do not work in isolation; they interact strongly. For example, poor physical health can lead to poor emotional health.

3. Exercise offers many health benefits. Regular exercise has been shown to reduce risk of CVD and diabetes, increase bone mass, and maintain physical working capacity as one ages.

4. The five major components of "total" health-related physical fitness are cardiorespiratory endurance, muscular strength, muscular endurance, flexibility, and body composition.

5. Used correctly, behavior modification strategies can be very helpful for changing health behaviors.

STUDY QUESTIONS

Find more review questions online at
www.pearsonhighered.com/powers.

REVIEW IT!
QUIZZES

1. _____ is any body movement produced by skeletal muscles that results in energy expenditure.
   - a. Exercise
   - b. Physical fitness
   - c. Physical activity
   - d. Health-related fitness

2. _____ is *not* a dimension of wellness.
   - a. Exercise
   - b. Spiritual health
   - c. Social health
   - d. Emotional health

3. Which of the following is *not* a component of health-related fitness?
   - a. muscular strength
   - b. body composition
   - c. agility
   - d. flexibility

4. Which of the following is a health benefit of regular physical activity?
   - a. reduced risk for osteoporosis
   - b. reduced risk for heart disease
   - c. improved mental health
   - d. all of the above

5. Which of the following is not a *Healthy People 2020* objective?
   - a. Increase the proportion of adults who get sufficient sleep.
   - b. Reduce the proportion of persons engaging in binge drinking of alcoholic beverages.
   - c. Increase the proportion of physician office visits that include counseling or education related to nutrition or weight.
   - d. All of the choices are *Healthy People 2020* objectives.

6. A person in the _____ stage of change has been fully participating in the new health behavior for less than 6 months.
   - a. maintenance
   - b. action
   - c. contemplation
   - d. new activity

7. Which of the following is an important step in initiating a health behavior change?
   - a. making a specific plan
   - b. mobilizing your support network
   - c. getting outside help if needed
   - d. all of the above

8. Which of the following should be considered when you are planning to make a behavior change?
   - a. number of behaviors you want to change and effort involved
   - b. motive for behavior change
   - c. current behavior patterns
   - d. all of the above

9. We discussed SMART goals in the chapter. What does the acronym SMART mean?
   - a. specific, manageable, accountability, revisable, time sensitive
   - b. sensitive, multiple, action-oriented, reasonable, time-stamped
   - c. specific, measurable, action-oriented, realistic, time-stamped
   - d. short-term, measurable, accountability, realistic, tough

10. What is wellness?

11. Name at least one behavior associated with each of the six components of wellness.

12. List and discuss the five components of health-related fitness.

13. Discuss the importance of the *Healthy People* goals and objectives.

HELPFUL WEBLINKS

For links to the organizations and websites listed, visit
www.pearsonhighered.com/powers.

DO IT!
WEBLINKS

American College of Sports Medicine
Comprehensive website providing information, articles, equipment recommendations, how-to articles, books, and position statements about all aspects of health and fitness. www.acsm.org

American Heart Association
Offers the latest information about ways to reduce your risk of heart and vascular diseases. Site includes information about exercise, diet, and heart disease. www.heart.org

Healthy People
Provides information about the U.S. government's initiative to improve health and wellness for the American people. www.healthypeople.gov

WebMD
Contains the latest information on a variety of health-related topics, including diet, exercise, and stress. Links to nutrition, fitness, and wellness topics. www.webmd.com

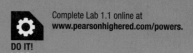

Name _____   Date _____

Lifestyle Assessment Inventory

The purpose of this lifestyle assessment inventory is to help you identify areas in your life that increase your risk of disease, injury, and possibly premature death. Awareness is the first step in making change.

Put a check by each statement that applies to you. You may select more than one choice per category.

Physical Health

A.   Physical Fitness

_____ I exercise for a minimum of 20 to 30 minutes at least 3 days per week.

_____ I walk for 15 to 30 minutes 3 to 7 days per week.

_____ I get lifestyle or occupational physical activity most days of the week.

B.   Body Fat

_____ There is no place on my body where I can pinch more than 1 inch of fat.

_____ I am satisfied with the way my body looks.

C.   Car Safety

_____ I always use a seat belt when I drive.

_____ I rarely drive above the speed limit.

_____ I do not drink and drive, and I do not ride in a car with someone who has been drinking.

D.   Sleep

_____ I always get 7 to 9 hours of sleep.

_____ I do not have trouble going to sleep.

_____ I generally do not wake up during the night.

E.   Diet

_____ I generally eat balanced meals and a variety of food.

_____ I eat fruits and vegetables daily.

_____ I rarely overeat.

_____ I rarely eat large quantities of fatty foods and sweets.

F.   Alcohol Use

_____ I consume fewer than two drinks per day.

_____ I never get intoxicated.

_____ I do not binge drink.

G.   Tobacco and Drug Use

_____ I never smoke (cigarettes, pipe, cigars, etc.) or use smokeless tobacco.

_____ I use prescription medications only for their intended purpose.

_____ I do not use illegal drugs.

H.   Sexual Practices

_____ I always practice safe sex (e.g., always using condoms or being involved in a monogamous relationship).

_____ I am not sexually active.

Social Health

_____ I have a happy and satisfying relationship with my spouse or boyfriend/girlfriend.

_____ I have good relationships with my close friends.

_____ I get a great deal of love and support from my family.

_____ I work to have good communication skills.

_____ I am able to express my feelings and emotions to people close to me.

Emotional Health

A. Stress Level

_____ I find it easy to relax.

_____ I rarely feel tense or anxious.

_____ I am able to cope with daily stresses without undue emotional stress.

_____ I have not experienced a major stressful life event in the past year.

B. Mental Health

_____ I do not suffer from depressive or anxiety disorders.

_____ I do not have an eating disorder.

Intellectual Health

_____ I attend class regularly.

_____ I keep informed about current events.

_____ I seek opportunities to learn new things.

_____ I have an open mind about ideas that might be different from mine.

Environmental Health

_____ I am not exposed to second-hand smoke on a regular basis.

_____ I use sunscreen regularly or limit my sun exposure.

_____ I carpool or use physical activity for transportation when possible.

_____ I recycle regularly.

_____ I limit my exposure to harmful environmental contaminants.

Spiritual Health

_____ I have a sense of meaning and purpose in my life.

_____ I am satisfied with my level of spirituality.

_____ I work to develop my spiritual health.

Evaluating Your Responses

1. What area of wellness is your strongest area? What do you do to maintain healthy behaviors for that wellness component?

    _____

    _____

2. What area of wellness is your weakest area? What behaviors can you change to improve that area?

    _____

    _____

3. Write a long-term goal for improving one wellness behavior you seriously want to change this semester. Write a short-term SMART goal that will help you reach your long-term goal.

    Long-term goal:

    _____

    _____

    Short-term SMART goal:

    _____

    _____

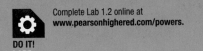
Name _____ **Date** _____

Changing Your Behavior

What is a health behavior for which your current stage of change is precontemplation, contemplation, or preparation? Now is the time to consider making a change. Select one of these health behaviors, and use the steps below to indicate how you will accomplish the change. Use additional paper if needed.

1. Select a behavior to change. _____

2. Use self-monitoring to assess your behavioral patterns. State at least one barrier you will face.

   _____

   _____

   State at least one thing that will support your change.

   _____

   _____

3. Name the people you will be able to count on for support and accountability. Will one of them be willing to sign the behavior change contract with you?

   _____

   _____

4. What behavior modification strategies will you use? For each strategy you list, write out a specific plan for how you will use it.

   _____

   _____

5. Write out your long-term goal and at least two short-term SMART goals that will help you get there.
   Long-term goal: _____

   _____

   Short-term SMART goals: _____

   _____

6. How will you reward yourself when you achieve your short- and long-term goals?

   _____

   _____

   _____

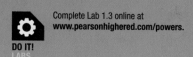
Name _____ **Date** _____

Medical History Check

Most people can safely begin an exercise program and significantly increase their physical activity. However, certain medical conditions require clearance from a physician or alternative prescriptions for exercise and physical activity. Therefore, it is important to assess your health before making significant physical activity changes. Respond honestly to the following questions to assess your medical history.

Do you currently have or have you ever had any of the following? Check any of the following that apply.

_____ Heart murmur

_____ Elevated cholesterol

_____ High blood pressure

_____ Irregular heart beat

_____ Coronary heart disease

_____ Chest pain

_____ Blood clots

_____ Abnormal rest or exercise electrocardiogram (ECG)

_____ Stroke

_____ Diabetes

_____ Heart attack

_____ Shortness of breath

_____ Family history of heart disease (blood relative)

_____ Arthritis

_____ Chronic back pain

_____ Obesity

_____ Asthma

_____ Any other heart, metabolic, or respiratory conditions

_____ Any other joint problems

Check any of the following that apply to you:

_____ 45 years or older

_____ Smoker or quit smoking within last 6 months

_____ Currently taking prescription medication

Please list: _____

Please explain any items you checked.

_____

_____

Please explain any reasons you feel it would be unsafe for you to exercise.

_____

Name _____ **Date** _____

Par-Q and You

The following questionnaire can also be used to determine your readiness to engage in a fitness program.

Physical Activity Readiness
Questionnaire - PAR-Q
(revised 2002)

PAR-Q & YOU

(A Questionnaire for People Aged 15 to 69)

Regular physical activity is fun and healthy, and increasingly more people are starting to become more active every day. Being more active is very safe for most people. However, some people should check with their doctor before they start becoming much more physically active.

If you are planning to become much more physically active than you are now, start by answering the seven questions in the box below. If you are between the ages of 15 and 69, the PAR-Q will tell you if you should check with your doctor before you start. If you are over 69 years of age, and you are not used to being very active, check with your doctor.

Common sense is your best guide when you answer these questions. Please read the questions carefully and answer each one honestly: check YES or NO.

YES	NO	
☐	☐	1. Has your doctor ever said that you have a heart condition <u>and</u> that you should only do physical activity recommended by a doctor?
☐	☐	2. Do you feel pain in your chest when you do physical activity?
☐	☐	3. In the past month, have you had chest pain when you were not doing physical activity?
☐	☐	4. Do you lose your balance because of dizziness or do you ever lose consciousness?
☐	☐	5. Do you have a bone or joint problem (for example, back, knee or hip) that could be made worse by a change in your physical activity?
☐	☐	6. Is your doctor currently prescribing drugs (for example, water pills) for your blood pressure or heart condition?
☐	☐	7. Do you know of <u>any other reason</u> why you should not do physical activity?

If

you

answered

YES to one or more questions

Talk with your doctor by phone or in person BEFORE you start becoming much more physically active or BEFORE you have a fitness appraisal. Tell your doctor about the PAR-Q and which questions you answered YES.

- You may be able to do any activity you want — as long as you start slowly and build up gradually. Or, you may need to restrict your activities to those which are safe for you. Talk with your doctor about the kinds of activities you wish to participate in and follow his/her advice.
- Find out which community programs are safe and helpful for you.

NO to all questions

If you answered NO honestly to <u>all</u> PAR-Q questions, you can be reasonably sure that you can:
- start becoming much more physically active – begin slowly and build up gradually. This is the safest and easiest way to go.
- take part in a fitness appraisal – this is an excellent way to determine your basic fitness so that you can plan the best way for you to live actively. It is also highly recommended that you have your blood pressure evaluated. If your reading is over 144/94, talk with your doctor before you start becoming much more physically active.

→ **DELAY BECOMING MUCH MORE ACTIVE:**
- if you are not feeling well because of a temporary illness such as a cold or a fever – wait until you feel better; or
- if you are or may be pregnant – talk to your doctor before you start becoming more active.

PLEASE NOTE: If your health changes so that you then answer YES to any of the above questions, tell your fitness or health professional. Ask whether you should change your physical activity plan.

<u>Informed Use of the PAR-Q</u>: The Canadian Society for Exercise Physiology, Health Canada, and their agents assume no liability for persons who undertake physical activity, and if in doubt after completing this questionnaire, consult your doctor prior to physical activity.

No changes permitted. You are encouraged to photocopy the PAR-Q but only if you use the entire form.

NOTE: If the PAR-Q is being given to a person before he or she participates in a physical activity program or a fitness appraisal, this section may be used for legal or administrative purposes.

"I have read, understood and completed this questionnaire. Any questions I had were answered to my full satisfaction."

NAME _____

SIGNATURE _____ DATE_____

SIGNATURE OF PARENT _____ WITNESS _____
or GUARDIAN (for participants under the age of majority)

Note: This physical activity clearance is valid for a maximum of 12 months from the date it is completed and becomes invalid if your condition changes so that you would answer YES to any of the seven questions.

Source: Physical Activity Readiness Questionnaire (PAR-Q) © 2002. Used with permission from the Canadian Society for Exercise Physiology www.csep.ca.

LABORATORY 1.5

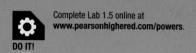

Complete Lab 1.5 online at
www.pearsonhighered.com/powers.

DO IT!
LABS

Name _____   **Date** _____

Evaluating Fitness Products

Complete this activity to evaluate fitness advertisements you see or hear regularly. Find three examples (from magazines, TV or radio ads, or online) of misleading or false claims on fitness or health products. Answer the following questions for each of your products.

1. What are two specific things (images or statements) that are false or misleading in the ad?

    _____

    _____

2. What makes them false? Support your answer with information you learned in class.

    _____

    _____

3. What are the credentials of the author or person endorsing the project? Is the information provided by an expert in the field of exercise science or physical fitness?

    _____

    _____

4. Are the benefits of the product realistic?

    _____

    _____

5. Does the ad contain gimmick words, such as "quick," "spot reduce," or "just minutes a day"?

    _____

    _____

6. Is the main purpose of the ad to provide useful information or only to sell a product?

    _____

    _____

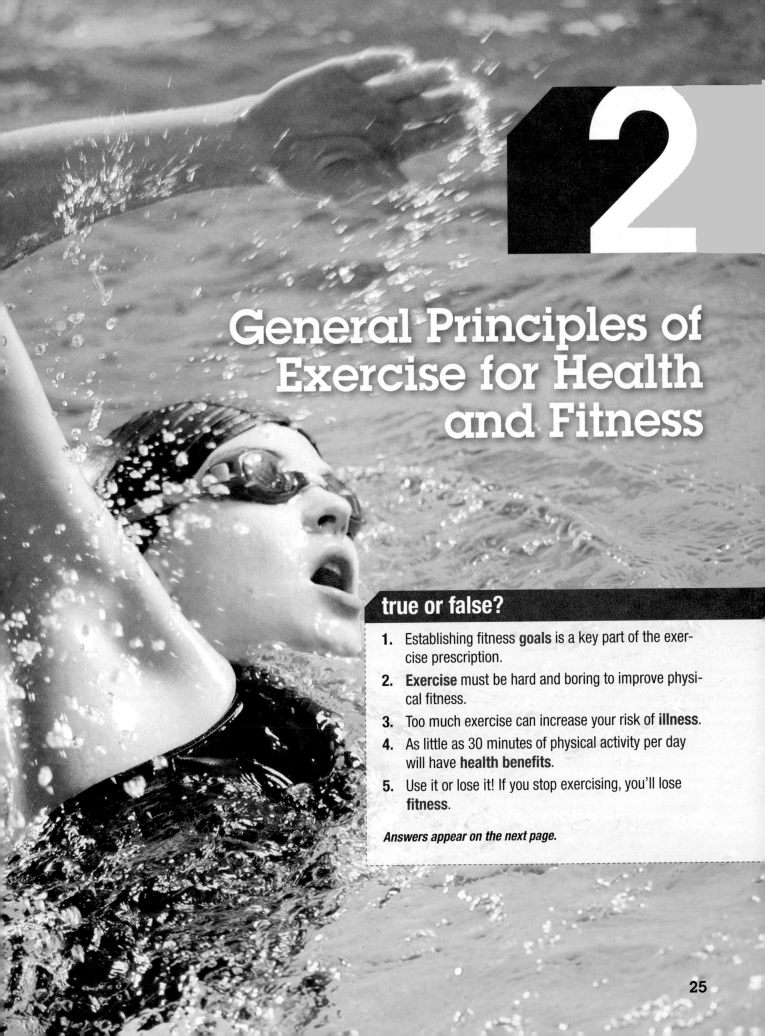

2

General Principles of Exercise for Health and Fitness

true or false?

1. Establishing fitness **goals** is a key part of the exercise prescription.
2. **Exercise** must be hard and boring to improve physical fitness.
3. Too much exercise can increase your risk of **illness**.
4. As little as 30 minutes of physical activity per day will have **health benefits**.
5. Use it or lose it! If you stop exercising, you'll lose **fitness**.

Answers appear on the next page.

Everyone can improve his or her level of physical fitness. Whether your idea of exercise is getting out of a chair to grab a soda or going for a daily run, you can improve your fitness level by analyzing your routine and making gradual improvements.

The purpose of this chapter is to discuss the general principles behind improving your physical fitness. The basic concepts presented here apply to both men and women of all ages and fitness levels. You will find out more about the individual components of health-related physical fitness—cardiorespiratory fitness, muscular strength and endurance, flexibility, and body composition—in the next four chapters and learn how to put these components together into a complete fitness program (Chapter 7).

Principles of Exercise Training to Improve Physical Fitness

Although everyone's exercise training program will vary according to personal needs, the general principles of physical fitness are universal. The more you exercise, and the greater the variety of activities you do, the more fit you'll be. In the following sections we describe the training concepts of overload, progression, specificity, recuperation, and reversibility, all of which affect the progress you'll make as you design and carry out your exercise training program.

Overload Principle

To improve physical fitness, systems of the body (e.g., the muscular and cardiorespiratory systems) must be stressed. For example, for a skeletal muscle to increase in strength, the muscle must work against a heavier load than normal. This concept is part of the **overload principle**, and it's a key component of all conditioning programs (1, 2) **(Figure 2.1)**. We achieve an overload by increasing the intensity of exercise, such as by using heavier weights.

You can also achieve overload by increasing the duration (or time) of exercise. For instance, to increase muscular endurance, a muscle must be worked over a longer duration than normal, such as by performing a greater number of exercise repetitions. To improve flexibility and increase the range of motion at a joint, we must either stretch the muscle to a longer length than normal or hold the stretch for a longer time.

Although overload is important to attaining physical fitness, your workouts should not be exhausting. The often-heard bodybuilding adage "No pain, no gain" is not accurate. In fact, you can improve your physical fitness without punishing training sessions.

FLEXIBILITY 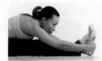 Stretch farther or longer

STRENGTH 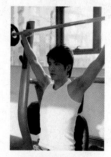 Increase weight loads

ENDURANCE 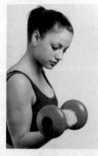 Perform more repetitions

CARDIO-RESPIRATORY 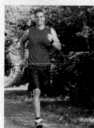 Run farther

FIGURE 2.1
You can use the overload principle to increase your fitness level in each of the key training areas.

Principle of Progression

The **principle of progression** is an extension of the overload principle. It states that overload should be increased gradually during the course of a physical fitness program. For example, Becky, a sedentary college-aged student who is slightly overweight, might begin her new fitness program with a daily 10-minute walk/jog, then move up to an 11-minute walk/jog in week 2, and by week 5, do a daily 16-minute jog.

The overload in a training program should generally be increased slowly during the first 1–6 weeks of the exercise program. After this initial period, the overload can be increased at a steady and progressive rate during the next 6–20 weeks of training. For best results, the overload should not be increased too slowly or too rapidly. Progressing too slowly may not result in the desired improvement in physical fitness, and progressing too quickly can increase your risk of muscular skeletal injuries.

What is a safe rate of progression during an exercise training program? Although people vary in their tolerance for exercise overload, a commonsense guideline to improve physical fitness and avoid overuse injuries is the **ten percent rule** (2). In short,

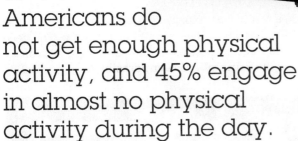

consider this!
More than 67% of Americans do not get enough physical activity, and 45% engage in almost no physical activity during the day.

this rule says that the training intensity or duration of exercise should be increased by no more than 10% per week. For example, a runner running 20 minutes per day could increase his or her daily exercise duration to 22 minutes per day (10% of 20 = 2) the following week.

Once you reach your desired level of physical fitness, you no longer need to increase the training intensity or duration of your physical conditioning. You should instead focus on designing a **maintenance program** to maintain your new fitness level with regular exercise **(Figure 2.2)**.

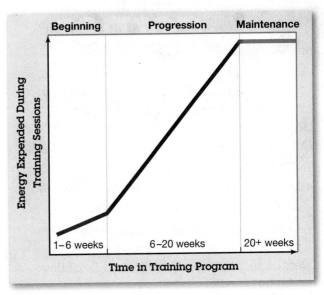

Key
— Beginning of program
— Slow progression during program
— Maintenance

FIGURE 2.2
If you're starting a new exercise training program, you'll begin slowly and progress toward doing more exercise at a greater intensity until you reach your desired fitness level. Then you'll develop a maintenance program to sustain your new level of fitness.

Principle of Specificity

Another key concept in training is the **principle of specificity**, which states that the exercise training effect is specific to those muscles involved in the activity (3). For example, if you perform leg curls, you wouldn't expect your upper arms to benefit, and likewise, your biceps curls aren't going to improve your calf muscles. This is part of the reason why a varied set of exercises is so important to overall physical fitness improvement.

overload principle A basic principle of physical conditioning that states that in order to improve physical fitness, the body or specific muscles must be stressed.

principle of progression A principle of training that states that overload should be increased gradually.

ten percent rule The training intensity or duration of exercise should not be increased by more than 10% per week.

maintenance program Exercising to sustain a desired level of physical fitness.

principle of specificity The effect of exercise training is specific to those muscles involved in the activity.

COACHING Corner

An important idea associated with a sound exercise program is consistency. If you have always considered fitness optional, it may be helpful to reframe that thought process. Consider adopting the mantra that fitness is nonnegotiable.

- Make a list of the obligations that may challenge your intentions to exercise.

- Create a schedule of fitness activities that includes several options for cardiorespiratory, strength, and flexibility training modes.

- Develop exercise bouts with friends—physical and social dimensions may flourish.

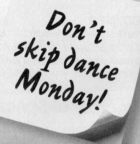

Don't skip dance Monday!

- Develop a backup plan for days when you are less motivated. Some activity is always better than no activity.

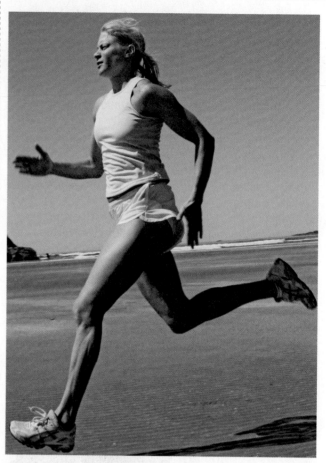

Because running involves the use of the leg muscles, doing it regularly will improve the endurance of those muscles. This is an example of specificity of training.

Specificity of training also applies to the types of adaptations that occur in the muscle. For instance, strength training, such as with free weights, results in an increase in muscle strength but does not greatly improve the endurance of the muscle. Therefore, strength training is specific to improving muscular strength (4). Similarly, endurance exercise training, such as distance running, results in improved muscular endurance without altering muscular strength significantly (5). Suppose you want to improve your ability to run a distance of 3 miles. In this case, specific training should include running 3 or more miles several times a week. This type of training would improve muscular endurance in your legs but would not result in large improvements in leg strength (3).

Principle of Recuperation

Overloading your muscles means stressing them, and they need a period of rest before your next workout. During the recovery period, the body adapts to the exercise stress by increasing endurance or becoming stronger. In fact, a rest period, usually 24 hours or more, is essential for achieving maximal benefit from exercise. The need for a rest period between exercise training sessions is called the **principle of recuperation** (2) **(Figure 2.3)**.

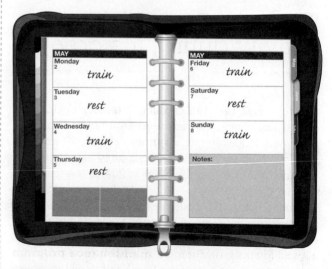

FIGURE 2.3
To avoid injury and maximize benefits, allow adequate rest periods between sessions in your exercise training program.

Choosing the Right Exercise Shoe

The right shoe can make it more comfortable for you to exercise and reduce your risk of injury, while the wrong shoe can cause you to avoid your workout or even contribute to injuries. Consider the following factors when buying a pair of workout shoes.

Exercise shoes vary in their design and function. For example, shoes designed for walking are often stiff compared to running shoes, which are more flexible and contain extra cushioning. Shoes for cross-training are designed for activities that involve lateral motion such as volleyball or kickboxing. A good rule of thumb to follow is that if you engage in an activity more than twice a week, buy a shoe designed for that activity.

Feet come in a variety of shapes, and knowing your foot's particular quirks is important in selecting the right shoe. For example, we all differ in the structure of our arch (i.e., the curvature of the bottom of your foot). You can determine your arch type by performing the "wet test." Wet your foot and step on a dry surface to trace your footprint. If you possess flat feet or a low arch, your footprint will reveal the entire sole of your foot, with little or no curve visible. If your footprint shows only a portion of your forefoot and heel with little or no connection between the two, you have high arches. Or you may have a neutral arch, in which case the wet test shows a distinct curve along the inside of your foot.

Here are some tips for choosing your optimal exercise shoe:

- Shop for shoes late in the day. The swelling your feet experience by the end of the day is similar to the swelling they experience during exercise (swelling is due to increased blood flow and fluid collection).

- Make sure that there is a full thumb length between the end of your longest toe and the end of the shoe. This ensures that the shoe is long enough for your foot.

- Make sure the front section of the shoe (the "toe box") allows the toes to move around.

- The shoe should not feel too tight, but the foot should not slide around in the shoe.

- Do not rely on a break-in period for your shoes to stretch— your shoes should feel good on the day you buy them.

- If in doubt about the correct size, buy the larger size.

consider this!
Among people who start an exercise program, 50% will drop out within 6 months.

Failure to get enough rest between sessions may result in a fatigue syndrome referred to as **overtraining**. Overtraining may lead to chronic fatigue and/or injuries. Common symptoms of overtraining include sore and stiff muscles or a feeling of general fatigue the morning after an exercise training session, sometimes called a "workout hangover." The cure is either to increase the duration of rest between workouts or to reduce the intensity of workouts, or both. Although too much exercise is the primary cause of the overtraining syndrome, an inadequate diet, particularly if it's short on carbohydrates, can also contribute. (We will cover more about the effects of good nutrition on exercise in Chapter 8.)

Principle of Reversibility

Although rest periods are important to maximizing your benefits from exercise, going too long between exercise sessions (such as days or weeks), or being too inconsistent in your routine, can result in losing the progress you've made (6). To maintain physical fitness, you need to exercise regularly. In other words, physical fitness

principle of recuperation The body requires recovery periods between exercise training sessions to adapt to the exercise stress. Therefore, a period of rest is essential for achieving maximal benefit from exercise.

overtraining The result of failure to get enough rest between exercise training sessions.

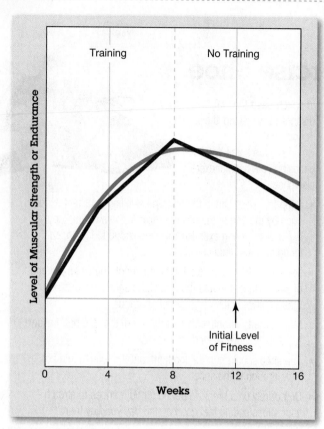

Key

━━━ Muscular endurance

━━━ Muscular strength

FIGURE 2.4
Stopping exercise training will reverse gains made in both muscular strength and muscular endurance.

cannot be stored. The loss of fitness due to inactivity is an example of the **principle of reversibility**.

How quickly is fitness lost after training has stopped? The answer depends on which component of physical fitness you are considering. For example, if you stop strength training, you will lose muscular strength relatively slowly (4, 7). In contrast, after you stop performing endurance exercise, you will lose muscular endurance relatively rapidly (6) **(Figure 2.4)**.

Note that 8 weeks after strength training is stopped, only 10% of muscular strength is lost (7). In contrast, 8 weeks after cessation of endurance training, 30–40% of muscular endurance is lost (6). Also, the health benefits of regular exercise are not stored forever and are lost within several months if you stop exercising on a regular basis. Therefore, to achieve a lifetime of health benefits from physical activity, it is important to maintain a regular routine of exercise throughout your lifespan.

MAKE SURE YOU KNOW...

- Five key principles of exercise training are the overload principle, principle of progression, specificity of exercise, principle of recuperation, and reversibility of training effects.

- The overload principle states that to improve physical fitness, the body or the specific muscle group used during exercise must be stressed.
- The principle of progression is an extension of the overload principle and states that overload should be increased gradually over the course of a physical fitness training program.
- The principle of specificity refers to the fact that exercise training is specific to those muscles involved in the activity.
- The requirement for a rest period between training sessions is called the principle of recuperation.
- The principle of reversibility refers to loss of physical fitness due to inactivity.

Designing Your Exercise Program

If you go to a doctor with a bacterial infection and she prescribes an antibiotic as treatment, chances are good that the dose you take is different from the dose that might be prescribed for your 10-year-old brother. Similarly, for each individual there is a correct "dose" of exercise to effectively promote physical fitness, called an **exercise prescription** (6). Exercise prescriptions should be tailored to meet the needs of the individual (3, 6, 8). They should include fitness goals, a mode of exercise (or type of activity), a warm-up, a primary conditioning period, and a cool-down. The following sections provide a general introduction to each of these components.

Setting Goals

Establishing fitness goals is the first step in designing your exercise program. If you don't know what you're working toward, you are not likely to achieve it. Thus, setting goals (both short-term and long-term goals) is an essential part of an exercise prescription. Visualizing goals such as a leaner, stronger body or an improved competitive performance would help motivate you to begin your exercise program. Further, attaining your fitness goals improves self-esteem and provides the incentive needed to make a lifetime commitment to regular exercise.

The importance of fitness goals cannot be overemphasized. Goals provide structure and motivation for a

principle of reversibility The loss of fitness due to inactivity.

exercise prescription The individualized amount of exercise that will effectively promote physical fitness for a given person.

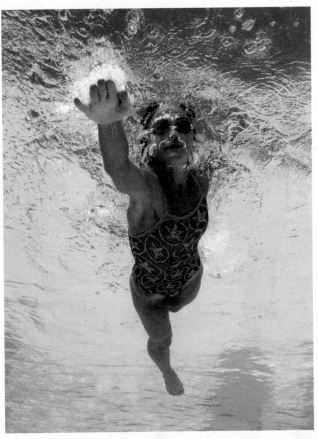
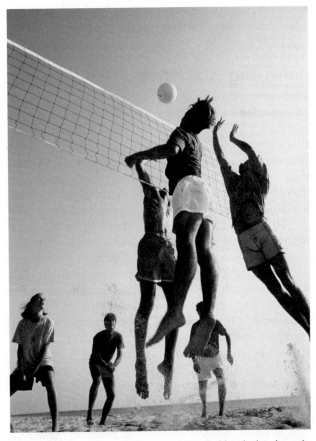

Swimming and volleyball are both excellent for the cardiovascular system. Swimming puts less stress on the joints and is considered a low-impact activity, whereas volleyball puts more stress on joints and is considered a high-impact activity.

A CLOSER LOOK

Too Much Exercise Increases Your Risk of Illness

Research indicates that intense exercise training (or overtraining) reduces the body's immunity to disease (13). In contrast, light to moderate exercise training boosts the immune system and reduces the risk of infections (28). The relationship between exercise training and the risk of developing an upper respiratory tract infection (e.g., a cold) is shown in the figure in this box. The J-shaped curve indicates that moderate exercise training reduces the risk of infection, whereas high-intensity and long-duration training increases the risk of infection.

The explanation for this relationship is complex, but it appears that too much exercise increases levels of stress hormones in the body that weaken the immune system. Depressed immune function increases your risk for developing an infection when you are exposed to bacteria or viruses.

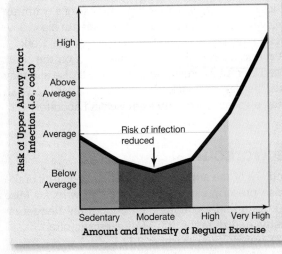

Key

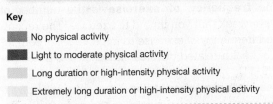

No physical activity

Light to moderate physical activity

Long duration or high-intensity physical activity

Extremely long duration or high-intensity physical activity

personal fitness program. (More details about the exercise goal-setting process will be provided later in Chapter 7.)

Selecting Activities

Every exercise prescription includes at least one **mode of exercise**—that is, a specific type of exercise to be performed. For example, to improve cardiorespiratory fitness, you could select from a wide variety of activities, such as running, swimming, or cycling. To ensure that you'll engage in the exercise regularly, you should choose activities that you will enjoy doing, that are available to you, and that carry little risk of injury.

Physical activities can be classified as being either high-impact or low-impact, based on the amount of stress placed on joints during the activity. Low-impact activities put less stress on the joints than high-impact activities. Because of the strong correlation between high-impact activities and injuries, many fitness experts recommend low-impact activities for fitness beginners or for people susceptible to injury (such as people who are older or overweight). Examples of low-impact activities include walking, cycling, swimming, and low-impact dance activities. High-impact activities include running, basketball, and high-impact dance (e.g., Zumba). (Chapter 7 will provide more details about activity selection in planning your exercise routine.)

The Importance of a Warm-Up

A **warm-up** is a brief (5–15-minute) period of exercise that precedes a workout. It generally involves light calisthenics or a low-intensity form of the exercise and often includes stretching exercises. The purpose of a warm-up is to elevate muscle temperature and increase blood flow to those muscles that will be engaged in the workout (1). A warm-up can also reduce the strain on the heart imposed by rapidly engaging in heavy exercise and may reduce the risk of muscle and tendon injuries. You can find some specific warm up exercises in Laboratory 2.1.

The Workout

Regardless of the activity, the major components of the exercise prescription that make up the workout (also called the primary conditioning period) are frequency, intensity, and duration (time) of exercise, often called the *FIT principle* (see **Figure 2.5**).

The **frequency of exercise** is the number of times per week that you intend to exercise. The recommended frequency of exercise to improve most components of health-related physical fitness is 3–5 times per week (9–11).

The **intensity of exercise** is the amount of physiological stress or overload placed on the body during the

An Example of the FIT Principle	
Frequency	3–5 times per week
Intensity	Moderate
Time (Duration)	30 minutes

FIGURE 2.5
An illustration of the FIT principle.

exercise. The method for determining the intensity of exercise varies with the type of exercise performed. For example, as you use more energy during exercise, your heart rate will increase, so measuring heart rate has become a standard means to determine exercise intensity during cardiorespiratory fitness training.

Whereas heart rate can be used to gauge exercise intensity during strength training, the number of repetitions performed before muscular fatigue occurs is more useful for monitoring intensity during weight lifting. For instance, a load that can be lifted only 5–8 times before complete muscular fatigue is an example of high-intensity weight lifting. In contrast, a load that can be lifted 50–60 times without resulting in muscular fatigue is an illustration of low-intensity weight training.

Finally, flexibility is improved by stretching muscles beyond their normal lengths. Intensity of stretching is monitored by the degree of tension felt during the stretch. Low-intensity stretching results in only minor tension on the muscles and tendons. In contrast, high-intensity stretching places great tension or moderate discomfort on the muscle groups being stretched.

A key aspect of the primary conditioning period is the **duration of exercise**—that is, the amount of time spent performing the primary workout. Note that the duration of exercise does not include the warm-up or cool-down. Research has shown that approximately 30 minutes per exercise session (performed 3 or more times per week) is the minimum amount of time required to significantly improve physical fitness. **Figure 2.6** (page 33) shows a physical activity pyramid that can help you identify types of physical activities that increase your fitness level, and how frequently you should perform them.

The Importance of the Cool-Down

The **cool-down** is a 5- to 15-minute period of low-intensity exercise that immediately follows the primary conditioning period. For instance, a period of slow walking might be used as a cool-down following a running

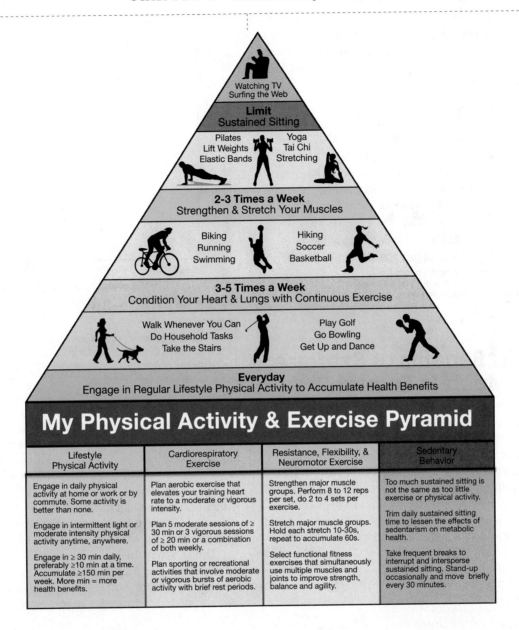

FIGURE 2.6
A physical activity and exercise pyramid like this one shows examples of activities you can incorporate into your fitness program; it can help guide the frequency and time you plan for each activity.

Source: Dr. Jerome Kotecki, Ball State University. Reprinted with permission of Ball State University © 2012.

workout. A cool-down period lowers body temperature after exercise and allows blood to return from the muscles toward the heart (3–6). During exercise, large amounts of blood are pumped to the working muscles. Once exercise stops, blood tends to pool in large blood vessels located around the exercised muscles. Failure to redistribute pooled blood after exercise could result in your feeling lightheaded or even fainting. You can prevent blood pooling by doing low-intensity exercise that uses the same muscles you used during the workout.

Personalizing Your Workout

Although the same general principles of exercise training apply to everyone, no two people are the same, and everyone's exercise prescription will be slightly different.

mode of exercise The specific type of exercise to be performed.

warm-up A brief (5- to 15-minute) period of exercise that precedes a workout.

frequency of exercise The number of times per week that one exercises.

intensity of exercise The amount of physiological stress or overload placed on the body during exercise.

duration of exercise The amount of time invested in performing the primary workout.

cool-down A 5- to 15-minute period of low-intensity exercise that immediately follows the primary conditioning period; sometimes called a *warm-down*.

Your exercise prescription should be based on your general health, age, fitness status, musculoskeletal condition, and body composition. (You will learn more about individualizing workouts in the next several chapters.)

MAKE SURE YOU KNOW...

- The "dose" of exercise required to effectively promote physical fitness is called the exercise prescription.

- The components of the exercise prescription include fitness goals, mode of exercise, the warm-up, the workout, and the cool-down. You can use the FIT principle (frequency, intensity, and duration or time of exercise) to help you design your fitness program.

- Exercise training programs should be individualized by considering such factors as your age, health, and fitness.

 What does it take to bring physical activity to two families' lives? Watch Personal Fitness and Exercise at **www.pearsonhighered.com/powers.**

SEE IT!
VIDEOS

Health Benefits of Exercise: How Much Is Enough?

Exercise training to improve sport performance differs from exercise performed to achieve health benefits (Chapter 1). Exercise training for sport performance typically includes long workouts (60–180 minutes/day) involving high-intensity exercise. In contrast, exercising to obtain health benefits does not need to be as high in intensity, or performed as long, as exercise to improve performance.

Although even low levels of physical activity can provide some health benefits, evidence indicates that moderate to high levels of physical activity are required to provide major health benefits (9, 11–16). The theoretical relationship between physical activity and health benefits is illustrated in **Figure 2.7**. Note that the mini-

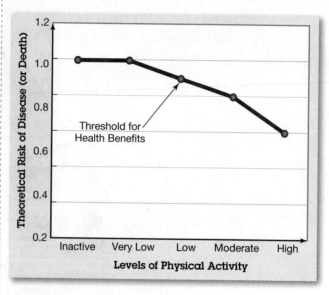

FIGURE 2.7
The relationship between physical activity and improved health benefits. Note that as the level of regular physical activity increases, the theoretical risk of disease (or death) decreases.
Source: Data are from References 15, 26, 27.

mum level of exercise required to achieve some of the health benefits is the **threshold for health benefits**. Most experts believe that 30–60 minutes of moderate- to high-intensity exercise performed 3–5 days per week will surpass the threshold for health benefits and will reduce the risk of all causes of death (15–21). (See Laboratory 2.3 for one way to determine whether you're engaging in enough physical activity to achieve health benefits—counting your steps with a pedometer.)

The U.S. government has provided physical activity guidelines for Americans. These guidelines recommend that adults aged 18–64 perform at least 150 minutes of moderate-intensity exercise or 75 minutes of

COACHING Corner

After deciding to begin an exercise routine, you begin to wonder which modes of exercise are best. Should you spend more time on the treadmill or the elliptical machine? Should you dance, walk, or run? Train with free weights or gym equipment?

Each of these exercise modalities will allow for adaptations if the principles of progressive overload and specificity are followed.

- Create a schedule that includes many different types of exercise. Variety in your

exercise choices can reduce the chances for overuse injury and boredom.

- Choose exercises based on what you enjoy. If you enjoy rock climbing, playing frisbee, and lifting free weights, add those activities to your schedule.

- Stick to your schedule: The best exercises are the ones you consistently perform.

Ideas for exercise

STEPS FOR ▸ BEHAVIOR CHANGE

Are you a couch potato?

Answer the following questions to find out whether you could use more daily physical activity.

Y N

☐ ☐ Do you usually drive to your destinations, even for short trips to the corner store?

☐ ☐ Do you tend to take the elevator instead of the stairs?

☐ ☐ Does your evening routine involve hours of inactivity (e.g., sitting in front of the computer or television)?

☐ ☐ When you drive to a store for shopping, do you tend to park as close to the store entrance as possible?

☐ ☐ Do you always use a remote control to adjust the volume on your stereo or change the channel on your television?

If you answered "yes" to more than one question, you may be a bit too sedentary.

TIPS TO INCORPORATE MORE PHYSICAL ACTIVITY INTO YOUR DAILY ROUTINE

Tomorrow, you will:

☑ Walk or ride your bike for short trips and errands; walk to class if you live close to or on campus.

☑ Get off the bus a stop early, and walk the rest of the way.

☑ Take the stairs instead of the elevator.

Within the next 2 weeks, you will:

☑ Go for a walk or a bike ride with a friend or family member instead of settling in with the television after dinner.

By the end of the semester, you will:

☑ Forgo an hour of Internet time every day to walk the dog, or play basketball or tennis with a friend.

---

vigorous-intensity aerobic physical activity per week (24). Fortunately, the activity doesn't need to be done all at once and can be divided into two to three segments of exercise throughout the day (18–25). If you walk briskly for 15 minutes to get to your class in the morning and then take a 15-minute bike ride to get to your job in the afternoon, you've attained the goal of incorporating 30 minutes of moderate exercise into your day.

However, this dose of exercise may be insufficient to prevent weight gain in some individuals who need additional exercise and calorie restriction to prevent weight gain. (See Chapter 9 for more details.) Further, people who get 30 minutes of moderate-intensity exercise per day are likely to achieve additional health benefits if they exercise for longer periods of time (19, 24).

Are some forms of exercise better than others for obtaining health benefits? There is no short answer to this question. Nonetheless, numerous activities, including running, swimming, cycling, and walking, can help achieve exercise-related health benefits. (Details on how to achieve health-related aspects of physical fitness will be discussed in Chapters 4 through 6.)

MAKE SURE YOU KNOW...

- Although low levels of physical activity can provide some health benefits, moderate-to-high levels of physical activity are required to provide major health benefits.

- The threshold for health benefits is the minimum level of exercise required to achieve some health benefits of exercise.

 Can Eric find the motivation he needs to start exercising? Listen to the online case study at **www.pearsonhighered.com/powers.**

HEAR IT!
CASE STUDY

Removing Barriers to Physical Activity

Despite the many benefits of an active lifestyle, the level of physical activity remains low for most Americans. For example, the Centers for Disease Control report that only 31% of Americans engage in some form of leisure time activity. Further, only 12% of Americans participate in a regular exercise program (i.e., >20 minutes of exercise per day/3 days week). There are four major barriers that contribute to this low level of exercise activity: lack of time, social and environmental influences, inadequate resources, and a lack of motivation/commitment. Without question, the most important of these barriers is the

threshold for health benefits The minimum level of physical activity required to achieve some of the health benefits of exercise.

lack of motivation and commitment to establish a regular exercise program. Completion of Laboratory 2.4 will assist you in identifying and overcoming personal barriers to physical activity.

Assess your physical activity with the *How Much Do I Move?* Take Charge Of Your Health! Worksheet online at **www.pearsonhighered.com/powers.**

**LIVE IT!
ASSESS
YOURSELF**

MAKE SURE YOU KNOW...

- Most Americans do not engage in leisure time activity or a regular program of exercise.
- Barriers to physical activity include a shortage of time and resources, social and environmental influences, inadequate resources, and inadequate motivation to participate in regular exercise.

SUMMARY

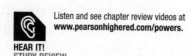

Listen and see chapter review videos at **www.pearsonhighered.com/powers.**

**HEAR IT!
STUDY REVIEW**

1. The overload principle, which is the most important principle of exercise training, states that to improve physical fitness, the body or muscle group used during exercise must be stressed.
2. The principle of progression states that overload should be increased gradually during the course of a physical fitness program.
3. The need for a rest period between exercise training sessions is called the principle of recuperation.
4. Physical fitness can be lost due to inactivity; this is often called the principle of reversibility.
5. The components of the exercise prescription include fitness goals, type of activity, the warm-up, the workout, and the cool-down.

6. All exercise training programs should be tailored to meet the objectives of the individual, taking into consideration the individual's age, health, fitness status, musculoskeletal condition, and body composition.
7. The minimum level of physical activity required to achieve some of the health benefits of exercise is called the threshold for health benefits.
8. There are four major barriers to performing physical activity: (1) lack of time; (2) social and environmental influences; (3) inadequate resources; and (4) a lack of motivation/commitment.

STUDY QUESTIONS

Find more review questions online at **www.pearsonhighered.com/powers.**

**REVIEW IT!
QUIZZES**

1. Which one of the following is NOT a key principle of exercise training?
   a. overload principle
   b. principle of progression
   c. principle of recuperation
   d. principle of supercompensation
2. The current public health recommendation is for adults to achieve a minimum of _____ minutes of moderate-intensity physical activity each day.
   a. 15
   b. 20
   c. 30
   d. 60
3. A primary purpose of a warm-up is to
   a. increase blood flow to the active muscles.
   b. remove lactic acid from the blood.
   c. reduce the level of stress hormones in the blood.
   d. reduce the length of conditioning time needed.
4. What is the difference between overtraining and the principle of recuperation?

5. What are the general purposes of a warm-up and a cool-down?
6. What are the components of the exercise prescription?
7. How does the principle of progression apply to the exercise prescription?
8. What is the overload principle, and what is one practical example?
9. Why is the threshold for health benefits an important concept?
10. What happens to physical fitness if you stop training?
11. Why should the exercise prescription be individualized?
12. What are the major barriers that prevent people from engaging in physical activity?

HELPFUL WEBLINKS

DO IT!
WEBLINKS

For links to the organizations and websites listed, visit
www.pearsonhighered.com/powers.

American College of Sports Medicine
Offers information about exercise, health, and fitness.
www.acsm.org

American Heart Association
Provides the latest news and research about ways
to reduce your risk of heart and vascular diseases.
Includes information about exercise, diet, and heart
disease. www.heart.org

Medline Plus
Contains up-to-date information on a variety of
health-related issues, including exercise and physical
fitness. www.nlm.nih.gov/medlineplus

U.S. Department of Health and Human Services
Provides the *2008 Physical Activity Guidelines for
Americans.* www.health.gov/paguidelines

WebMD
Gives the latest information on a variety of
health-related topics, including diet, exercise, and
stress. Includes links to nutrition, fitness, and wellness
topics. www.webmd.com

Name _____ Date _____

Warming Up

Use the following activities to warm up your body for aerobic activities such as jogging, walking, or cycling. Perform the stretching exercises slowly, holding each stretch for 20 to 30 seconds. Do not bounce or jerk the muscle. Do each stretch at least once and up to three times.

CARDIOVASCULAR WARM-UP

Walk briskly or jog slowly for 5 minutes.

STRETCHES

Calf Stretch for Gastrocnemius and Soleus

Stand with your right foot about 1 to 2 feet in front of your left foot, with both feet pointing forward. Keeping your left leg straight, lunge forward by bending your right knee and pushing your left heel backward. Hold this position. Then pull your left foot in slightly and bend your left knee. Shift your weight to your left leg and hold. Repeat this entire sequence with the left leg forward.

Scan to view a demonstration video of the calf stretch. ▶

Sitting Toe Touch for Hamstrings

Sit on the ground with your right leg straight and your left leg tucked close to your body. Reach toward your outstretched right foot as far as possible with both hands. Repeat with the left leg.

Scan to view a demonstration video of the hamstring stretch. ▶

Step Stretch for Quadriceps and Hip

Step forward and bend your front knee about 90 degrees, keeping your knee directly above your ankle. Stretch the opposite leg back so that it is parallel to the floor. Rotate your hips forward and slightly down to stretch. Your arms can be at your sides or resting on top of your forward thigh. Repeat on the other side.

Scan to view a demonstration video of the hip flexor stretch. ▶

Leg Hug for the Hip and Back Extensors

Lie flat on your back with both legs straight. Bending your knees, bring your legs up to your torso, and grasp both legs behind the thighs. Pull both legs in to your chest and hold.

Scan to view a demonstration video of the knee-to-chest stretch. ▶

Side Stretch for the Torso

Stand with feet shoulder-width apart, knees slightly bent, and pelvis tucked under. Raise one arm over your head, and bend sideways from the waist toward your raised arm. Support your torso by placing the hand of your resting arm on your hip or thigh for support. Repeat on the other side.

Scan to view a demonstration video of the side stretch. ▶

You can also repeat these same exercises after a workout to cool down.

1. Did you notice an increase in heart rate during the cardiovascular warm-up? _____

2. In which stretch did you feel the most tightness? _____

3. Do you think the sample warm-up is adequate for the activities you plan to do as part of your exercise program? If not, what exercises would you add?

_____

_____

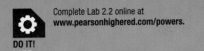

Name _____ Date _____

Which Physical Activities Work Best for You?

As you design your personal fitness program, think about the activities you currently enjoy most and least and about new activities you would like to try. Which can you incorporate into your program?

Answer the following questions in the spaces provided.

1. List the fitness/wellness activities in which you have participated or are currently participating.

   _____

2. Which of these activities did you enjoy the most? Why?

   _____

3. What are some new activities you might enjoy? (See the list at the end of the lab for additional options.)

   _____

   _____

4. What components of physical fitness do you think these activities affect? For instance, jogging improves cardiovascular fitness, whereas weight lifting increases muscular strength.

   _____

   _____

5. What areas of physical health would you like to improve? Can you think of any activities that would aid in this goal?

   _____

   _____

Examples of Exercise and Physical Activity

- Walking or jogging on a treadmill
- Walking or cycling to work
- Cycling on an upright or recumbent exercise bike
- Walking, jogging, or cycling outdoors
- Zumba, kickboxing class, or martial arts
- Weight or resistance training
- Yoga
- Pilates
- Hiking
- Rock climbing
- Elliptical trainer
- Sport activities (e.g., soccer, basketball, tennis, racquetball)

LABORATORY 2.3

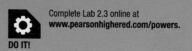

Complete Lab 2.3 online at
www.pearsonhighered.com/powers.

DO IT!
LABS

Name _____ Date _____

Using a Pedometer to Count Your Steps

One way to determine your level of daily physical activity is to use a pedometer to measure the number of steps you take in a day. A pedometer is a small portable device that contains a sensor and, often, software applications to estimate the distance walked and the number of calories expended. The accuracy of pedometers can vary from device to device, but many pedometers are reasonably accurate if they are worn in the optimal position (such as on a belt clip). However, carrying a pedometer in a pocket or handbag tends to reduce its accuracy. Moreover, some pedometers record movement other than walking (e.g., bending to tie your shoes), and therefore some "false steps" may show up on your daily step count.

   Experts currently recommend 10,000 steps per day to reach a level of physical activity that is considered to be an active lifestyle with positive health benefits. Do you think you meet this goal?

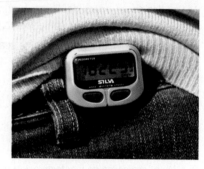

A pedometer worn at the waist.

Directions:

Wear a pedometer for a day and note your number of steps. Write in the total number below. Then set a goal for the number of steps you want to take per day, and list some strategies for incorporating more steps into your day. Track the number of steps you take every day for the next 2 weeks, and note your progress toward your goal.

Goal number of steps/day: _____

Number of steps for day 1: _____   **Number of steps for day 8:** _____

Number of steps for day 2: _____   **Number of steps for day 9:** _____

Number of steps for day 3: _____   **Number of steps for day 10:** _____

Number of steps for day 4: _____   **Number of steps for day 11:** _____

Number of steps for day 5: _____   **Number of steps for day 12:** _____

Number of steps for day 6: _____   **Number of steps for day 13:** _____

Number of steps for day 7: _____   **Number of steps for day 14:** _____

Analysis:

1. Did you meet your goal for number of daily steps on most days? Yes/No

2. Are you walking at least the recommended 10,000 steps per day? Yes/No

3. If not, think about how you can incorporate more steps into your daily routine. List below four ways to increase the amount of walking you do daily:

_____

_____

_____

_____

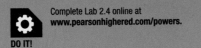
Name _____   Date _____

Identifying Barriers to Physical Activity

This lab will assist you in identifying the major barriers that prevent you from participating in regular physical activity and exercise. Listed below are the primary reasons why most people do not engage in regular physical activity and exercise. Please read each statement and select the number in the answer box that best applies to you. At the end of this exercise, add up the total number of points in each of the four major categories of barriers to physical activity.

Barrier category 1: Lack of time

How likely are you to say this?	Unlikely	Likely	Very Likely
My day is too busy for exercise. I cannot find the time to include regular physical activity.	0	1	2
Physical activity takes too much time away from work and my family commitments.	0	1	3
My periods of free time during the day are too short to exercise.	0	1	3

Barrier category 2: Social and environmental influences

How likely are you to say this?	Unlikely	Likely	Very Likely
None of my friends or family members are interested or involved in physical activity.	0	1	2
I am embarrassed to exercise in front of other people.	0	1	3
My school or place of work does not provide an environment that permits exercising.	0	1	3

Barrier category 3: Lack of resources

How likely are you to say this?	Unlikely	Likely	Very Likely
I do not have access to walking/jogging trails, swimming pools, or bike paths.	0	1	2
It is too expensive to join a health club or purchase exercise equipment.	0	1	3
My school or place of work does not provide shower facilities or an exercise facility.	0	1	3

Barrier category 4: Lack of motivation

How likely are you to say this?	Unlikely	Likely	Very Likely
I have been considering exercise but I can't seem to get started.	0	1	2
It is easy for me to find an excuse not to exercise.	0	1	3
I would like to exercise but I have difficulty sticking to a commitment.	0	1	3

Scoring and Using Your Results

Add up the total number of points scored in each of the four barrier categories and record your scores in the space provided below. If you scored 2 or more points in any category, this indicates that this category represents one of your major barriers to becoming physically active.

Barrier category 1. Lack of time: Total points =_____

Barrier category 2. Social and environmental influences: Total points =_____

Barrier category 3. Lack of resources: Total points =_____

Barrier category 4. Lack of motivation: Total points =_____

Planning Your Next Steps

Now that you've identified your major barriers to becoming physically active, your next move is to develop strategies to remove each barrier. The chart below provides suggestions for strategies that can assist you in eliminating barriers.

Barrier	Suggestions for overcoming physical activity barriers
Lack of time	1. Identify available time slots in your day that could be used to exercise. 2. Select a time during your day to replace a sedentary activity with physical activity, such as riding a bike instead of driving. 3. Increase the length of your day to include a time slot for exercise.
Social and environmental influences	1. Encourage your family and friends to exercise. 2. Identify new friends who are already physically active, and make plans to exercise with them. 3. Plan social activities that involve exercise.
Lack of resources	1. Select activities that do not require expensive equipment, such as walking, calisthenics, or jumping rope. 2. Identify inexpensive exercise facilities that are available in your community (park and recreation programs, worksite programs, etc.) 3. Use commonplace areas to incorporate exercise, such as the stairs in your apartment building.
Lack of motivation	1. Write down your exercise goals and put them in a place where you see them every day. 2. Plan your day around a time to exercise. 3. Join an exercise class. 4. Pack a bag with your exercise clothes and place it somewhere you will see it before leaving for work or school.

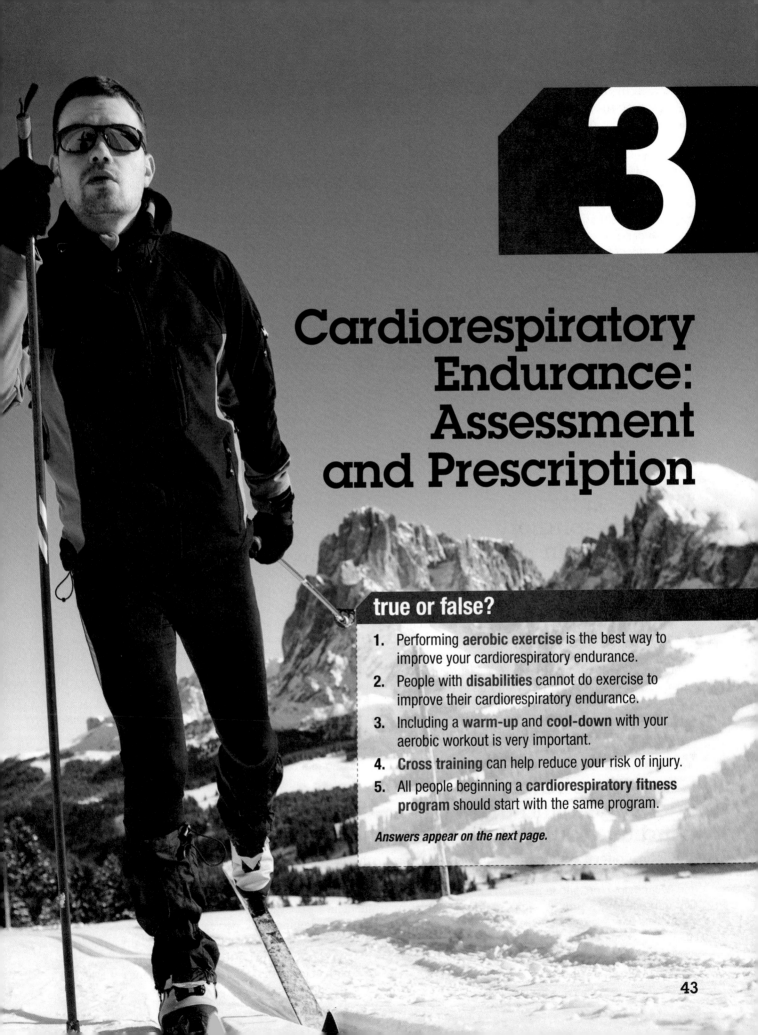

3

Cardiorespiratory Endurance: Assessment and Prescription

true or false?

1. Performing **aerobic exercise** is the best way to improve your cardiorespiratory endurance.
2. People with **disabilities** cannot do exercise to improve their cardiorespiratory endurance.
3. Including a **warm-up** and **cool-down** with your aerobic workout is very important.
4. **Cross training** can help reduce your risk of injury.
5. All people beginning a **cardiorespiratory fitness program** should start with the same program.

Answers appear on the next page.

Are there any hills on your campus? Have you ever trudged up one of them, only to be winded and out of breath by the time you got to the top? Do you notice that some of your fellow students, and probably many of your professors, can perform the activity without exertion? If you answered yes to these questions, you are already familiar with the concept of cardiorespiratory endurance. The low cardiorespiratory endurance that often accompanies a lack of regular exercise can make even common everyday tasks difficult. In this chapter, we will explore the basics of cardiorespiratory endurance and the types of exercise that will improve it.

We discussed the health benefits of exercise and the general principles of exercise training in Chapters 1 and 2. In this chapter (and in the next three chapters) we describe how to assess your level of each health-related fitness component and show you how to begin designing a comprehensive, scientifically based exercise program to meet your health and fitness goals. Before we discuss the assessment and prescription for cardiovascular fitness, we need to define cardiorespiratory endurance and to cover some basic cardiovascular physiology.

The Need for Cardiorespiratory Endurance in Daily Living

Developing cardiorespiratory endurance is beneficial for a number of everyday activities. Walking around your campus to get to class or the library requires cardiorespiratory fitness. Other everyday activities, such as cleaning your dorm room or apartment, or yard work if you live in a house, are easier when you have a higher level of cardiorespiratory fitness. Your leisure time and social activities, such as a weekend hiking or camping trip with friends or a night out dancing, are more enjoyable with higher cardiorespiratory fitness.

What Are Cardiorespiratory Endurance and the Cardiovascular System?

Cardiorespiratory endurance is the ability to perform **aerobic exercises,** such as swimming, jogging, and cycling, for a prolonged period of time, and is effective in promoting weight loss and reducing the risk of cardiovascular disease. Because of this, many exercise scientists consider cardiorespiratory endurance the most important component of health-related physical fitness (1, 2).

answers

1. **TRUE** Aerobic exercises such as walking, participating in aerobics classes, and swimming will improve or maintain cardiorespiratory endurance.

2. **FALSE** There are many activities that persons with disabilities can do to improve their cardiorespiratory fitness. The Closer Look box on page 55 and the Appreciating Diversity box on page 59 discuss some exercise options for people with temporary or permanent disabilities.

3. **TRUE** A warm-up and cool-down will help reduce your risk of injury and muscle soreness. Both should be included with your workouts even if you are exercising for a short duration or at moderate intensity.

4. **TRUE** Cross training means using multiple types of exercise, and this practice can reduce the risk for overuse injuries, especially if you perform high-impact exercises.

5. **FALSE** Your program should be based on your initial fitness level. The sample programs on pages 61–64 provide examples for beginners of initial low, average, and high fitness levels.

The most valid measurement of cardiorespiratory fitness is $\dot{V}O_2$ **max**, or maximal aerobic capacity, which is the maximum amount of oxygen the body can take in and use during exercise. In simple terms, $\dot{V}O_2$ max is a measure of the endurance of both the cardiorespiratory system and exercising skeletal muscles.

The cardiorespiratory system is made up of the cardiovascular system (the heart and blood vessels) and the respiratory system (the lungs and muscles involved in respiration). Together these systems deliver oxygen and nutrients throughout the body and remove waste products (e.g., carbon dioxide) from tissues. Exercise challenges the cardiorespiratory system because it increases the demand for oxygen and nutrients in the working muscles.

The Cardiovascular System

The heart is a pump, about the size of your fist, that contracts and generates pressure to move blood through the blood vessels throughout the body. Actually, the heart is considered two pumps in one. The right side pumps oxygen-depleted (deoxygenated) blood to the lungs in a pathway called the **pulmonary circuit,** and the left side pumps oxygen-rich (oxygenated) blood to tissues throughout the body through a pathway called the **systemic circuit.** Figure 3.1 (page 46) illustrates the path of blood through the heart and lungs.

consider this!
Up to 50% of college students do not get the recommended amount of exercise.

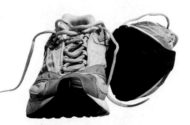

There are different types of blood vessels in the circulatory system. With the exception of the pulmonary artery (which carries oxygen-depleted blood from the heart to the lungs), **arteries** carry oxygen-rich blood away from the heart to the rest of the body. Except for the pulmonary vein (which carries oxygen-rich blood from the lungs to the heart), **veins** carry oxygen-depleted blood from the body's tissues back to the heart.

Blood is pumped from the left side of the heart into the aorta, the largest artery in the body. From the aorta, arteries branch into smaller vessels called *arterioles,* which further branch into **capillaries.** The capillaries have walls that are one cell thick, through which oxygen and nutrients can easily pass. Through the capillaries, oxygen and nutrients are delivered to the tissues, and carbon dioxide and waste are picked up from the tissues and taken back to the heart. The capillaries branch into bigger vessels called *venules,* and then into veins. From the veins the blood enters the right side of the heart and is pumped to the lungs.

Every time your heart pumps (or beats), you can feel a pulse. People often measure the number of times their heart beats per minute (commonly called the *heart rate*) to gauge their exercise intensity (more on this later in the chapter). When people say they are "taking their pulse," they are referring to their heart rate. The easiest places to take your heart rate are your radial and carotid arteries. The radial artery is located on the inside of your wrist just below your thumb, and the carotid artery can be found along the neck (see **Figure 3.2** on page 47). The amount of blood that is pumped with each heartbeat is called **stroke volume.** The product of heart rate and stroke volume is **cardiac output,** which is the amount of blood that is pumped per minute.

The Respiratory System

The respiratory system controls our breathing. In the lungs, carbon dioxide and waste from the oxygen-depleted blood pass into tiny air sacs called **alveoli.** When we exhale, the carbon dioxide and waste are released into the air. Then, as we inhale, we bring oxygen into the lungs, where oxygen enters the alveoli and passes into the capillaries. From the lungs the oxygen-rich blood travels to the left side of the heart to start the process again.

MAKE SURE YOU KNOW...

- Cardiorespiratory endurance, which refers to how well you can perform aerobic exercises, is considered one of the most important health-related fitness components.
- $\dot{V}O_2$max is a measure of cardiorespiratory endurance.
- The cardiorespiratory system consists of the cardiovascular and respiratory systems.
- The heart and blood vessels make up the cardiovascular system, and the lungs and muscles used for breathing make up the respiratory system.
- The pulmonary circuit pumps blood to the lungs, and the systemic circuit pumps blood throughout the body.

How Do We Get Energy for Exercise?

We have discussed the importance of getting oxygen to the muscles and having energy for prolonged exercise. But why is it important to get more oxygen to the

---

cardiorespiratory endurance The ability to perform aerobic exercises for a prolonged period of time.

aerobic exercise A common term to describe all forms of exercises that primarily use the aerobic energy system and that are designed to improve cardiorespiratory fitness.

$\dot{V}O_2$ max The maximum amount of oxygen the body can take in and use during exercise.

pulmonary circuit The vascular system that circulates blood from the right side of the heart, through the lungs, and back to the left side of the heart.

systemic circuit The vascular system that circulates blood from the left side of the heart, throughout the body, and back to the right side of the heart.

arteries The blood vessels that carry blood away from the heart.

veins The blood vessels that transport blood toward the heart.

capillaries Thin-walled vessels that permit the exchange of gases (oxygen and carbon dioxide) and nutrients between the blood and tissues.

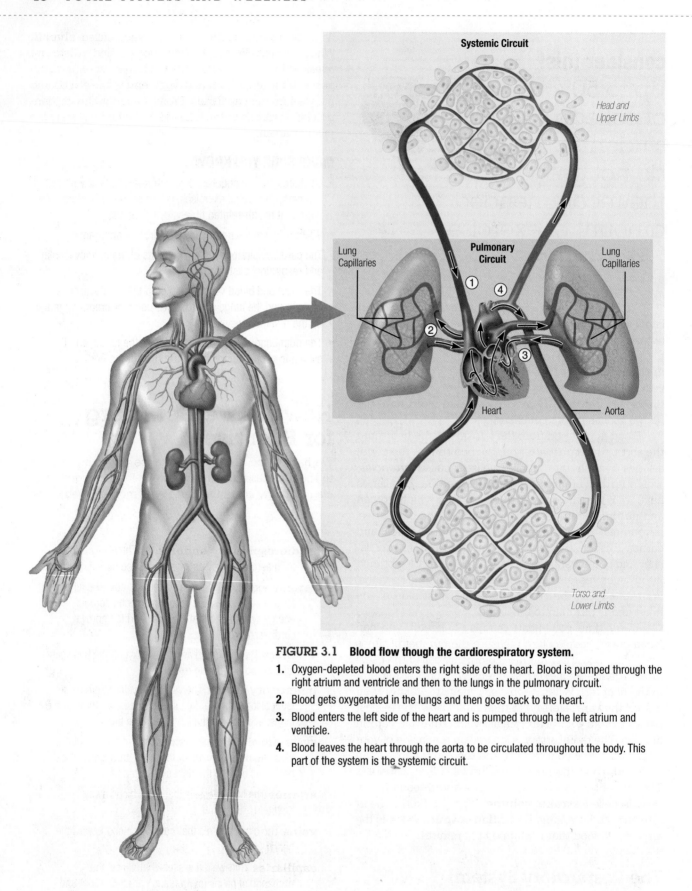

FIGURE 3.1   Blood flow though the cardiorespiratory system.

1. Oxygen-depleted blood enters the right side of the heart. Blood is pumped through the right atrium and ventricle and then to the lungs in the pulmonary circuit.

2. Blood gets oxygenated in the lungs and then goes back to the heart.

3. Blood enters the left side of the heart and is pumped through the left atrium and ventricle.

4. Blood leaves the heart through the aorta to be circulated throughout the body. This part of the system is the systemic circuit.

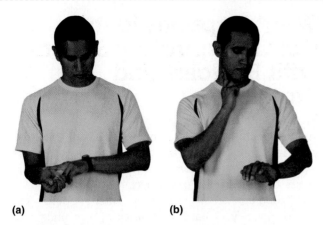

(a)   **(b)**

FIGURE 3.2
You can measure heart rate at either the radial artery in the wrist just under the thumb **(a)** or at the carotid artery in the neck below the jawline **(b)**. See Laboratory 3.3 at the end of the chapter for detailed instructions and links to demonstration videos.

muscles, and what do we mean by *energy*? Energy is the fuel needed to make the muscles move for activity, and we get that energy from the breakdown of food. However, food energy cannot be used directly by the muscles. Instead, the energy released from the breakdown of food is used to make a biochemical compound called **adenosine triphosphate (ATP).** ATP is made and stored in small amounts in muscle and other cells. The breakdown of ATP releases energy that your muscles can use to contract and make you move and it is the only compound in the body that can provide this immediate source of energy. Therefore, for muscles to contract during exercise, a supply of ATP must be available.

The body uses two "systems" in muscle cells to produce ATP. One system does not require oxygen and is called the **anaerobic** ("without oxygen") system. The second requires oxygen and is called the **aerobic** ("with oxygen") system. The aerobic system is the primary system for developing cardiorespiratory endurance, which is why we need to get oxygen to the muscles.

Anaerobic Energy Production

Most of the anaerobic ATP production in muscle occurs during **glycolysis,** the process that breaks down carbohydrates in cells. In addition to ATP, glycolysis often results in the formation of **lactic acid,** and this pathway for ATP production is often called the *lactic acid system*. This system uses only carbohydrates as an energy source. Carbohydrates are supplied to muscles from blood sugar (glucose) and from muscle stores of glucose called *glycogen*.

The anaerobic pathway provides ATP at the beginning of exercise and for short-term (30–60 seconds)

high-intensity exercise. Exercise that is intense and less than 2 minutes in duration, such as a 60- to 80-second 400-meter sprint, relies primarily on this system. During this type of intense exercise, muscles produce large amounts of lactic acid because the lactic acid system is operating at high speed.

Aerobic Energy Production

After about a minute of high-intensity exercise, anaerobic production of ATP begins to decrease, and aerobic production of ATP starts to increase. The aerobic system requires oxygen for the chemical reactions to make ATP. Activities of daily living and many types of exercise depend on ATP production from the aerobic system.

Whereas the anaerobic system uses only carbohydrates as a food source, aerobic metabolism can use fats, carbohydrates, and protein to produce ATP, though for a healthy person who eats a balanced diet, proteins have a limited role during exercise—carbohydrates and fats are the primary sources. In general, at the beginning of exercise, carbohydrates are the main fuel broken down during aerobic ATP production. During prolonged exercise (i.e., longer than 20 minutes), there is a gradual shift from carbohydrates to fats as an energy source (see **Figure 3.3** on page 48).

stroke volume The amount of blood pumped per heartbeat (generally expressed in milliliters).

cardiac output The amount of blood the heart pumps per minute.

alveoli Tiny air sacs in the lungs that receive carbon dioxide and other wastes from oxygen-depleted blood.

adenosine triphosphate (ATP) A high-energy compound that is synthesized and stored in small quantities in muscle and other cells. The breakdown of ATP results in a release of energy that can be used to fuel muscular contraction.

anaerobic "Without oxygen"; in cells, pertains to biochemical pathways that do not require oxygen to produce energy.

aerobic "With oxygen"; in cells, pertains to biochemical pathways that use oxygen to produce energy.

glycolysis A process during which carbohydrates are broken down in cells. Much of the anaerobic ATP production in muscle cells occurs during glycolysis.

lactic acid A by-product of glucose metabolism, produced primarily during intense exercise (i.e., greater than 50%–60% of maximal aerobic capacity).

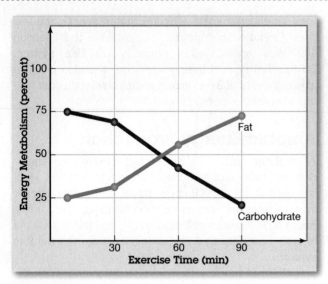

FIGURE 3.3
After about 60 minutes of exercise, the body begins to use more fat and fewer carbohydrates for ATP production.

The Energy Continuum

Although we often speak of aerobic versus anaerobic exercise, in reality many types of exercise use both systems. Figure 3.4(a) (page 49) illustrates the anaerobic–aerobic energy continuum as it relates to exercise duration. Anaerobic energy production is dominant during short-term exercise, and aerobic energy production predominates during long-term exercise. For example, a 100-meter dash uses anaerobic energy sources almost exclusively. At the other end of the energy spectrum, running a marathon uses mostly aerobic production of ATP, because the exercise involves 2 or more hours of continuous activity. Running a maximal-effort 800-meter race (exercise of 2–3 minutes' duration) is an example of an exercise that uses almost an equal amount of aerobic and anaerobic energy sources.

Figure 3.4(b) (page 49) applies the anaerobic–aerobic energy continuum to various sports activities. Weight lifting, gymnastics, and wrestling are examples of sports that use anaerobic energy production almost exclusively. Boxing and skating (1500 meters) require an equal contribution of anaerobic and aerobic energy production. During cross-country skiing and jogging, on the other hand, aerobic energy production dominates.

MAKE SURE YOU KNOW...

- ATP is used for energy during exercise.
- Anaerobic energy production does not require oxygen, uses carbohydrates for fuel, and supplies energy for short-term, high-intensity exercises.
- Aerobic energy production requires oxygen to make ATP; can use carbohydrates, fats, or proteins for fuel; and is used for longer-duration exercises.
- Many activities use both energy systems.

What Happens to the Cardiorespiratory System with Exercise and Training?

You have probably noticed that when you go for a run or spend more than a few minutes on an exercise bike, your heart rate increases and you start to sweat. These reactions are due to specific needs of your body during exercise. We'll discuss these next.

During an exercise session and after a regular exercise program, your cardiorespiratory system undergoes several **responses** and **adaptations.** Responses are the changes that occur during and immediately after exercise. For example, your increased heart rate and heavy breathing after you walk up a hill are responses. Adaptations are the changes you will see if you stick with a regular exercise program. Your ability to walk up that hill without getting winded after a few weeks of regular aerobic exercise is the result of adaptations to the cardiorespiratory system. As the cardiorespiratory system gets stronger, it does not have to work as hard for the same level of exercise.

Responses to Exercise

When you exercise, the exercising muscles need more oxygen and nutrients to maintain their activity, so your cardiac output has to increase. The faster heart rate you experience during exercise contributes to the increased cardiac output. Increases in stroke volume also increase cardiac output, enabling your working muscles to get enough oxygen to produce energy. The arteries going to the working muscles dilate (expand) to deliver the increased blood and oxygen to the exercising muscles.

The respiratory system also has to respond to the demands of exercise by maintaining constant levels of oxygen and carbon dioxide in the blood. Exercise increases the amount of oxygen the body uses and the amount of carbon dioxide produced. Therefore, breathing rate increases to bring more oxygen into the body and to remove the carbon dioxide, so that as you exercise at higher intensities, breathing increases rapidly, which enhances the removal of carbon dioxide.

Adaptations to Exercise

Regular endurance exercise training results in adaptations in the cardiovascular and respiratory systems, skeletal muscles, and the energy-producing systems.

Endurance training results in several adaptations in the cardiovascular system (3). One thing you will notice as your cardiorespiratory fitness level increases is that your resting heart rate decreases. This occurs because

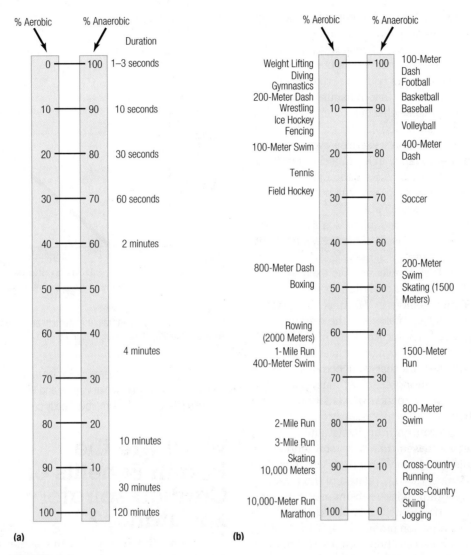

FIGURE 3.4
Contributions of aerobically and anaerobically produced ATP to energy metabolism during exercise.
(a) Contributions as a function of exercise duration. **(b)** Contributions for various sport activities.

your heart is able to pump more blood per heartbeat, so it does not have to beat as many times per minute to get the same amount of blood throughout the body. The maximum number of times your heart beats per minute does not increase with aerobic exercise training, but your maximal stroke volume does, and as stroke volume increases, maximal cardiac output increases. Remember that cardiac output is the amount of blood that is pumped through the body per minute. Because the maximal amount of blood your heart can pump per minute increases, the maximal amount of oxygen you can use during exercise (your $\dot{V}O_2$ max) increases.

Aerobic exercise training does not alter the structure or function of the respiratory system, but it does increase the endurance of the muscles involved in the breathing process (3). The diaphragm, located below the lungs, and other key muscles of respiration can work harder and longer without fatigue. This improvement in respiratory muscle endurance may reduce the feeling of being out of breath during exercise and eliminate the pain in the side

responses The changes that occur during exercise to help you meet the demands of the exercise session. These changes return to normal levels shortly after the exercise session.

adaptations Semipermanent changes that occur over time with regular exercise. Adaptations can be reversed when a regular exercise program is stopped for an extended period of time.

(often called a stitch) that people sometimes experience when beginning an aerobic exercise program.

Endurance training also increases the muscles' capacity to produce aerobic energy. The practical results of this adaptation are that the body is better able to use fat to produce energy and that muscular endurance increases (3). Note that these changes occur only in those muscles used for exercise or activity. For example, endurance training using a stationary exercise cycle results in improved muscular endurance in leg muscles, but it has little effect on arm muscles. Also, although endurance training improves muscle tone, you will not see significant increases in muscle size or strength.

Recall that many exercise physiologists consider $\dot{V}O_2$ max the best single measure of cardiorespiratory fitness. Therefore, improved $\dot{V}O_2$ max is an important adaptation resulting from regular aerobic exercise training. In general, 12 to 15 weeks of endurance exercise produce a 10%–30% improvement in $\dot{V}O_2$ max (3), the result of a combination of the adaptations of the cardiorespiratory system, improved aerobic capacity of the aerobic muscles, and increased maximal cardiac output. The benefits of the increase are that your body can deliver and use more oxygen during exercise, muscular endurance improves, and you experience less fatigue during routine daily activities.

In general, a person with an initial low $\dot{V}O_2$ max will have greater increases than a person who starts an aerobic exercise program with a high $\dot{V}O_2$ max. The increase in $\dot{V}O_2$ max is directly related to the intensity of the training program, with high-intensity training programs producing greater increases than low-intensity and short-duration programs (4) **(Figure 3.5)**. Note, though, that poor nutritional habits will impede improvements in $\dot{V}O_2$ max. (You will learn more about developing a healthy diet in Chapter 8.)

Body Composition

Endurance training generally produces a loss of body fat and healthier body composition (3). However, a loss of body fat is not guaranteed. If you begin an aerobic exercise program with the goal of losing weight, you also need to consider the amount of exercise you do and your dietary habits. (You will learn more about body composition and weight management in Chapters 6 and 9.)

MAKE SURE YOU KNOW...

- Responses are the short-term changes that occur during exercise, and adaptations are the changes that occur over time as a result of regular exercise.
- Responses to exercise include increases in heart rate, stroke volume, cardiac output, and breathing rate.

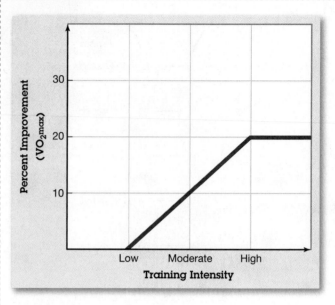

FIGURE 3.5
The relationship between training intensity and improvements in $\dot{V}O_2$max following a 12-week training period.

- Adaptations to regular aerobic exercise include decreased resting heart rate, increased stroke volume and $\dot{V}O_2$max, improved ability to use fats for fuel, and improved body composition.

What Are the Health Benefits of Cardiorespiratory Endurance?

Health and fitness are not the same, and there are differences between physical activity and exercise (as you learned in Chapter 1). Regular physical activity can lead to health improvements (e.g., reduced risk for heart disease) even if you do not have a structured exercise program. However, without a structured program, you probably will not see significant changes in your cardiorespiratory endurance level.

Among the most significant health benefits of cardiorespiratory fitness are a lower risk of cardiovascular disease (CVD) and increased longevity. Also, people who exercise to improve their cardiorespiratory fitness have a reduced risk of type 2 diabetes, lower blood pressure, and increased bone density in weight-bearing bones (5).

In addition to physical health benefits, there are also psychological health benefits associated with regular aerobic exercise training, including a higher level of self-esteem and a more positive body image (6). This relationship is due to multiple factors. First, there is a sense of accomplishment that comes from starting and maintaining a regular exercise program and meeting personal goals. Regular exercise also improves muscle tone and helps with weight management, both of which can have positive impact on appearance. Improved sleep quality is another psychological benefit of regular exercise (7). Fit individuals tend to sleep longer without interruptions (i.e., they enjoy more restful sleep) than do less-fit people. A better night's rest will likely translate to a more complete feeling of being mentally restored.

Benefits of cardiorespiratory endurance also extend to activities of daily living. More energy for work and play is a commonly reported benefit; fit individuals can perform more work with less fatigue. People with high levels of cardiorespiratory fitness often say they exercise because it makes them feel better.

MAKE SURE YOU KNOW...

- Regular exercise is needed to improve your cardiorespiratory endurance.
- There are numerous physical and psychological health benefits of regular aerobic exercise, including reduced risk of CVD, increased longevity, and improved self-esteem and body image.

Evaluation of Cardiorespiratory Endurance

The most accurate means of measuring cardiorespiratory fitness is the laboratory assessment of $\dot{V}O_2 max$ (3, 8). However, direct measurement of $\dot{V}O_2 max$ requires expensive equipment and is very time-consuming, so it is not practical for general use. Fortunately, there are numerous field tests for estimating $\dot{V}O_2 max$ (9–11). Each of these tests has a margin of error, but they are valid measures, and the practical advantages outweigh the disadvantages. This section will explain some of the common ways you can easily estimate your $\dot{V}O_2 max$, and you can use Laboratory 3.1A–D at the end of the chapter for this purpose.

One of the simplest and most accurate assessments of cardiorespiratory fitness is the **1.5-mile run test.** This test is based on the idea that people with a higher level of cardiorespiratory fitness can run 1.5 miles faster than those with a lower level (9, 10).

The objective of the test is to complete a 1.5-mile run in the shortest possible time. Regular exercisers and people with active lifestyles can probably complete the 1.5-mile distance running or jogging. Because this test requires you to run the 1.5 miles as fast as you can, it is not the best option for sedentary people over age 30, for people who have a very low fitness level due to medical reasons, for individuals with joint problems, or for obese individuals. For less active individuals, a 1.5-mile run/walk test is better suited. Laboratory 3.1A at the end of the chapter provides instructions for performing the test and recording the score.

The 1-mile walk test is another common field test to estimate cardiorespiratory fitness. The walk test is based on the same idea as the 1.5-mile run test: that people who have higher cardiorespiratory fitness will be able to complete the test faster than those with low cardiorespiratory fitness. This test is particularly good for sedentary individuals (12–14). However, people with joint problems should consider a non–weight-bearing test, such as the cycle test described next. See Laboratory 3.1B for instructions on how to perform the 1-mile walk test and how to determine your score.

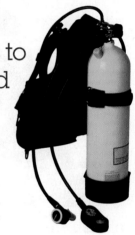

consider this!
$\dot{V}O_2 max$ begins to decrease around the age of 25 and decreases at a rate of approximately 1% per year.

Two other tests that can be used to assess your cardiorespiratory endurance are the cycle ergometer test and the step test. A **cycle ergometer** test (see **Figure 3.6** on page 52) is ideal for people with joint problems because, unlike walking or jogging, it does not involve weight bearing. The cycle ergometer test is a submaximal cycle test based on the principle that individuals with high cardiorespiratory fitness levels have a lower exercise heart rate at a standard workload than less-fit individuals (11). You can use Laboratory 3.1C to estimate your $\dot{V}O_2 max$ according to your heart rate and the workload used during the cycle ergometer test.

Finally, the step test can be performed by people at all fitness levels. Additionally, this test does not require expensive equipment, and it can be performed

1.5-mile run test One of the simplest and most accurate assessments of cardiorespiratory fitness.

cycle ergometer A stationary exercise cycle that provides pedaling resistance so the amount of work can be measured.

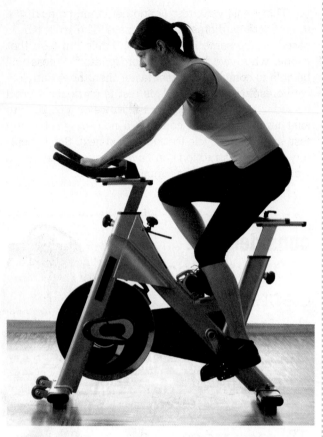

FIGURE 3.6
A cycle ergometer can be used to assess cardiorespiratory endurance.

in a short amount of time. However, the step test is not recommended for overweight individuals or for people with joint problems. The step test is based on the principle that your heart rate "recovers," or returns to resting levels, faster after exercise when you have a high level of cardiorespiratory fitness. Therefore, individuals with a higher cardiorespiratory fitness will have a lower heart rate during a 3-minute period immediately following the test compared to less-fit individuals (3). Also, be aware that this test requires stepping at a consistent rate and accurately taking your heart rate multiple times, so there is more chance for error. You can use Laboratory 3.1D to perform the step test and to find the norms for step test results in a college-aged population (18–25 years).

MAKE SURE YOU KNOW...

- Common tests to assess cardiorespiratory fitness include the 1.5-mile run, the 1-mile walk, the cycle ergometer test, and the step test.
- Obese individuals and people with joint problems should avoid weight-bearing cardiorespiratory assessment tests. Sedentary individuals should avoid the 1.5-mile run test.

Designing Your Aerobic Exercise Program

After you know your level of cardiorespiratory fitness, you can design an appropriate exercise plan to meet your goals. (We will discuss some of the basics for getting started in this chapter, but you will get more details about planning your exercise program in Chapter 7.) Setting goals and developing an action plan to meet long- and short-term goals is key to making healthy behavior changes (Chapter 1). Starting and maintaining your aerobic exercise program will be much easier if you set goals first and then plan your program specifically to meet those goals. Many fitness experts agree that lack of goals is a major contributor to the high dropout rates seen in many organized fitness programs (15,16).

Each exercise session will include the warm-up, workout, and cool-down phases (as you learned in Chapter 2). Within the workout phase you need to consider the frequency, intensity, time, and type (mode) of exercise. Also, it is important to consider the stage of the program—the initial conditioning, progression, or maintenance phase.

The Warm-Up

Every workout should begin with a warm-up of 5 to 10 minutes of low-intensity exercise and some light stretching. If you take a class such as step aerobics or spinning, your instructor will lead you though an appropriate warm-up. If you do other aerobic exercises, such as jogging or swimming, then you will need to plan your own warm-up. Typically, the warm-up will include a lower-intensity activity that is similar to or the same as your activity of choice for your workout. For example, you might walk or jog as warm-up for a run or swim a couple of laps more slowly than you would for the rest of your swim workout. You might also include some light stretching (see Chapter 5). Then, as you start the workout phase, you will gradually increase your intensity to the desired level.

The Workout

The components of an exercise prescription to improve cardiovascular fitness include the components of the FITT principle: frequency, intensity, time (or duration), and type of exercise.

Frequency The general recommendation for exercise frequency is 3 to 5 sessions per week to achieve near-optimal gains in cardiorespiratory fitness with minimal risk of injury. However, cardiorespiratory fitness gains can be achieved with as few as 2 exercise sessions per week (8). You typically will not see significantly greater improvements in your cardiorespiratory fitness if you exercise more than 5 days per week. Additionally, greater exercise frequency entails a greater risk of injury, which generally does not outweigh any added benefit of a greater frequency.

You might have to start with 2 or 3 days per week and increase the frequency as you progress through your program. You should also consider the rest between exercise sessions. A general rule is to exercise no more than 3 days in a row and to rest no more than 3 days in a row, especially if you are doing the same exercise each session.

Intensity Cardiorespiratory fitness improves when the training intensity is at least 50% of $\dot{V}O_2$ max (this level is often called the **training threshold**). Training at exercise intensities close to $\dot{V}O_2$ max does not produce significantly greater benefits and increases risk for injury. Therefore, the recommended range of exercise intensity for improving health-related physical fitness is between 50% and 85% $\dot{V}O_2$ max.

You cannot readily assess your percent $\dot{V}O_2$ max during exercise, but you can use heart rate to monitor exercise intensity. $\dot{V}O_2$ max and heart rate both increase linearly as exercise intensity increases. We also know that maximal heart rate is reached at $\dot{V}O_2$ max. This relationship, coupled with the fact that heart rate is easily monitored, makes heart rate a practical way to monitor exercise intensity.

How do you know what your heart rate should be during exercise? We can calculate a **target heart rate (THR)** range. **Figure 3.7** illustrates the pattern of heart rate during an exercise session. Because the tests we described to assess cardiorespiratory endurance are submaximal tests, we have to estimate maximal heart rate.

TABLE 3.1	Heart Rate Classifications
Heart Rate	**Classification**
<60 BPM	Bradycardia*
60–100 BPM	Normal range
>100 BPM	Tachycardia

*Many people, especially those who participate in regular aerobic exercise, have a resting heart rate below 60 BPM.

Before we explain how to determine your target heart rate range, let's discuss how to take your heart rate. Figure 3.2 (page 47) shows how to locate the radial and carotid pulse, and Lab 3.3 will provide the opportunity to practice taking your heart rate. When you find your pulse, make sure you use your index and middle finger. Do not use your thumb to take your heart because it also has a pulse and you will not be able to distinguish between the two pulses for an accurate heart rate. If you find your heart rate from your neck, be careful to press lightly. There is a receptor in the carotid artery that responds to changes in pressure, and too much pressure will make your heart rate slow down. It is best to take your resting heart rate for 30 or 60 seconds when you are very relaxed (e.g., first thing in the morning). However, your heart rate drops quickly when you stop exercising, especially as your fitness level increases, so you should take your exercise heart rate for a shorter time frame, 10 or 15 seconds. Lab 3.3 provides instructions for determining the number of beats per minute when you take you heart rate for less than full minute. If you are timing your heart rate with a stop watch, the first beat is counted as zero, but you count the first beat as 1 if you are timing with a running watch (e.g., the second hand on your wrist watch). See Table 3.1 for the typical heart rate ranges.

Maximal heart rate (HR_{max}) decreases with age and can be estimated by this formula:

$$HR_{max} = 206.9 - (.67 \times \text{age in years})$$

For example, we can estimate a 20-year-old college student's maximal heart rate by the formula

$$HR_{max} = 206.9 - (.67 \times 20) = 194 \text{ bpm}$$

training threshold The training intensity above which there is an improvement in cardiorespiratory fitness. This intensity is approximately 50% of $\dot{V}O_2$max.

target heart rate (THR) The range of heart rates that corresponds to an exercise intensity of approximately 50%–85% $\dot{V}O_2$max. This is the range of training heart rates that results in improvements in aerobic capacity.

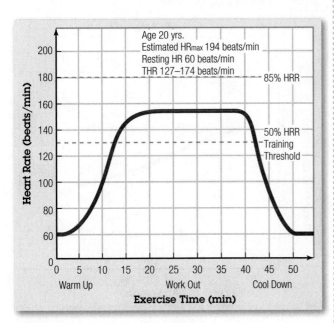

FIGURE 3.7
Sample workout in the target heart rate range.

COACHING Corner

Do you have a difficult time taking your pulse while doing your cardiovascular workout to check whether you're meeting your target heart rate range? Achieving an intensity that is greater than your normal daily activities and sustaining that intensity for a period of time is ideal as you work toward physical adaptations. Gauge your intensity with the following strategies:

- Recite your address or another familiar phrase out loud. If you find that you are beginning to breathe with your mouth open as you talk, you are likely approaching an appropriate intensity for your exercise.

- Reflect on how the intensity feels for you. Can you sustain low- to moderate-intensity movements for at least a 10-minute bout? If you feel as if you are going to have to stop exercising within a couple of minutes or less, you may be working at too high an intensity.

Achieve target heart range!

To determine your THR, we next have to determine your **heart rate reserve (HRR).** Heart rate reserve is the difference between your maximal heart rate and resting heart rate:

$$HRR = HR_{max} - resting\ HR$$

Let's assume that our 20-year-old college student's resting heart rate is 60 beats per minute (bpm). Then,

$$HRR = 194 - 60 = 134\ bpm$$

After determining the HRR, we can calculate 50% and 85% of his HRR. This range will place him at the desired percentage of his $\dot{V}O_2$ max.

$$0.50 \times 134 = 67\ bpm$$
$$0.85 \times 134 = 114\ bpm$$

The final step in determining the THR is to add the resting heart rate back to the values just calculated. This step is done because the resting heart rate is the starting point. Our student's THR is calculated as follows:

$$67 + 60 = 127\ bpm$$
$$114 + 60 = 174\ bpm$$
$$THR = 127 - 174\ bpm$$

You can calculate your THR using Laboratory 3.3 at the end of the chapter. Because your maximal heart rate decreases with age, your THR will change as you get older (**Figure 3.8**). Also, remember that a lower resting heart rate is an adaptation of aerobic exercise training. As you get older and see changes in your resting heart rate, you should recalculate your THR.

Another way to estimate exercise intensity is the **Borg Rating of Perceived Exertion (RPE)** scale (17). Perceived exertion is how hard you think you are working during exercise. To determine your RPE, take into consideration your efforts in breathing, how much you are sweating, and feelings in your muscles. Do not focus on just one these aspects of your effort, but consider how they contribute to your overall effort. Because your heart rate increases as your exercise intensity increases, your perception of effort assessed using the RPE scale typically correlates with heart rate during exercise. The RPE scale is a 15-point scale, ranging from 6 to 20. Consider that a resting heart rate might be around 60 beats per minute and a maximal heart rate around 200 beats per minute. So, if you multiply your rating on the RPE scale by 10, it will likely be close to your exercise heart rate. To provide some guidance for using the scale, a value of 6 on the scale

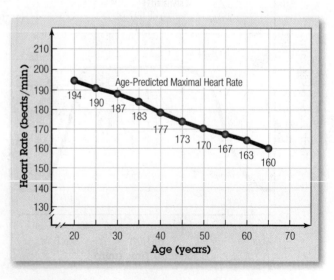

FIGURE 3.8
As you age, your maximal heart rate will decrease.

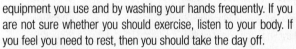

Aerobic Workouts—FAQS

Which is better, exercising for a brief period several times, or exercising for one longer period?

Both approaches can work. If you choose multiple sessions, your total workout time should be the same as for one longer session. Also, shorter sessions should not be less intense. You still have to maintain your prescribed exercise intensity to maximize the benefits. And regardless of the session length, you do need to warm up for 5 to 10 minutes and cool down for 5 to 10 minutes. Short sessions last typically at least 10 minutes for the workout phase. After you add the time for the warm-up and cool-down, you are looking at a 20-minute session.

What is the best time of day to exercise?

It doesn't matter whether you exercise in the morning or afternoon, but it does matter that you stick with your routine. So the best time of day to exercise is whenever you're most likely to do it consistently.

Should I train if I'm sick?

Generally, if the sickness is above the neck (e.g., sinus problem, headache, sore throat), light exercise might not be a problem. Just take it easy, and be sure to respect others who are not sick by wiping off any equipment you use and by washing your hands frequently. If you are not sure whether you should exercise, listen to your body. If you feel you need to rest, then you should take the day off.

Can I do aerobic exercise if I have asthma?

People with asthma can, in general, safely participate in all types of exercise. However, it is important to have a prescribed medication program to control your asthma (18). When asthma is under control, your exercise prescription need not be different from those for individuals without asthma. Exercise with other people present, and keep your inhaler readily available while exercising in case of an asthma attack. Additionally, you should avoid exercise in cold weather and in polluted environments. If you live in an area with a high level of pollution, exercising in a place with properly filtered indoor air may be preferable to exercising outdoors.

---

means that there is no level of exertion (e.g., standing on the treadmill before your run). Values in the range of 8–11 are common during the warm-up or cool-down phase of the workout. An RPE value between 12 and 16 will correspond with the target heart rate range for most people. Ratings of 12 to 13/14 are typical for moderate-intensity exercise, while 13/14 to 16 are common for vigorous-intensity workouts.

Time (Duration)   Recall that the duration of exercise does not include the warm-up or cool-down. In general, exercise durations most effective in improving cardiorespiratory fitness are between 20 and 60 minutes (8). The time you need to obtain your desired benefits will be specific to your initial level of fitness and your training intensity. For example, a poorly conditioned individual may see improvement in his cardiorespiratory endurance with 20 to 30 minutes of exercise 3 to 5 days per week at his THR. In contrast, a highly trained person may need regular exercise sessions of 40 to 60 minutes duration to improve cardiorespiratory fitness.

When determining your exercise duration, you also have to consider your exercise intensity. If you choose lower-intensity exercise rather than higher-intensity exercise, you will need to factor in a longer duration. For example, training at the lower end of your target heart rate range, around 50% of HRR, might require an exercise duration of 40 to 50 minutes to improve cardiorespiratory fitness. However, if you exercise at a moderate or higher intensity, such as 70% of HRR, you might see similar improvements with only 20 to 30 minutes.

Type   Any type of aerobic activities that you enjoy enough to do consistently will help improve and maintain your cardiorespiratory fitness. Also, any activity that uses a large muscle mass (e.g., the legs) in a slow, rhythmic pattern can improve cardiorespiratory endurance. These activities can be performed for a duration and at an intensity that will use the aerobic energy system. Table 3.2 (page 56) lists several activities that have been shown to improve cardiorespiratory fitness.

Because there are many exercises and activities that will improve your cardiorespiratory endurance, it is important to select activities you will enjoy.

---

heart rate reserve (HRR) The difference between your maximal heart rate and resting heart rate.

Borg Rating of Perceived Exertion (RPE) A subjective way of estimating exercise intensity based on a numerical scale of 6 to 20.

TABLE 3.2 Exercises and Activities That Can Improve Cardiorespiratory Fitness and the Number of Calories Expended per 30-Minute Workout*

Activity	Calories Expended per 30 Minutes
Aerobics classes (moderate intensity step aerobics)	250–400
Bicycling (moderate intensity)	225–375
Bicycling (mountain biking)	250–400
Bicycling (stationary cycle – moderate intensity)	200–325
Brisk walking (~3.5 mph)	150–250
Circuit training	225–375
Cross-country skiing (moderate intensity)	250–400
Elliptical (moderate intensity)	250–400
Hiking	175–300
Rowing machine (moderate intensity)	200–350
Running (8.5-minute mile)	350–500
Skipping rope (moderate pace)	300–450
Spinning classes (moderate intensity)	150–300
Swimming (fast, freestyle)	300–450
Water aerobics	125–300
Zumba (moderate intensity)	250–400

*These numbers are estimates; the actual numbers will vary depending on body weight.

Another consideration is the risk of injury associated with high-impact activities, such as running. Listen to your body when it comes to choosing a high-impact exercise. If you experience joint pain or discomfort, you should see a health-care provider. You might need to find lower-impact exercises, such as swimming or cycling. Cross training, discussed later in the chapter, is another option to reduce your risk of injury if you enjoy a high-impact exercise. For an example of how to use the FITT principle in designing an exercise program, see **Figure 3.9.**

Assess your fitness with the *At-Home Fitness Test* Take Charge of Your Health! Worksheet online at **www.pearsonhighered.com/powers.**

**LIVE IT!
ASSESS
YOURSELF**

Frequency	3–5 times per week
Intensity	50%–85% of HRmax
Time	20–60 minutes per session
Type	Jogging

FIGURE 3.9
An example of the FITT principle for improving cardiorespiratory fitness.

The Cool-Down

Every training session should conclude with a cool-down of light exercises and stretching. Allowing your cardiovascular system to slow down gradually is important: Stopping your workout abruptly can cause blood to pool in the arms and legs, which could result in dizziness and/or fainting. A cool-down may also decrease the muscle soreness and cardiac irregularities that sometimes occur after a vigorous workout. Although cardiac irregularities are rare in healthy individuals, a cool-down period is still wise to minimize the risk.

A general cool-down of at least 5 minutes (e.g., light exercise such as walking, or a lighter intensity of the activity you did for your exercise session) should be followed by 5 to 30 minutes of flexibility exercises. If you take an exercise class, your instructor will lead you through the cool-down. In general, stretching exercises should focus on the muscles used during training. The type and duration of the stretching session depend on your flexibility goals (Chapter 5).

MAKE SURE YOU KNOW...

- Establishing both short-term and long-term fitness goals is essential before beginning a fitness program.
- Each workout should include warm-up, workout, and cool-down phases.
- You need to consider the exercise frequency, intensity, time (duration), and type (mode) for the workout phase.
- Intensity can be monitored using the target heart rate range or Rating of Perceived Exertion.
- Aerobic exercise performed 3 to 5 days per week at 50%–85% of your heart rate reserve for 20–60 minutes is recommended to improve your cardiorespiratory endurance.

Developing an Individualized Exercise Prescription

Anyone beginning a new aerobic exercise program, regardless of initial fitness level or exercise mode, will usually go through three stages: initial conditioning, improvement, and maintenance (as discussed in Chapter 2). In this section we will show you how you can individualize these stages to meet your specific needs and goals. You can use the sample programs for cardiorespiratory endurance on pages 61–64 and Laboratory 3.4 to design your aerobic exercise program.

Should You Ditch the Shoes?

When Abebe Bikila ran barefoot in the 1960 Olympics and Zola Budd Pieterse followed suit in 1984, people thought it was a bit strange that world-class athletes were competing without shoes. Now it is not uncommon to see runners of all levels kicking off their shoes and hitting the streets. Barefoot running or running with five-finger shoes is becoming quite popular. Most report running without traditional running shoes because they want to prevent injury or alleviate pain.

However, the jury is still out as to whether barefoot running does prevent common running injuries or pain. You will find researchers and physicians who support it and those who oppose it. So what do we know? Proponents of barefoot running say that since the advances in running shoes in the 1960s there has not been a significant decrease in the number of running-related injuries. Also, they report that there are changes in stride length, foot strike patterns, and force on the joints that seem to be healthier.

Opponents of barefoot running agree that there are changes in the mechanics of running without shoes. However, they argue that there is not strong evidence that changes are associated with less pain or fewer injuries. They also argue that there are still unknown factors in the relationship between barefoot running and injury, and say it is premature to make general recommendations.

Although there are different perspectives, both sides agree on a few points:

- Trauma to the foot is a serious potential risk. Minimalist or five-finger shoes are preferred over barefoot running to protect against trauma, extreme temperatures, and infection.

- Running injuries and pain are influenced by a number of internal (e.g., strength, body size, flexibility) and external (e.g. mileage, type of workout, terrain) factors. It is important to understand your individual problem. Seek help from a qualified medical professional before trying to find a solution to your problem on your own.

- Start slowly when trying barefoot running. Try it for just a few days a week and for short time periods and gradually increase to your typical routine.

- Discontinue barefoot running and seek medical attention if you experience new pain or injuries or if your previous pains and injuries persist or worsen.

- More research is needed to determine who is likely to benefit most from barefoot running.

Sources: Collier, R. The rise of barefoot running. *Canadian Medical Association Journal* 183(1):E37–38, 2011; Krabak, B. J., M. D. Hoffmann, and G. Y. Millet. Barefoot running: point/counterpoint. *Physical Medicine and Rehabilitation* 3(12):1142–1149, 2011.

Initial Conditioning Phase

The initial conditioning stage is to your program what the warm-up is to your workout. Starting slowly will allow the body to adapt gradually to exercise and to avoid soreness, injury, and discouragement. Generally this stage lasts 4 weeks, but it can be as short as 2 weeks or as long as 6 weeks, depending on your initial fitness level (8). For example, if your cardiorespiratory fitness is poor, the initial conditioning stage will likely last closer to 6 weeks, but if you start at a relatively high cardiorespiratory fitness level, 2 weeks might be sufficient.

You should include 10- to 15-minute warm-up and cool-down phases with each workout. In the initial conditioning period of your workout, exercise intensity will be low, typically 40%–60% HRR or RPE of 11–13 (8). For people who have never been involved in a regular exercise program or who have very low fitness, the initial intensity might even be less than the 50% HHR we calculated earlier. It is acceptable to start at an intensity of 40%–50% HRR if that is comfortable for you (8). The duration of the session will likely be short. Initial sessions for a person with very low fitness might be as short as 10 to 15 minutes. At these intensity and duration levels, an exercise frequency of 3 or 4 days is ideal (8).

Here are some key points to remember for your initial conditioning stage:

- Start at an exercise intensity that is comfortable for you.

- Increase your training duration or intensity when you are comfortable, but do not increase intensity and duration at the same time. Gradually increase your duration, and then work on increasing the intensity. Your goal should be 20 to 30 minutes of continuous low to moderate (40%–60% HHR) activity at the end of the initial conditioning phase (8).

- Be aware of new aches or pains. Pain is a symptom of injury and indicates that the body needs rest to repair itself.

STEPS FOR ▶ BEHAVIOR CHANGE

How good is your level of cardiorespiratory fitness?

Answer the following questions to assess your level of cardiorespiratory fitness.

Y N

☐ ☐ Do you participate in recreational or competitive sports?

☐ ☐ Can you perform at least 20 minutes of continuous aerobic exercise?

☐ ☐ Can you do your regular household chores without getting out of breath (e.g., cleaning your apartment, walking your dog, mowing the lawn)?

☐ ☐ Can you walk across campus to your classes with little effort?

If you answered yes to either of the first two questions, your cardiorespiratory fitness level is probably above average. If you answered yes only to the last two questions or to none of the questions, you might need to make some improvements.

TIPS TO BECOME MORE ACTIVE

Tomorrow, you will:

☑ Take the stairs when possible.

☑ Walk to class instead of driving or taking the bus.

☑ Find a friend to take a walk with you.

Within the next 2 weeks, you will:

☑ Join a club or intramural sport team.

☑ Visit your campus recreation center for options for activity and exercise programs.

☑ Get a pedometer to see how many steps per day you walk. Fewer than 5000 per day indicates a sedentary lifestyle.

By the end of the semester, you will:

☑ Try at least three different types of aerobic activities.

☑ Participate in at least 30 minutes of moderate intensity aerobic at least 5 days per week.

Improvement Phase

The improvement phase can range from 12 to 40 weeks, and your program will progress more rapidly during this period than in the initial conditioning phase (8). Duration and frequency are increased first, and then the intensity is increased toward the upper end of the THR (60%–85% HRR or RPE of 13–16). The changes should be gradual, with increases in duration of no more than 20% per week until you can do 20 to 30 minutes at a moderate to vigorous intensity (8). Frequency of 3 to 4 days might still be appropriate, but if you want greater changes in your cardiorespiratory endurance, increasing to 5 days might be necessary. A general recommendation is to increase the intensity by no more than 5% of your HRR every sixth exercise session (8). If you are exercising 3 days per week, that means an increase every 2 weeks. As you can see, the changes are gradual, and you should not feel pressure to make increases faster than you feel comfortable doing.

Maintenance Phase

The average college-aged student will generally reach the maintenance phase of the exercise prescription after 16 to 28 weeks of training, but it might take longer for those who started at a low fitness level. In the maintenance stage, you have achieved your fitness goal, and your new goal is to maintain this level of fitness. You still need to exercise regularly, but you do not need to keep increasing all of the components of your exercise prescription.

Several studies have shown that the key factor in maintaining cardiorespiratory fitness is exercise intensity (4). If you keep your intensity at the same level you reached in the final weeks of the improvement stage, you can reduce your frequency. Exercising as few as 2 days per week can still maintain your fitness level. If you keep to the same frequency and intensity as you achieved during the final weeks of the improvement stage, you can reduce duration to 20 to 25 minutes per session. However, if you hold frequency and duration constant, decreasing

Don't Let A Disability Stop You!

A temporary or permanent disability can discourage you from exercising, but you can take comfort in knowing that even with most disabilities you can obtain all of the benefits of cardiovascular exercise. If you have an injury that temporarily keeps you from performing your exercise of choice, your physical therapist or physician can help you find suitable alternative exercises to maintain your fitness level. Consulting a physical therapist, physician, or exercise specialist for the best exercise options is also recommended if you have a permanent disability. Additionally, these health professionals will be able to make you aware of any medical complications associated with your disability and how you can address them.

In general, swimming and other water activities are excellent ways to decrease the need to support your body weight and safely exercise capable muscle groups. Other benefits of water exercise include the following:

- They pose little to no risk of falling.
- Flexibility exercises are much easier to do in water.
- Water provides resistance to capable muscle groups. This resistance enables you to progressively overload the intensity and improve the cardiorespiratory system.
- A variety of water aids, including hand paddles, pull-buoys, flotation belts, and kickboards, can be used to help maintain buoyancy and balance as well as help you work in the water.

Basic water safety rules still apply, so be sure to perform water activities with a workout partner or with a lifeguard present.

intensity by even one-third can significantly decrease your cardiorespiratory endurance. So if you keep up your exercise intensity, you can cut back the duration or frequency and keep your hard-earned benefits.

MAKE SURE YOU KNOW...

- Regardless of your initial fitness level, an exercise prescription to improve cardiorespiratory fitness has three phases: initial conditioning, improvement, and maintenance.

- Your exercise program should be tailored to your individual needs and should take into account your current fitness level.

Training Techniques

Endurance training is a generic term that refers to any type of exercise aimed at improving cardiorespiratory endurance. However, there are numerous endurance training methods that you can use for this purpose. Most

People are very motivated to exercise during the New Year, but motivation often decreases after several weeks. Similarly, you may notice a decrease in gym usage just after spring break. Try the following strategies if getting active after a break is a struggle for you:

- Reframe your break. Instead of thinking you've fallen off the wagon, view the break as a natural part of your training routine. Reduce your intensity and duration for the first several bouts to ease back into your activity routine.

- Plan ahead for school breaks if you know you will be less likely to exercise. Actively plan a

return to activity by putting your workouts in your calendar.

- Participate in a new or different type of exercise during the break. This is a wonderful opportunity to cross-train in creative ways.

- Remember that the pursuit of fitness is a lifelong endeavor. Anchor your fitness plans as an unchanging part of your life and plan the rest of your life around those intentions—including the breaks.

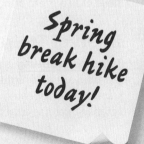

Spring break hike today!

Spinning—Rev It Up?

Do you like to exercise with a group? Do you like biking but find it hard to do around campus or in your city? Find a spinning class! Spinning is an aerobic exercise performed on stationary bikes in an indoor group ride led by an instructor. The bike is specially designed so you can quickly change the speed and resistance of pedaling. Being able to make quick changes enables you to mimic cycling in outdoor settings, such as a long country road or up a mountain. The spinning bikes also are designed to be much more comfortable than typical stationary bikes and feature multiple ways to adjust the seats and handlebars.

Spinning is led by an instructor, so you have the benefit of someone guiding you through your session. The instructor's direction is especially important if you are a beginner, because the instructor can tell you how to make the changes in intensity to fit your experience and fitness level. The classes usually last 30 to 60 minutes, have music for motivation, and use visualization techniques so you can feel as though you were cycling over hills and through valleys.

Spinning is an excellent exercise for improving cardiorespiratory endurance. You can burn up to 600 calories in an hour

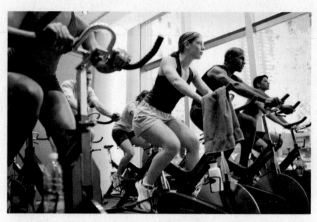

Cycling, whether outside or at the gym, is one popular type of exercise that will improve cardiorespiratory endurance.

depending on the speed and resistance, and it is a low-impact activity that is easy on your joints. Additional benefits of spinning include a group setting for support and encouragement and an indoor setting so weather is not a barrier.

---

common is the use of a continuous activity, such as walking or jogging at a constant intensity. Cross training and interval training are two techniques for people who need some variety or want to make faster gains.

Cross Training

Cross training is the use of multiple training modes. To cross-train, you might take an aerobic class one day, run one day, and swim another day. Some people use cross training to reduce the boredom of performing the same kind of exercise day after day. Cross training also might reduce the risk and occurrence of overuse injuries. However, cross training does not provide training specificity. Your cardiorespiratory endurance will improve, but jogging will not improve your swimming, because jogging does not train the arm muscles. Cross training might not be ideal if you are looking to improve your ability in a specific activity, but if you like variety and simply want to increase your cardiorespiratory fitness, it is a great option.

Interval Training

Interval training is typically used by athletes and others who are at a higher fitness level. This type of training includes repeated sessions, or intervals, of relatively intense exercise alternated with lower-intensity periods

to rest or recover. Runners, swimmers, and cyclists use interval training to improve their times in competition. People exercising to improve fitness might use interval training to make more rapid increases in their exercise intensity during the improvement stage. Interval workouts are intense training sessions and should not be used on a daily basis; rather, they should be alternated with continuous moderate-intensity exercise sessions.

The duration of the intervals can vary, but a 1- to 5-minute duration is common. Each interval is followed by a rest period, which should be equal to or slightly longer than the interval. For example, if you are running 400-meter intervals on a track and it takes you approximately 90 seconds to complete each run, your rest period between efforts should be at least 90 seconds. An "active rest" period is recommended. If you are running, your rest would be an easy jog or brisk walk to prevent muscle tightness. You do not have to use a track for interval training. You can use a stop watch and do an interval workout anywhere you usually train.

MAKE SURE YOU KNOW...

- Cross training can prevent you from becoming bored with an exercise program and reduce your risk of injury.
- Interval training is used by athletes and more advanced exercisers to produce faster gains in cardiorespiratory endurance.

How Can You Get Motivated to Be Active?

Every year, millions of people make the decision to start an exercise program. Unfortunately, over half of those who begin such a program quit within the first 6 months (16). There are many reasons for this high dropout rate, but lack of time is the most commonly cited reason (16). Although finding time for exercise in a busy schedule is difficult, it is not impossible. The key is to schedule a regular time for exercise and to stick with it. A small investment in time to exercise can reap large improvements in fitness and health.

Think about how much time you have in a week and how much of that time is needed to improve your cardiorespiratory endurance. There are 168 hours in every week, and all you need is three 30-minute workouts to improve cardiorespiratory fitness. Of course, you need to add warm-ups, cool-downs, and showers, which still totals only about 3 hours per week. That leaves you with 165 hours per week to accomplish all of the other things you need to do. The bottom line is that with proper time management, anyone can find time to exercise.

Consider the strategies you learned for behavior change (Chapter 1) and apply them to your aerobic exercise program. Setting long- and short-term goals is important. Changes happen slowly, and short-term goals will help you monitor your progress to stay on track. Keeping a record of your training program will help you see the small changes that occur on the way to your long-term goal. Keeping your program enjoyable is also important. Exercising with a partner can make your workout more fun and maintain your commitment to a regular exercise routine. Just make sure you choose a partner who is committed and is a good exercise role model.

Finally, some discomfort and soreness is normal after your first several exercise sessions. Do not let these feelings discourage you. In a short time the soreness will fade, and the discomfort associated with exercise will disappear. As your fitness level improves, you will feel better and look better. Although reaching and maintaining a healthy level of cardiorespiratory fitness requires time and effort, the rewards are well worth the labor.

MAKE SURE YOU KNOW...

- You should apply behavior strategies (Chapter 1) to help maintain your new aerobic exercise program.
- Discomfort and soreness are normal with a new exercise routine but will last only for a brief period.

cross training The use of a variety of activities for training the cardiorespiratory system.

interval training Type of training that includes repeated sessions or intervals of relatively intense exercise alternated with lower-intensity periods to rest or recover.

Sample Exercise Prescriptions for Cardiorespiratory Training

Scan to plan your individualized program for cardiorespiratory training. ▶

Your exercise program should be tailored to your individual needs to meet the goals you set. An important consideration in designing a personal training program is your current fitness level. People with good or excellent cardiorespiratory fitness can start at a higher level and progress more rapidly than people with low cardiorespiratory endurance.

The sample cardiorespiratory training programs below present examples to get help get you started. (You can also use Laboratory 3.4 at the end of this chapter to develop your personal exercise prescription.) These programs are designed for college-aged people with varying initial cardiorespiratory fitness levels. Note that in each program, the exercise duration and intensity increase as the program progresses. It is recommended to increase the exercise duration first and then to increase the exercise intensity once you are comfortable with the new duration. One you reach the maintenance phase, the exercise duration decreases. Research indicates that the benefits achieved during the improvement phase can be maintained with a shorter duration or with few days per week when the exercise intensity is maintained. So, in this example the frequency increased and the duration is decreased.

The only component missing from this program example is the mode of exercise. That choice is up to you. Just make sure you are participating in aerobic exercise (e.g., waking, jogging, swimming, cycling), and that you select exercises that you will enjoy. To maximize benefits and reduce the risk for injury, you can follow the recommendation of "no more than 3 days on; no more than 3 days off." Also, keep in mind that you can break the workout up into smaller sessions within a day of at least 10–15 minutes if time is an issue.

Beginner Cardiorespiratory Training Program

	Monday	Tuesday	Wednesday	Thursday	Friday	Saturday	Sunday
Initial Conditioning							
Week 1	10 min		10 min		10 min		
Week 2	10 min		10 min		10 min		
Week 3	12 min		12 min		12 min		
Week 4	12 min		12 min		12 min		
Week 5	15 min		15 min		15 min		
Week 6	15 min		15 min		15 min		
Improvement							
Week 7	20 min		20 min		20 min		
Week 8	20 min		20 min		20 min		
Week 9	25 min		25 min		25 min		
Week 10	25 min		25 min		25 min		
Week 11	30 min		30 min		30 min		
Week 12	30 min		30 min		30 min		
Week 13	35 min		35 min		35 min		
Week 14	35 min		35 min		35 min		
Week 15	40 min		40 min		40 min		
Week 16	40 min		40 min		40 min		
Week 17	40 min		40 min		40 min		
Week 18	40 min		40 min		40 min		
Maintenance							
Week 19	40 min		40 min		40 min		
Week 20	40 min		40 min		40 min		40 min
Week 21	40 min		40 min		40 min		40 min
Week 22	30 min		30 min		30 min		30 min
Week 23	30 min		30 min		30 min		30 min
Week 24	30 min		30 min		30 min		30 min
Week 25	30 min		30 min		30 min		30 min
Week 26	30 min		30 min		30 min		30 min

Intensity Key

60% of HRmax

70% of HRmax

75% of HRmax

Intermediate Cardiorespiratory Training Program

	Monday	Tuesday	Wednesday	Thursday	Friday	Saturday	Sunday
Initial Conditioning							
Week 1	10 min		10 min		10 min		
Week 2	15 min		15 min		15 min		
Week 3	15 min		15 min		15 min		
Week 4	20 min		20 min		20 min		
Improvement							
Week 5	25 min		25 min		25 min		
Week 6	25 min		25 min		25 min		
Week 7	25 min		25 min		25 min		
Week 8	30 min		30 min		30 min		
Week 9	30 min		30 min		30 min		
Week 10	35 min		35 min		35 min		
Week 11	35 min		35 min		35 min		
Week 12	40 min		35 min		40 min		
Week 13	40 min		35 min		40 min		
Week 14	40 min		35 min		40 min		
Week 15	40 min		40 min		40 min		
Week 16	40 min		40 min		40 min		40 min
Week 17	40 min		40 min		40 min		40 min
Week 18	40 min		40 min		40 min		40 min
Maintenance							
Week 19	30 min		30 min		30 min		30 min
Week 20	30 min		30 min		30 min		30 min
Week 21	30 min		30 min		30 min		30 min
Week 22	30 min		30 min		30 min		30 min

Intensity Key
70% of HRmax
75% of HRmax
80% of HRmax

Advanced Cardiorespiratory Training Program

	Monday	Tuesday	Wednesday	Thursday	Friday	Saturday	Sunday
Initial Conditioning							
Week 1	15 min		15 min		15 min		
Week 2	20 min		20 min		20 min		
Improvement							
Week 3	25 min		25 min		25 min		
Week 4	30 min		30 min		30 min		
Week 5	35 min		35 min		35 min		
Week 6	40 min		40 min		40 min		40 min
Week 7	40 min		40 min		40 min		40 min
Week 8	40 min		40 min		40 min		40 min
Week 9	*40 min*		*40 min*		*40 min*		*40 min*
Week 10	*40 min*		*40 min*		*40 min*		*40 min*
Week 11	*40 min*		*40 min*		*40 min*		*40 min*
Week 12	*40 min*		*40 min*		*40 min*		*40 min*
Week 13	*40 min*		*40 min*		*40 min*		*40 min*
Week 14	*40 min*		*40 min*		*40 min*		*40 min*
Maintenance							
Week 15	*30 min*		*30 min*		*30 min*		*30 min*
Week 16	*30 min*		*30 min*		*30 min*		*30 min*
Week 17	*30 min*		*30 min*		*30 min*		*30 min*
Week 18	*30 min*		*30 min*		*30 min*		*30 min*

Intensity Key
75% of HRmax
80% of HRmax
80%-85% of HRmax

SUMMARY

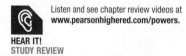

Listen and see chapter review videos at
www.pearsonhighered.com/powers.

HEAR IT!
STUDY REVIEW

1. Benefits of cardiorespiratory fitness include a lower risk of disease, feeling better, increased capacity to perform everyday tasks, and improved self-esteem and body image.

2. Adenosine triphosphate (ATP) provides the energy muscles need to move. It is produced by two systems: anaerobic (without oxygen) and aerobic (with oxygen).

3. Anaerobic energy production is the primary source of energy for short-term exercise, and aerobic energy production dominates during prolonged exercise.

4. The term *cardiorespiratory system* refers to the cooperative work of the circulatory and respiratory systems. The primary function of the circulatory system is to transport blood carrying oxygen and

nutrients to body tissues. The principal function of the respiratory system is to load oxygen into and remove carbon dioxide from the blood.

5. Responses to exercise are the short-term changes that occur during exercise to meet the immediate demands of exercise. Adaptations are developed over the long term through regular exercise training and will persist if you continue your exercise program.

6. Many exercise physiologists consider $\dot{V}O_2$ max (the maximum capacity of the cardiorespiratory system to transport and use oxygen during exercise) to be the most valid measurement of cardiorespiratory endurance.

7. Cardiac output, stroke volume, and heart rate increase as a function of exercise intensity. Breathing rate also increases in proportion to exercise intensity.

8. There are many field tests that can be used to estimate $\dot{V}O_2$ max. These tests are practical and can be performed with little equipment.

9. Establishing both short-term and long-term fitness goals is essential before beginning a fitness program.

10. These primary elements make up the exercise prescription: warm-up, workout (primary conditioning period), and cool-down.

11. The components of the workout are the frequency, intensity, time (duration), and type (mode) of exercise (FITT).

12. In general, the FITT principle for improving cardiorespiratory endurance calls for a type of exercise that uses large-muscle groups in a slow, rhythmic pattern for 20 to 60 minutes, 3 to 5 times per week.

13. The target heart rate is the range of exercise heart rates that lies between 50% and 85% of heart rate reserve.

14. Regardless of your initial fitness level, an exercise prescription for improving cardiorespiratory fitness has three phases: initial conditioning, improvement, and maintenance.

15. Cross training and interval training provide alternatives to a continuous workout of the same mode. Cross training can be done by individuals of all fitness levels, but interval training is for those who are more experienced with exercise.

16. Maintaining a regular exercise routine requires proper time management and choosing physical activities that you enjoy.

STUDY QUESTIONS

Find more review questions online at
www.pearsonhighered.com/powers.

REVIEW IT!
QUIZZES

1. Which of the following is not an example of an aerobic exercise?
   a. running
   b. swimming
   c. abdominal toning class
   d. spinning class

2. The anaerobic energy pathway is predominantly responsible for production of ATP during which of the following activities?
   a. wrestling
   b. 800-meter run
   c. 400-meter swim
   d. 30-minute brisk walk

3. _____ is an adaptation of a regular aerobic exercise program.
   a. Lower maximal heart rate
   b. Lower resting heart rate
   c. Faster breathing rate
   d. All of the above

4. Exercise intensity should be at least _____%
   of heart rate reserve to improve cardiorespiratory endurance.
   a. 85   b. 70   c. 50   d. 25

5. _____ is a response during exercise.
   a. Faster heart rate
   b. Increased cardiac output
   c. Faster breathing
   d. All of the above

6. _____ are the blood vessels that take blood away from the heart.
   a. Arteries
   b. Veins
   c. Capillaries
   d. Venules

7. What is meant by the term *cardiorespiratory system*?

8. List the major functions of the circulatory and respiratory systems.

9. Why is the heart considered "two pumps in one"?

10. Define the following terms:
    adenosine triphosphate (ATP)
    cross training
    target heart rate

HELPFUL WEBLINKS

DO IT!
WEBLINKS

For Links to the organizations and websites listed, visit **www.pearsonhighered.com/powers.**

American College of Sports Medicine
Comprehensive website providing information, articles, equipment recommendations, how-to articles, books, and position statements about all aspects of health and fitness. www.acsm.org

Meriter Fitness
Offers information on injury prevention and treatment, weight training, flexibility, exercise prescriptions, and more. www.meriter.com

The Running Page
Contains information about racing, running clubs, places to run, running-related products, magazines, and treating running injuries. www.runningpage.com

WebMD
General information about exercise, fitness, and wellness. Great articles, instructional information, and updates. www.webmd.com

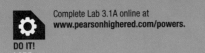
Name _____   Date _____

Measuring Cardiorespiratory Fitness: The 1.5-Mile Run Test

The objective of this test is to complete the 1.5-mile distance as quickly as possible. You can complete the run on an oval track or on any properly measured course. If the run will take place outside, the test is best conducted in moderate weather conditions; avoid running it on very hot or very cold days. A good strategy is to try to keep a steady pace over the entire distance. Performing a practice test is a good way to get familiar with the distance and determine the ideal pace you can maintain. You should use a stopwatch to get an accurate time. You should attempt this test only if you have met the medical clearance criteria (discussed in Chapter 1).

Before the test, perform a 5- to 10-minute warm-up. If you become extremely fatigued during the test, slow your pace or walk—do not overstress yourself! If you feel faint or nauseated or experience any unusual pains in your upper body, stop and notify your instructor.

After you complete the test, cool down and record your time and fitness category from Table 3.3 included in this lab. Locate your time range according to your sex and age group. The fitness classifications are along the top of the table.

Test date: _____   Finish time: _____   Fitness category: _____

1. Is your fitness classification what you expected based on your current level of activity? If not, why do you think it was higher or lower than expected?

   _____

   _____

2. Write fitness goals for maintaining or improving your cardiorespiratory endurance.

   _____

   _____

TABLE 3.3   **Fitness Categories for Cooper's 1.5-Mile Run Test**

Estimated Run Time Ratings				
Men	**Excellent**	**Good**	**Fair**	**Poor**
20–29 yrs	<10:10	10:10–11:29	11:30–12:38	>12:38
30–39 yrs	<10:47	10:47–11:54	11:55–12:58	>12:58
40–49 yrs	<11:16	11:16–12:24	12:25–13:50	>13:50
50–59 yrs	<12:09	12:09–13:35	13:36–15:06	>15:06
60–69 yrs	<13:24	13:24–15:04	15:05–16:46	>16.46
Women	**Excellent**	**Good**	**Fair**	**Poor**
20–29 yrs	<11:59	11:59–13:24	13:25–14:50	>14:50
30–39 yrs	<12:25	12:25–14:08	14:09–15:43	>15:43
40–49 yrs	<13:34	13:24–14:53	14:54–16:31	>16:31
50–59 yrs	<14:35	14:35–16:35	16:36–18:18	>18:18
60–69 yrs	<16:34	16:34–18:27	18:28–20:16	>20:16

Source: Reprinted with permission from The Cooper Institute®, Dallas, Texas from a book called *Physical Fitness Assessments and Norms for Adults and Law Enforcement*. Available online at www.CooperInstitute.org.

LABORATORY 3.1B

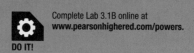

Name _____   Date _____

Measuring Cardiorespiratory Fitness: The 1-Mile Walk Test

The objective of this test is to walk the 1-mile distance as quickly as possible. You can complete the walk on an oval track or on any properly measured course. You should attempt this test only if you have met the medical clearance criteria (discussed in Chapter 1).

Before the test, perform a 5- to 10-minute warm-up. If you become extremely fatigued during the test, slow your pace—do not over-stress yourself! If you feel faint or nauseated or experience any unusual pains in your upper body, stop and notify your instructor.

After you complete the test, cool down and record your time and fitness category from Table 3.4 included in this lab. Locate your time range according to your sex and age group. The fitness classifications are along the top of the table.

Test date: _____

Finish time: _____

Fitness category: _____

1. Is your fitness classification what you expected based on your current level of activity? If not, why do you think it was higher or lower than expected?

_____

_____

2. Write fitness goals for maintaining or improving your cardiorespiratory endurance.

_____

_____

_____

TABLE 3.4   Fitness Classification for 1-Mile Walk Test

Men	Excellent	Good	Average	Poor	Very Poor
13–19 yrs	<12:30	12:30–14:00	14:01–16:00	16:01–17:30	>17:30
20–29 yrs	<13:00	13:00–14:30	14:31–16:30	16:31–18:00	>18:00
30–39 yrs	<13:30	13:30–15:30	15:31–17:30	17:31–19:00	>19:00
40+ yrs	<14:00	14:00–16:00	16:01–18:30	18:31–21:30	>21:30
Women	Excellent	Good	Average	Poor	Very Poor
13–19 yrs	<13:30	13:31–14:30	14:31–16:30	16:31–18:00	>18:01
20–29 yrs	<13:30	13:31–15:00	15:01–17:00	17:01–18:30	>18:31
30–39 yrs	<14:00	14:01–16:00	16:01–18:00	18:01–19:30	>19:31
40+ yrs	<14:30	14:31–18:00	18:01–19:30	19:31–20:00	>20:01

Because the 1-mile walk test is designed primarily for older or less-conditioned individuals, the fitness categories listed here do not include a "superior" category.

Source: From Rockport Fitness Walking Test. Copyright © 1993 The Rockport Company, Inc.

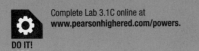
Name _____ **Date** _____

Measuring Cardiorespiratory Fitness: Submaximal Cycle Test

This test is performed with a partner. While you are exercising, your partner will help by setting the workload for the test, checking your pedal rate, and taking your heart rate. The work performed on a cycle ergometer is commonly expressed either in *kilopond meters per minute (KPM)* or in watts. Your instructor will explain how to use the KPM and watts settings to adjust the workload.

Warm up for 3 minutes without using any resistance (unloaded pedaling). Your instructor will tell you how to adjust the workload. Set the appropriate load for your age, sex, and level of conditioning (Table 3.5), and begin pedaling at the rate of 50 revolutions per minute (RPM). Your instructor will set a metronome so you know how fast to pedal. Exercise for a 5-minute period. Your partner will take your heart rate during a 15-second period between minutes 4.5 and 5 of the test.

Cool down for 3 to 5 minutes without resistance. Record your heart rate (15-second count) below, and calculate your relative $\dot{V}O_2$max using Table 3.6 (page 70). After calculating your relative $\dot{V}O_2$max, locate your fitness category in Table 3.7 (page 70).

Test date: _____

Heart rate (15-second count) during minute 5 of test: _____

Fitness category: _____

1. Is your fitness classification what you expected based on your current level of activity? If not, why do you think it was higher or lower than expected?

   _____

   _____

2. Write fitness goals for maintaining or improving your cardiorespiratory endurance.

   _____

   _____

TABLE 3.5 **Work Rates for Submaximal Cycle Ergometer Fitness Test**

Men	Pedal Speed (RPM)	Load	(watts)
Up to 29 yrs	50	150	(900 KPM)
30 + yrs	50	50	(300 KPM)
Women	**Pedal Speed (RPM)**	**Load**	**(watts)**
Up to 29 yrs (or well conditioned)	50	100	(600 KPM)
30 + yrs (or poorly conditioned)	50	50	(300 KPM)

To calculate your relative $\dot{V}O_2$max using Table 3.6, locate your 15-second heart rate in the left-hand column; then find your estimated $\dot{V}O_2$max in the appropriate column on the right. For example, the second column from the left contains the absolute $\dot{V}O_2$max (expressed in mL/min) for male subjects using the 900-KPM work rate. The third column from the left contains the absolute $\dot{V}O_2$max (expressed in mL/min) for women using the 600-KPM work rate, and so on. After determining your absolute $\dot{V}O_2$max, calculate your relative $\dot{V}O_2$max (mL/kg/min) by dividing your $\dot{V}O_2$max expressed in mL/min by your body weight in kilograms (1 kilogram = 2.2 pounds). For example, if your body weight is 70 kilograms and your absolute $\dot{V}O_2$max is 2631 mL/min, your relative $\dot{V}O_2$max is approximately 38 mL/kg/min (2631 ÷ 70 = 37.6). After computing your relative $\dot{V}O_2$max, use Table 3.7 to identify your fitness category.

TABLE 3.6 Cycle Ergometer Fitness Index for Men and Women

15-Second Heart Rate	Estimated Absolute VO₂max (mL/min)		
	Men: 900-KPM Work Rate (mL/min)	Women: 600-KPM Work Rate (mL/min)	Men or Women: 300-KPM Work Rate (mL/min)
28	3560	2541	1525
29	3442	2459	1475
30	3333	2376	1425
31	3216	2293	1375
32	3099	2210	1325
33	2982	2127	1275
34	2865	2044	1225
35	2748	1961	1175
36	2631	1878	1125
37	2514	1795	1075
38	2397	1712	1025
39	2280	1629	—
40	2163	1546	—
41	2046	1463	—
42	1929	1380	—
43	1812	1297	—
44	1695	1214	—
45	1578	1131	—

After determining your relative V̇O₂max (mL/kg/min) in Table 3.6, find your appropriate fitness category.

TABLE 3.7 Cardiorespiratory Fitness Norms for Men and Women Based on Estimated V̇O₂max

	Estimated V̇O₂max Fitness Ratings (ml/kg · min)					
Men	Superior	Excellent	Good	Fair	Poor	Very Poor
18–29 yrs	>56.1	51.1–56.1	45.7–51.0	42.2–45.6	38.1–42.1	<38.1
30–39 yrs	>54.2	48.9–54.2	44.4–48.8	41.0–44.3	36.7–40.9	<36.7
40–49 yrs	>52.8	46.8–52.8	42.4–46.7	38.4–42.3	34.6–38.3	<34.6
50–59 yrs	>49.6	43.3–49.6	38.3–43.2	35.2–38.2	31.1–35.1	<31.1
60–69 yrs	>46.0	39.5–46.0	35.0–39.4	31.4–34.9	27.4–31.3	<27.4
Women	Superior	Excellent	Good	Fair	Poor	Very Poor
18–29 yrs	>50.1	44.0–50.1	39.5–43.9	35.5–39.4	31.6–35.4	<31.6
30–39 yrs	>46.8	41.0–46.8	36.8–40.9	33.8–36.7	29.9–33.7	<29.9
40–49 yrs	>45.1	38.9–45.1	35.1–38.8	31.6–35.0	28.0–31.5	<28.0
50–59 yrs	>39.8	35.2–39.8	31.4–35.1	28.7–31.3	25.5–28.6	<25.5
60–69 yrs	>36.8	32.3–36.8	29.1–32.2	26.6–29.0	23.7–26.5	<23.7

Source: Reprinted with permission from The Cooper Institute®, Dallas, Texas from a book called *Physical Fitness Assessments and Norms for Adults and Law Enforcement.* Available online at www.CooperInstitute.org.

Name _____   **Date** _____

Measuring Cardiorespiratory Fitness: Step Test

To complete this test, you need a step or bench that is approximately 18 inches high, such as a locker room bench or a sturdy chair. The step test lasts for 3 minutes, and then heart rate is assessed in the 3.5 minutes following the test. You will need a metronome to help you maintain the step rate.

To perform this test, you will step up and down at a rate of 30 complete steps per minute. If you set the metronome to 60 tones per minute, you will step with each tone, making a complete step (up, up, down, down) every 2 seconds. Note that it is important that you straighten your knees during the "up" phase of the test. After you complete the test, sit quietly in a chair or on the step bench, and take your heart rate for 30 seconds at the following times:

1 to 1.5 minutes post exercise

2 to 2.5 minutes post exercise

3 to 3.5 minutes post exercise

Maintaining the 30-step-per-minute cadence and accurately taking your heart rate are very important for getting a good estimate from the step test. To determine your fitness category, add the three 30-second heart rates obtained during the period after exercise.

Record your heart rates below, and use Table 3.8 on this page to determine your fitness category.

Test date: _____

Recovery heart rate post exercise (bpm)

1–1.5 min: _____   **Total (recovery index):** _____

2–2.5 min: _____   **Fitness category:** _____

3–3.5 min: _____

Throughout the test, make sure to maintain correct form with your back straight.

Scan to view a demonstration video of the step test. ▶

1. Is your fitness classification what you expected based on your current level of activity? If not, why do you think it was higher or lower than expected?

    _____

    _____

2. Write fitness goals for maintaining or improving your cardiorespiratory endurance.

    _____

    _____

TABLE 3.8   Norms for Cardiorespiratory Fitness Using the Sum of Three Recovery Heart Rates Obtained Following the Step Test

	3-Minute Step Test Recovery Index					
	Superior	Excellent	Good	Average	Poor	Very Poor
Men	95–117	118–132	133–147	148–165	166–192	193–217
Women	95–120	121–135	136–153	154–174	175–204	205–233

Fitness categories are for college-aged men and women (aged 18–25 years) at the University of Florida who performed the test on an 18-inch bench.

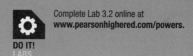
Name _____   Date _____

Assessing Cardiorespiratory Fitness for Individuals with Disabilities

This test uses arm exercise and is for people who cannot perform exercise that requires use of the legs (people in wheelchairs or with leg or foot injuries). To perform this assessment, you will need an arm crank ergometer. Your instructor will adjust the ergometer to the correct height and position for the test.

First, do a warm-up with no resistance. Then your instructor will increase the resistance, and you will perform a 2-minute stage. Rest 5 to 10 minutes. Then, after your instructor increases the workload, perform another 2-minute period of arm exercise. Repeat this cycle until you cannot complete 2 minutes of exercise at a given workload. Your instructor will tell you the workload for the last stage in which you completed the full 2 minutes of exercise. You can use that number and the calculation below to determine your $\dot{V}O_2$max.

$$\dot{V}O_2 \text{ max} = 3 \times (\text{work rate}*)/\text{body weight in kg}^\dagger + 3.5$$

Table 3.7 (page 70) in Laboratory 3.1C has the fitness classifications that correspond to your $\dot{V}O_2$max. Because this test uses arm exercise, which involves a smaller muscle mass than leg or whole-body exercise, your $\dot{V}O_2$max estimate will be a slight underestimate.

Fitness category: _____

1. Is your fitness classification what you expected based on your current level of activity? If not, why do you think it was higher or lower than expected?

   _____

   _____

2. Write fitness goals for maintaining or improving your cardiorespiratory endurance.

   _____

   _____

* Your instructor will give you this value.
† Weight in kg = weight in lbs ÷ 2.2.

Name _____   **Date** _____

Determining Target Heart Rate

Practice taking your heart rate at both the carotid and radial locations. You can feel the carotid pulse next to the larynx, beneath the lower jaw. The radial pulse is located on the inside of the wrist, directly in line with the base of the thumb. Use a stopwatch to count for 15, 30, and 60 seconds. To determine your heart rate in beats per minute (bpm), multiply your 15-second count by 4, and your 30-second count by 2.

Try locating and taking the heart rate of a classmate at both the radial and carotid locations. Record your resting pulse counts in the spaces provided.

Carotid Pulse Count (self)	Heart Rate (bpm)	Radial Pulse Count (self)	Heart Rate (bpm)
15 seconds × 4		× 4	
30 seconds × 2		× 2	
60 seconds × 1		× 1	

Carotid Pulse Count (partner)	Heart Rate (bpm)	Radial Pulse Count (partner)	Heart Rate (bpm)
15 seconds × 4		× 4	
30 seconds × 2		× 2	
60 seconds × 1		× 1	

The target heart rate (THR) range is calculated in steps.

STEP 1: Calculate your estimated maximal heart rate (HR_{max}).

$HR_{max} = 206.9 - (.67 \times$ age)

STEP 2: Calculate your heart rate reserve (HRR) by subtracting your resting heart rate from your HR_{max} (use the 60-second count from above).

HRR = HR_{max} − resting heart rate

HRR = _____ - _____

HRR = _____

STEP 3 : Calculate 50% and 85% HRR (use decimal values).

Lower end of THR = 0.5 (HRR) = _____

Upper end of THR = 0.85 (HRR) = _____

STEP 4: Add your resting heart rate back to these values.

50% HRR + resting heart rate = _____

85% HRR + resting heart rate = _____

THR = _____ bpm to _____ bpm

1.   Which of the resting pulses did you find easiest to locate on yourself?

_____ Carotid _____ Radial

2.   Which resting pulse was easiest to locate on your partner?

_____ Carotid _____ Radial

3.   Which of the two locations would you prefer to use when counting exercise heart rate?

_____ Carotid _____ Radial

Why? _____

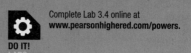

Complete Lab 3.4 online at
www.pearsonhighered.com/powers.

DO IT!
LABS

Name _____   Date _____

Developing Your Personal Exercise Prescription

Develop your personal exercise program based on your current fitness level and goals. Record the appropriate information in the spaces provided below.

Week	Phase	Intensity (% of HHR or RPE)	Exercise Mode	Duration (min/day)	Monday	Tuesday	Wednesday	Thursday	Friday	Saturday	Sunday
1											
2											
3											
4											
5											
6											
7											
8											
9											
10											
11											
12											
13											
14											
15											
16											

Review the behavior change strategies (discussed in Chapter 1), and write two strategies that can help you begin or maintain your aerobic exercise program (e.g., substituting behaviors—I will take a walk and talk with my friend Mary after class instead of having a text conversation with her).

_____

_____

_____

_____

_____

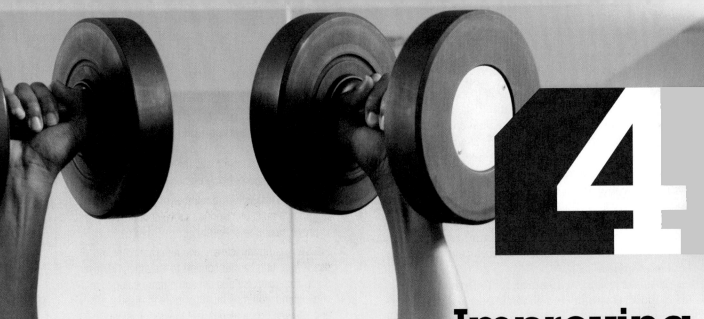

4

Improving Muscular Strength and Endurance

true or false?

1. Women who lift weights will quickly develop **"bulky"** muscles.
2. Increasing **muscle endurance** will always increase **muscle strength**.
3. Muscle turns to **fat** if you don't use it regularly.
4. Weight lifters should take protein or other **supplements** to get bigger faster.
5. Strength training is important only when you are **young**.

Answers appear on the next page.

Can you imagine running the 26 continuous miles of a marathon or biking the 2241 miles in the Tour de France? Or would you consider competing in the Iron Man triathlon, in which you swim 2.4 miles, bike 112 miles, and then run 26.2 miles, all in less than 9 hours? These extraordinary feats of human performance are all possible because of the human body's great capacity for muscular strength and endurance. And although not everyone will compete in a bike race, marathon, or triathalon, improved muscular strength and endurance offers numerous everyday benefits for everyone.

In this chapter you'll learn about the everyday benefits of muscle strength and endurance, the anatomy and physiology behind them, how to assess your own level of muscle fitness, and how to develop an exercise plan to improve your strength and endurance.

The Need for Muscular Strength and Endurance in Daily Living

When you climb a flight of stairs or carry a heavy book bag across campus, you're relying on your muscular strength and endurance to perform the task without becoming exhausted. If you've ever worked in a job that required you to shuttle loaded trays of food among tables or move boxes from point A to point B, you've relied on strength and endurance to earn your living. And if you play competitive or recreational sports, your skill level is determined in large part by the strength and endurance of your muscles. Whether we're aware of it or not, the strength and endurance of our muscles affects our physical performance numerous times every day.

Muscular strength and endurance are related, but they are not the same thing (Chapter 1). Muscular strength is the ability of a muscle to generate maximal force. In simple terms, muscular strength is the amount of weight that an individual can lift during one maximal effort. In contrast, muscular endurance is the ability to generate force over and over again. In general, increasing muscular strength by exercise training will also increase muscle endurance. However, training to improve muscular endurance does not significantly improve muscular strength.

Muscle strength and endurance can be increased and maintained with strength-training and endurance-training programs. In addition, regular strength training promotes numerous health benefits. For example, incidence of low back pain, a common problem in both men and women, can be reduced with appropriate strengthening exercises for the lower back and abdominal muscles (1). Further, studies demonstrate that muscle-strengthening exercises may reduce the occurrence of joint and/or muscle abnormalities and injuries

answers

1. **FALSE** The male sex hormone testosterone affects muscle size. With the same amount of training, men will gain more muscle mass than women because they produce more testosterone.

2. **FALSE** The intensity and number of exercises you do to improve muscular endurance will not necessarily improve muscular strength.

3. **FALSE** Fat and muscle are two different types of tissue, and one cannot convert to the other. However, if you stop exercise and consume more calories than you expend, you may build up more fat tissue, and you will probably notice it in your physical appearance.

4. **FALSE** Buying supplements such as protein powders or pills is mostly a waste of your hard-earned funds. Although athletes do need slightly higher amounts of protein than less active people, their needs can easily be met through a healthy diet, so supplements are unnecessary.

5. **FALSE** Muscle strength and endurance are needed throughout the lifespan. Strength training for older individuals has been shown to help prevent falls and allow for independent living.

that occur during physical activity (2). Strength training can also delay the decrease in muscle strength experienced by sedentary older individuals (3) and may help prevent osteoporosis.

Another important benefit of strength training is that it increases **resting energy expenditure** in larger muscles (4). Resting energy expenditure (also called *resting metabolic rate*) includes the energy required to drive the heart and respiratory muscles and to build and maintain body tissues. An elevated metabolic rate allows the body to burn more calories throughout the day. Conversely, a lower metabolic rate burns fewer calories, thereby leading to weight gain.

How does strength training influence resting metabolic rate? One of the primary results of strength training is an increase in muscle mass in relation to body fat. An increase of 1 pound of muscle elevates resting metabolism by approximately 2%–3%. This increase can be magnified with larger gains in muscle. For instance, a 5-pound increase in muscle mass results in a 10%–15% increase in resting metabolic rate. Changes of this magnitude can play an important role in helping you lose weight or maintaining desirable body composition throughout life. Although overall body weight may increase slightly as muscle mass increases, fat mass should decrease. Clothing may fit better, and self-image is likely to improve.

You now know that strength training will increase muscle mass. But how does this work, and how do muscles, in general work? We'll discuss this next.

MAKE SURE YOU KNOW...

- Muscular strength and endurance are important for numerous daily tasks. Strength training can reduce low back pain, reduce the incidence of exercise-related injuries, decrease the incidence of osteoporosis, and help maintain functional capacity that normally decreases with age.

- Muscular strength is the ability to generate maximal force, whereas muscular endurance is the ability to generate force over and over again.

- Strength training can improve a muscle's resting energy expenditure.

How Muscles Work: Structure and Function

There are about 600 skeletal muscles in the human body, and their primary function is to provide force for physical movement. When the muscles shorten or lengthen during a **muscle action**, they apply force to the bones, causing the body to move.

The skeletal muscles also are responsible for maintaining posture and regulating body temperature through the mechanism of shivering (which results in heat production). Because all fitness activities require the use of skeletal muscles, anyone beginning a physical fitness program should understand basic muscle structure and function.

Muscle Structure

Skeletal muscle is a collection of long, thin cells called *fibers*. These fibers are surrounded by a dense layer of connective tissue called **fascia** that holds the individual fibers together and separates muscle from surrounding tissues **(Figure 4.1)**.

Muscles are attached to bones by connective tissues known as **tendons**. Muscular action causes the tendons to pull on the bones, thereby causing movement. Muscles cannot push the bones; they can only pull them. Many of the muscles involved in movement are illustrated in **Figure 4.2** on page 78.

Muscle Function

Muscle actions are regulated by electrical signals from motor nerves, which originate in the spinal cord and send messages to individual muscles throughout the body. A motor nerve and an individual muscle fiber make contact at a neuromuscular junction (see **Figure 4.3** on page 79). Note from the figure that each motor nerve branches and then connects with numerous individual muscle fibers.

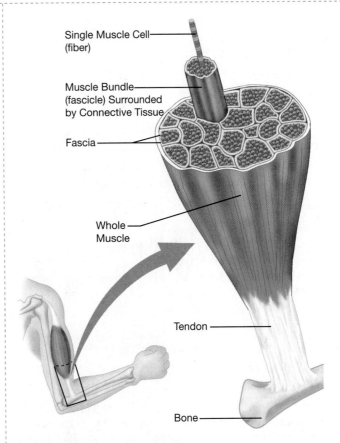

Single Muscle Cell (fiber)

Muscle Bundle (fascicle) Surrounded by Connective Tissue

Fascia

Whole Muscle

Tendon

Bone

FIGURE 4.1

The structure of skeletal muscle.

Source: Johnson, Michael D., *Human Biology: Concepts and Current Issues*, 4th Ed., © 2008. Reprinted and Electronically reproduced by permission of Pearson Education, Inc., Upper Saddle River, New Jersey.

The motor nerve and all of the muscle fibers it controls comprise a **motor unit**. Motor units come in various sizes, depending on how many muscle fibers they contain. A motor nerve can innervate a few muscle fibers for fine motor control, such as blinking the eye, or it can innervate many muscle fibers for gross motor movement, such as kicking a ball.

---

resting energy expenditure The amount of energy expended during all sedentary activities. Also called *resting metabolic rate*.

muscle action The shortening of a skeletal muscle (causing movement) or the lengthening of a skeletal muscle (resisting movement).

fascia A thin layer of connective tissue that surrounds the muscle.

tendons A fibrous connective tissue that attaches muscle to bone.

motor unit A motor nerve and all of the muscle fibers it controls.

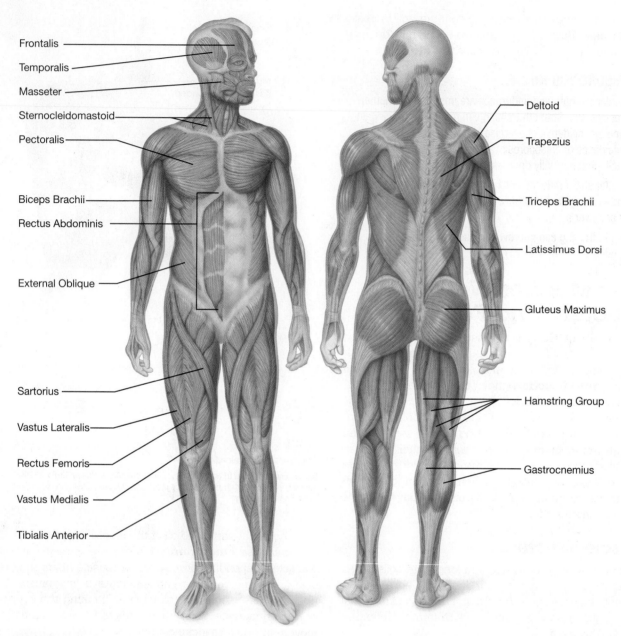

FIGURE 4.2
Major muscles of the human body.

Source: Johnson, Michael D., *Human Biology: Concepts and Current Issues*, 4th Ed., © 2008. Reprinted and Electronically reproduced by permission of Pearson Education, Inc., Upper Saddle River, New Jersey.

A muscle action begins when a message to develop tension (called a nerve impulse) reaches the neuromuscular junction. The arrival of the nerve impulse triggers the action process by permitting the interaction of contractile proteins in muscle. Just as the nerve impulse initiates the contractile process, the removal of the nerve signal from the muscle "turns it off." That is, when a motor nerve ceases to send signals to a muscle, the muscle action stops. Occasionally, however, an uncontrolled muscular action occurs, which results in a muscle cramp or a muscle twitch.

Muscle Exercise and Muscle Actions

Skeletal muscle exercise is classified into three major categories: **isotonic**, **isometric**, and **isokinetic**. Isotonic (also called *dynamic*) exercise results in movement of a body part at a joint. Most exercise or sports activities are isotonic. For example, lifting a dumbbell involves movement of the forearm and is therefore classified as an isotonic exercise.

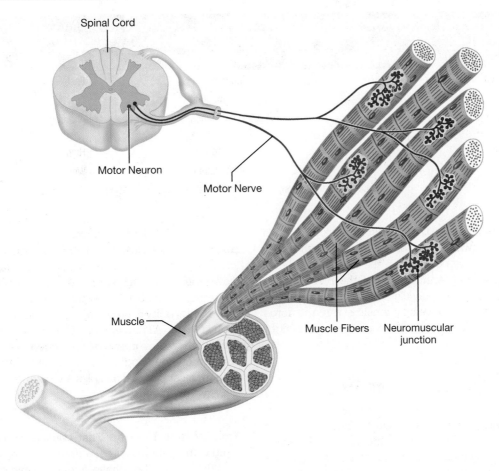

Spinal Cord

Motor Neuron

Motor Nerve

Muscle

Muscle Fibers

Neuromuscular
junction

FIGURE 4.3
A motor unit. Two motor nerves from the central nervous system are shown innervating several muscle fibers. With one impulse from the motor
nerve, all fibers respond.

An isometric (also called *static*) exercise requires
the development of muscular tension but results in no
movement of body parts. A classic example of isometric
exercise is pressing the palms of the hands together.
Although there is tension within the muscles of the
arms and chest, the arms do not move. Isometric exercises are an excellent way to develop strength during
the early stages of an injury rehabilitation program.

Isokinetic exercises are performed at a constant
velocity; that is, the speed of muscle shortening or
lengthening is regulated at a fixed, controlled rate. This
is generally accomplished by using a machine that
provides an accommodating resistance throughout the
full **range of motion**.

Muscle actions can similarly be classified as isometric, concentric, or eccentric, depending on the activity
the muscle needs to perform. Like isometric exercise,
isometric muscle actions are static and do not involve
any joint movement. An isometric muscle action occurs
during isometric exercises.

A **concentric muscle action** causes movement
of the body part against resistance or gravity; it occurs
when the muscle shortens. Concentric muscle actions

(also called *positive work*) can be performed during isotonic or isokinetic exercise. For example, the upward
movement of the arm during a bicep curl (see **Figure 4.4**,
top, on page 80) is an example of a concentric muscle
action.

isotonic A type of exercise in which there is movement
of a body part. Most exercise or sports skills are
isotonic exercise. Also called *dynamic* exercise.

isometric A type of exercise in which muscular tension
is developed but the body part does not move. Also
called *static* exercise.

isokinetic A type of exercise that can include concentric
or eccentric muscle actions performed at a constant
speed using a specialized machine.

range of motion The amount of movement possible
at a joint.

concentric muscle action Action in which the muscle develops tension as it shortens against resistance
and/or gravity. Also called *positive work*.

TABLE 4.1 Properties of Human Skeletal Muscle Fiber Types			
	Fiber Type		
Property	Slow-Twitch	Intermediate	Fast-Twitch
Contraction speed	Slow	Intermediate	Fast
Resistance to fatigue	High	Intermediate	Low
Predominant energy system	Aerobic	Combination aerobic and anaerobic	Anaerobic
Force generation	Low	Intermediate	High
Color	Red	White (pink)	White
Best suited for	Endurance events (marathon)	Middle-distance events (5–10 K)	Fast events (100-m sprint)

In contrast, **eccentric muscle actions** (also called *negative work*) control movement with resistance or gravity; they occur when the muscle lengthens. The downward or lowering phase of the bicep curl is controlled as the biceps muscle lengthens (**Figure 4.4**, bottom); the muscle develops tension, but the force developed is not great enough to prevent the weight from being lowered.

Types of Muscle Fibers

There are three types of skeletal muscle fibers: slow-twitch, intermediate, and fast-twitch. These fiber types differ in their speeds of action and in fatigue resistance (5). Because most human muscles contain a mixture of all three fiber types, it is helpful to understand each of them before beginning the strength-training process.

Concentric Action

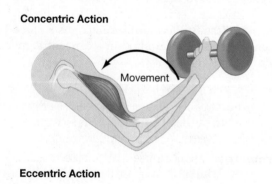

Movement

Eccentric Action

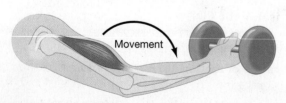

Movement

FIGURE 4.4
Concentric and eccentric muscle actions in an isotonic exercise. The muscle shortens during a concentric action and lengthens during an eccentric action.

Slow-Twitch Fibers As the name implies, **slow-twitch fibers** contract slowly and produce small amounts of force; however, these fibers are highly resistant to fatigue. Slow-twitch fibers appear red or darker in color because of the numerous capillaries that supply the fibers. They have the capacity to produce large quantities of adenosine triphosphate (ATP) aerobically, which makes them ideally suited for low-intensity, prolonged exercise, such as walking or slow jogging. Because of their resistance to fatigue, most postural muscles are composed primarily of slow-twitch fibers.

Fast-Twitch Fibers **Fast-twitch fibers** contract rapidly and generate great amounts of force, but fatigue quickly. These fibers have a low aerobic capacity and appear white because they are supplied by only a few capillaries. Fast-twitch fibers are well equipped to produce ATP anaerobically, but only for a short time. With their ability to shorten rapidly and produce large amounts of force, fast-twitch fibers are used during activities requiring rapid or forceful movement, such as jumping, sprinting, and weight lifting. These fibers are most easily damaged in strenuous exercise, causing soreness.

Intermediate Fibers **Intermediate fibers** have a combination of characteristics found in fast- and slow-twitch fibers. They contract rapidly, produce great force, and resist fatigue because they have a well-developed aerobic capacity. Intermediate fibers contract more quickly and produce more force than slow-twitch fibers, but they contract more slowly and produce less force than fast-twitch fibers. They are slightly redder in appearance than fast-twitch fibers but are not as red as the slow-twitch fibers. Table 4.1 summarizes the properties of the three fiber types.

You can see the differences in fiber types during your next chicken or turkey dinner. The dark meat of a chicken drumstick contains primarily slow-twitch fibers. Because these fibers are slow to fatigue, a living bird is able to walk around most of the day. The white meat in the chicken breast is composed mostly of fast-twitch fibers. Fast-twitch fibers allow the bird to fly, but only for short distances before fatiguing. The intermediate fibers found in the bird's wings exhibit the beneficial characteristics of each fiber type—they resist fatigue and generate high force.

Individual Variations in Fiber Type

People vary in the number of slow-twitch, intermediate, and fast-twitch fibers their muscles contain; however, the average nonathlete generally has equal numbers of all three fiber types. Research has shown a relationship between muscle fiber type and athletic success. For example, champion endurance athletes, such as marathon runners, have a predominance of slow-twitch fibers. This finding makes sense, because endurance sports require muscles with high fatigue resistance. In contrast, elite sprinters, such as 100-meter runners, have more fast-twitch fibers.

Muscle fiber type has also been suggested as a link to obesity and diabetes (6, 7). Individuals with a predominance of fast-twitch muscle fibers may be more susceptible to obesity and diabetes than those with a predominance of slow-twitch muscle fibers.

Some evidence has shown that fibers can be converted from one type to another. For example, endurance training has been shown to cause some fiber conversion between the intermediate- and fast-twitch fibers. However, there is limited evidence of fast- or intermediate-twitch fibers converting to slow-twitch fibers (8). This means that athletes who do well in short distances can stretch their careers by moving to intermediate distances, and athletes who do well at long distances can also move to the intermediate distances. But a long-distance athlete would not be able to switch to a short-distance event. Lance Armstrong, for example, started doing Iron Man for Kids triathlons when he was 13. He has had a great career as a long-distance bicyclist and has run several marathons.

Although endurance exercise training has been shown to cause some fiber conversion, the number and percentage of skeletal muscle fiber types are strongly influenced by genetics (5).

Recruitment of Muscle Fibers during Exercise

Many types of exercise use only a small fraction of the muscle fibers available in a muscle group. For example, walking at a slow speed may use fewer than 30% of the muscle fibers in the legs. More intense types of exercise, however, require more force. To generate this force, a greater number of muscle fibers must be made to contract.

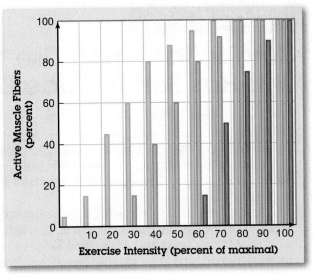

Key
- Slow-Twitch Fibers
- Intermediate Fibers
- Fast-Twitch Fibers

FIGURE 4.5
The relationship between exercise intensity and recruitment of muscle-fiber type.

The process of involving more muscle fibers to produce increased muscular force is called **fiber recruitment**. **Figure 4.5** illustrates the order in which muscle fibers are recruited as the intensity of exercise increases. Note that during low-intensity exercise, only slow-twitch fibers are used. As the exercise intensity increases, fibers are progressively recruited, from slow-twitch to

eccentric muscle action Action in which the muscle develops tension as it lengthens while controlling the movement with gravity. Also called *negative work*.

slow-twitch fibers Red muscle fibers that contract slowly and are highly resistant to fatigue. These fibers have the capacity to produce large quantities of ATP aerobically.

fast-twitch fibers White muscle fibers that contract rapidly but fatigue quickly. These fibers have a low aerobic capacity and produce ATP anaerobically.

intermediate fibers Muscle fibers with a combination of the characteristics of fast- and slow-twitch fibers. They contract rapidly and are fatigue resistant because they have a well-developed aerobic capacity.

fiber recruitment The process of involving more muscle fibers to increase muscular force.

Anabolic Steroid Use Increases Muscle Size But Has Serious Side Effects

The abuse of *anabolic steroids* (synthetic forms of the hormone testosterone) and their precursors has mushroomed over the past several decades. The fierce competition in body building and other sports that require strength and power has driven both men and women to risk serious health consequences in the quest to develop large muscles.

The large doses of steroids needed to increase muscle mass produce several health risks. A partial list of the side effects caused by abusing steroids and their precursors includes liver cancer, increased blood pressure, increased levels of "bad" cholesterol, severe depression, and prostate cancer. Prolonged use and high doses of steroids can be lethal.

One of the most popular chemical precursors to testosterone, androstenedione, is used to increase blood testosterone with the intent to increase strength, lean body mass, and sexual performance. However, research indicates that androstenedione does not significantly increase strength and/or lean body mass.

Another precursor to testosterone production in the body, dehydroepiandrosterone (DHEA), has also been used to increase testosterone in the body. DHEA is also advertised as a weight-loss and anti-aging supplement capable of improving libido, vitality, and immunity levels. However, the best evidence demonstrates that DHEA supplementation does not increase testosterone concentrations or increase strength in men, and it may have masculinizing effects in women.

intermediate fibers and finally to fast-twitch fibers. High-intensity activities, such as weight training, recruit large numbers of fast-twitch fibers. Why does this matter? By understanding which types of fibers are used for various exercises, you will better understand why you are working a particular muscle, or muscle group, in a particular way.

Muscular Strength

Two physiological factors determine the amount of force that a muscle can generate: the size of the muscle and the number of fibers recruited during the contraction. Muscle size is the primary factor. The larger the muscle, the greater the force it can produce.

Although there is no difference in the chemical makeup of muscle in men and women, men tend to have more muscle mass and are therefore generally stronger. The larger muscle mass is due to higher levels of the hormone testosterone in men, which helps build muscle. The fact that testosterone promotes an increase in muscle size has led some athletes to use drugs in an attempt to improve muscular strength (see A Closer Look above).

The other significant factor that determines how much force is generated is the number of fibers recruited for a given movement. The more muscle fibers that are stimulated, the greater the total muscle force generated, because the force generated by individual fibers is additive (Figure 4.6).

Muscle fiber recruitment is regulated voluntarily through the nervous system. That is, we decide how much effort to put into a particular movement. For instance, when we choose to make a minimal effort to lift an object, we recruit only a few motor units, and the

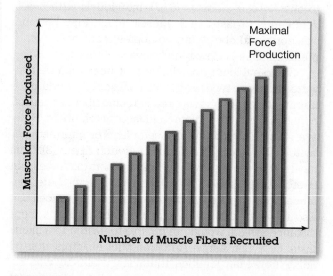

FIGURE 4.6
The relationship between recruitment of motor units and production of muscular force.

muscle develops limited force. However, if we decide to exert maximal effort to lift a heavy object, many muscle fibers are recruited, and a larger force is generated. Have you ever tried to open a locked door? If you didn't know the door was locked, your first attempt might involve minimal effort and few muscle fibers, because you hadn't anticipated having to use much force. However, once your first attempt didn't work, you might try again and recruit more muscle fibers to call upon more force to open the door. This process might continue until you either exerted enough force to yank the door open or gave up and looked for the key.

MAKE SURE YOU **KNOW…**

- Skeletal muscle is composed of various types of fibers that are attached to bone by tendons.

- Skeletal muscle actions are regulated by signals coming from motor nerves. A motor unit consists of a motor nerve and all the muscle fibers it controls.

- Exercise can be isometric, isotonic, or isokinetic. Isometric actions do not result in movement, whereas isotonic actions move a body part.

- Isometric exercise involves isometric muscle actions. Isotonic and isokinetic exercises use concentric actions (muscle shortens) and eccentric actions (muscle lengthens).

- Slow-twitch muscle fibers shorten slowly but are fatigue resistant. Fast-twitch fibers shorten rapidly but fatigue rapidly. Intermediate fibers shorten quickly but fatigue slowly.

- The process of involving more muscle fibers to produce increased muscular force is called fiber recruitment.

- Two factors determine muscle force: the size of the muscle and the number of fibers recruited.

Evaluation of Muscular Strength and Endurance

Muscular strength can be assessed by the **one-repetition maximum (1 RM) test**, which measures the maximum amount of weight that can be lifted one time. Although the 1 RM test for muscular strength is widely accepted, it has been criticized as unsuitable for use by older individuals or highly deconditioned people (9), for whom the major concern is the risk of injury. The 1 RM test should therefore be attempted only after several weeks of strength training, which will improve both skill and strength and thus reduce the risk of injury. An older or sedentary individual would probably require 6 weeks of exercise training prior to the 1 RM test, whereas a physically active college-aged person could probably perform the 1 RM test after 1 to 2 weeks of training. See Laboratory 4.1 for a step-by-step walk-through of the 1 RM test.

To further reduce the possibility of injury during strength testing, researchers have developed a method to estimate the 1 RM using a series of submaximal lifts. Although this method is slightly less accurate, it does reduce the risk of injury. You can read instructions for performing this test in Laboratory 4.2.

Muscular endurance is usually evaluated with two simple tests: the **push-up test** and either the **sit-up test** or the **curl-up test**. Push-ups require endurance in the shoulder, arm, and chest muscles, whereas sits-ups and curl-ups primarily require endurance in the abdominal muscles. To learn how to perform these tests and assess your own muscular endurance, turn to Laboratory 4.3 at the end of the chapter.

MAKE SURE YOU **KNOW…**

- The 1 RM test can be used to evaluate muscular strength.

- To reduce the possibility of injury, the estimated 1 RM test can be performed instead of the 1 RM test.

- The push-up and sit-up (or curl-up) tests are used to evaluate muscular endurance.

Principles for Designing a Strength and Endurance Program

We discussed the general principles for developing training programs to improve physical fitness in Chapter 2. Before we discuss the specifics of how to develop a strength-training program, let's discuss how two training principles, overload and specificity, factor into the design of a muscular strength- and endurance-training program.

Progressive Resistance Exercise

The concept of **progressive resistance exercise (PRE)** is an application of the overload principle to strength and endurance exercise programs. If your goal is to develop strong biceps muscles, you must progressively increase the resistance that you lift. For example, you may begin your program using 10-pound dumbbells and perform one set of 8 repetitions 3 times a week. As this exercise becomes easier, you can progressively increase the workload by increasing the weight, increasing the number of sets up to 3, and/or increasing the number of repetitions up to 12.

Specificity of Training

The principle of **specificity of training** states that development of muscular strength and endurance is

one-repetition maximum (1 RM) test Measurement of the maximum amount of weight that can be lifted one time.

push-up test A fitness test designed to evaluate endurance of shoulder and arm muscles.

sit-up test A test to evaluate abdominal and hip muscle endurance.

curl-up test A test to evaluate abdominal muscle endurance.

progressive resistance exercise (PRE) Application of the overload principle to strength and endurance exercise programs.

specificity of training The concept that the development of muscular strength and endurance, as well as cardiorespiratory endurance, is specific to both the muscle group exercised and the training intensity.

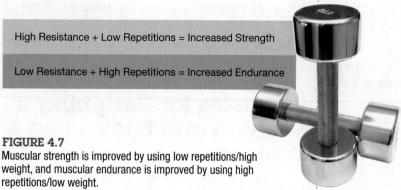

High Resistance + Low Repetitions = Increased Strength

Low Resistance + High Repetitions = Increased Endurance

FIGURE 4.7
Muscular strength is improved by using low repetitions/high weight, and muscular endurance is improved by using high repetitions/low weight.

specific to both the muscle group that is exercised and the training intensity. Only those muscles that are trained will improve in strength and endurance. To improve the strength of the back muscles, for example, you need to train the specific muscles involved with movement of the lower back.

The intensity of training will determine whether the muscular adaptation is primarily an increase in strength or in endurance (Figure 4.7). High-intensity training (e.g., lifting heavy weights 6 to 8 times) increases muscular strength but yields only limited improvements in muscular endurance. Conversely, high-repetition, low-intensity training (e.g., lifting light weights 20–25 times or more) increases muscular endurance but yields only limited improvements in muscular strength.

MAKE SURE YOU KNOW...

- In the context of strength and endurance training, the PRE principle means you need to progressively increase the amount of resistance with which you train.

- The intensity of training determines whether you primarily increase muscular strength or endurance. High-intensity training will increase muscle strength and size; low-intensity training will increase muscular endurance.

Strength Training: How the Body Adapts

What physiological changes result from strength training? How quickly can you gain muscular strength? Do men and women differ in their responses to weight-training programs? Let's address these questions next.

Physiological Changes Due to Weight Training

You now know that programs designed to improve muscular strength can do so only by increasing muscle size and/or by increasing the number of muscle fibers recruited. Strength training alters both these factors (10). Research has shown that strength-training programs

increase muscular strength first by altering fiber recruitment patterns, and then by increasing muscle size.

Increase in muscle size is due primarily to an increase in fiber size, called **hypertrophy** (10). Most research has shown that strength training has little effect on the formation of new muscle fibers, a process called **hyperplasia**. The role that hyperplasia plays in the increase in muscle size due to strength training remains controversial (11). Regardless, the increase in muscle size depends on diet, the muscle fiber type (fast-twitch fibers may hypertrophy more than slow-twitch fibers), blood levels of testosterone, and the type of training program.

Although strength training does not result in significant improvements in cardiorespiratory fitness (12), a regular weight-training program can provide positive changes in both body composition and flexibility. For most men and women, rigorous weight training results in an increase in muscle mass and a loss of body fat, both of which decrease the percentage of body fat.

Performing weight-training exercises over the full range of motion at a joint can improve flexibility (9). In fact, many diligent weight lifters have excellent flexibility. Thus, the notion that weight lifting causes inflexibility is generally incorrect.

Rate of Strength Improvement with Weight Training

How rapidly does strength improvement occur? The answer depends on your initial strength level. Strength gains occur rapidly in untrained people, and more gradually in individuals with relatively higher strength levels. In fact, for a novice lifter, strength gains can occur very quickly (13). These rapid gains tend to motivate the lifter to stick with a regular weight-training program.

Gender Differences in Response to Weight Training

Men and women do not differ in their initial responses to weight-training programs (14). On a percentage basis, women gain strength as rapidly as men during the first 12 weeks of a strength-training program. However, with long-term weight training, men generally exhibit a greater increase in muscle size than do women. The reason is that men have 20 to 30 times more testosterone than do women.

MAKE SURE YOU KNOW...

- Muscle size increases primarily because of hypertrophy (increase in size) of muscle fibers.

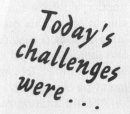

COACHING **Corner**

Whether you choose to train for strength, endurance, or for gains in both it may be helpful to make note of your successes along the way. Identifying adaptations that occur is a helpful way to maintain consistency. Once each month consider trying the following reflective activity. Respond to the following questions succinctly on an index card or other medium and file it away for comparison next month.

- What was challenging for you during today's workout?

- What was the most pleasurable part of today's workout?
- What would you consider changing to make this workout more enjoyable?
- What is one of the most important things you noticed about yourself during today's workout?
- What is different during this workout than you experienced one month ago?

Today's challenges were . . .

- Strength training promotes positive changes in both body composition and flexibility.
- The rate of improvement in weight training depends on initial strength level.
- Early in a weight-training program, women gain strength as quickly as men.

Designing a Training Program for Increasing Muscle Strength

There are numerous approaches to designing weight-training programs. Any program that adheres to the basic principles described earlier will improve strength and endurance. However, the type of weight-training program that you develop for yourself depends on your goals and the types of equipment available to you. There are several other factors to consider in developing a weight-training program; we discuss those next.

Safety Concerns

Before beginning any weight-training program, you need to think about safety. Follow these safety guidelines when weight training:

- When using free weights (such as barbells), have spotters (helpers) help you perform the exercises. The purpose of a spotter is to help you complete a lift if you are unable to do it on your own. Using weight machines reduces the need for spotters.
- Be sure that the collars on the ends of the bars of free weights are tightly secured to prevent the weights from falling off. Dropping weight plates on toes and

feet can result in serious injuries. Again, many weight machines have safety features that reduce the risk of dropping weights.

- Warm up properly before doing any weight-lifting exercise. Stretching the intended muscles and lifting very light weight is a good way to start.
- Do not hold your breath during weight lifting. Instead, follow this breathing pattern: Exhale while lifting the weight, and inhale while lowering it. Also, breathe through both your nose and mouth.
- Although debate continues as to whether high-speed weight lifting yields greater strength gains than slow-speed lifting, slow movements may reduce the risk of injury. A general rule of thumb is to lift the weight on the count of 2 and to lower the weight on the count of 4.
- Use light weights in the beginning so that you can maintain the proper form through the full range of motion in each exercise. This is particularly important when you are lifting free weights.

Types of Weight-Training Programs

Weight-training programs specifically designed to improve strength and those designed to improve muscular endurance differ mainly in the number of repetitions and the amount of resistance (10). A combination

hypertrophy An increase in muscle fiber size.
hyperplasia An increase in the number of muscle fibers.

of low repetition and high resistance appears to be the optimal training method to increase strength; moreover, this type of training improves muscular endurance as well. In contrast, a program of high repetition and low resistance improves endurance but results in only small strength increases, particularly in less-fit individuals.

As with types of weight-training exercise, weight-training programs can be divided into three general categories: isotonic, isometric, and isokinetic.

Isotonic Programs Isotonic programs involve contracting a muscle against a movable load (usually a free weight or weights on a weight machine). The load is lifted on the up phase using concentric muscle actions and then lowered on the down phase using eccentric muscle actions. Isotonic programs are the most common type of weight-training program in use today.

Weight-training machines are ideal for the beginning exerciser because the weight is mounted to a cable or chain. If you were unable to complete a lift using a heavy weight and accidentally let go of the bar, the weights would slam down on the weight stack without injuring you or anyone else. In addition, machines allow a single joint to be isolated and exercised.

Free weights are preferred by many serious weight lifters because they can be used to exercise multiple joints. For example, the squat exercise involves muscles of the hip, knee, and ankle, thus allowing three joints to be exercised during one movement.

Isometric Programs An isometric strength-training program is based on the concept of contracting a muscle at a fixed angle against an immovable object, using an isometric muscle action. Interest in strength training increased dramatically during the 1950s with the finding that maximal strength could be increased by contracting a muscle for 6 seconds at two-thirds of maximal tension once per day for 5 days per week. Although subsequent studies suggested that these claims were exaggerated, it is generally agreed that isometric training can increase muscular strength and endurance (15).

Two important aspects of isometric training make it different from isotonic training. First, in isometric training, the development of strength and endurance is

STEPS FOR BEHAVIOR CHANGE

Are you reluctant to strength train?

Answer the following questions to assess the barriers that prevent you from starting a strength-training program.

Y N

☐ ☐ I feel intimidated by other people in the strength-training facility.

☐ ☐ I cannot find time in my schedule to exercise.

☐ ☐ I do not know how to use the various machines or free weights.

☐ ☐ I do not know how to begin a strength-training program.

If you answered yes to more than one question, check out the following tips to help you break through the barriers.

TIPS TO EASE YOURSELF INTO A STRENGTH-TRAINING ROUTINE

Tomorrow, you will:

☑ Research the fitness facilities in your area. Fitness facilities cater to a wide range of clients, from beginners to professional body builders. Try to find one that is convenient, affordable, and contains enough of the basic equipment to meet your strength-training goals.

Within the next 2 weeks, you will:

☑ Join a fitness facility. After doing your research for a facility, join the one that meets the criteria above and also makes you feel welcome and comfortable.

☑ Take an orientation tour through the fitness facility to familiarize yourself with the machines and equipment.

☑ Consider hiring a personal trainer at the facility if you feel you need more individualized instruction. Most facilities have fitness professionals who will assess your overall strength and suggest a starting program.

By the end of the semester, you will:

☑ Make a commitment to set aside 30–60 minutes a day for training, and do not allow others to interfere with your personal time. Personal fitness does require a time commitment, but you are worth the investment.

specific to the joint angle at which the muscle group is trained (15). Therefore, if you use isometric techniques, you will need to perform isometric contractions at several different joint angles if you want to gain strength and endurance throughout a full range of motion. In contrast, because isotonic contractions generally involve the full range of joint motion, strength is developed over the full movement pattern.

Second, the static nature of isometric muscle actions can lead to breath holding (called a **Valsalva maneuver**), which can reduce blood flow to the brain and cause dizziness and fainting. In an individual at high risk for coronary disease, the maneuver could be extremely dangerous and should always be avoided. Remember: Continue to breathe during any type of isometric or isotonic exercise.

Isokinetic Programs Recall that isokinetic exercise involves concentric or eccentric muscle actions performed at a constant speed (*isokinetic* refers to constant speed of movement). Isokinetic training is a relatively underused strength-training method, so limited research exists to describe its strength benefits compared with those of isometric and isotonic programs.

Isokinetic exercises require the use of machines that govern the speed of movement during muscle actions. The first isokinetic machines available were very expensive and were used primarily in clinical settings for injury rehabilitation. Recently, less expensive machines use a piston device (much like a shock absorber on a car) to limit the speed of movement throughout the range of the exercise.

MAKE SURE YOU KNOW...

- The greatest strength gains are made with a training program using low repetitions and high resistance, whereas the greatest improvements in endurance are made using high repetitions and low resistance.

- Isotonic programs include exercises with movable loads. Isometric training includes exercises in which a muscle contracts at a fixed angle against an immovable object. Isokinetic exercises involve machines that govern the speed of movement during muscle contraction.

Assess your exercise I.Q. with the *Test Your Exercise I.Q.* Take Charge of Your Health! Worksheet online at **www.pearsonhighered.com/powers**.

**LIVE IT!
ASSESS
YOURSELF**

Exercise Prescription for Weight Training

The general concepts of the frequency, intensity, and duration (or time) of exercise are required to improve physical fitness (Chapter 2). Although these same concepts apply to improving muscular strength and endurance through weight training, the terminology used to monitor the intensity and duration of weight training is unique. For example, the intensity of weight training is measured not by heart rate but by the number of *repetition maximums*. Similarly, the duration of weight training is measured not by actual time but by the number of sets performed. Let's discuss these two concepts briefly.

The intensity of exercise in both isotonic and isokinetic weight-training programs is measured by the repetition maximum (RM). Recall from earlier in the chapter that 1 RM is the maximal load that a muscle group can lift one time. Similarly, 6 RM is the maximal load that can be lifted six times. Therefore, the amount of weight lifted is greater when you perform a low number of RM than a high number of RM; that is, the weight lifted while you perform 4 RM is greater than the weight lifted while you perform 15 RM.

The number of repetitions (reps) performed consecutively without resting is called a **set**. For example, if you lift 6 RM, 1 set = 6 reps. Because the amount of rest required between sets will vary among individuals depending on how fit they are, the duration of weight training is measured by the number of sets performed, not by actual time.

Although experts disagree as to the optimum number of reps and sets required to improve strength and endurance, they do agree on some general guidelines. To improve strength, 3 sets of 6 reps for each exercise are generally recommended. Applying the concept of progressive resistance to a strength-training program involves increasing the amount of weight to be lifted a specific number of reps. For example, suppose that 3 sets of 6 reps were selected as your exercise prescription for increasing strength. As the training progresses and you become stronger, the amount of weight you lift must be increased. A good rule of thumb is that once you can perform 10 reps easily, you should increase the load to a level at which 6 reps are again maximal. **Figure 4.8** on page 88 illustrates the relationship between strength improvement and various combinations of reps and sets.

A key point in Figure 4.8 is that programs involving 3 sets result in the greatest strength gains. The reason is that the third set requires the greatest effort and thus is the greatest overload for the muscle. Although it may seem that adding a fourth set would elicit even greater

Valsalva maneuver Breath holding during an intense muscle contraction; can reduce blood flow to the brain and cause dizziness and fainting.

set The number of repetitions performed consecutively without resting.

A CLOSER LOOK

Do Weight Lifters Need Large Amounts of Protein in Their Diets?

Although many nutritional supplement companies claim that weight lifters require large quantities of protein in their diets, organizations such as the American College of Sports Medicine (ACSM), Academy of Nutrition and Dietetics (AND), and Dietitians of Canada (DC) have concluded that athletes have only slightly higher protein requirements than nonathletes. These organizations have also found that most athletes consume protein far in excess of any increased protein requirement. Provided that sound nutrition principles are followed and energy intake is sufficient to maintain body weight, athletes require about 10%–15% of their total caloric intake from protein and do not need to fortify their diets with expensive protein powders or amino acid supplements. The table below illustrates the daily energy and protein requirements for the average endurance or strength athlete.

Daily Protein Requirement for a 154-lb Active Individual*				
Type of Athlete	Energy (Calories per day)	Grams of Protein per lb Body Weight per Day[†]	Total Grams of Protein per Day	% of Daily Calories
Endurance	3800	0.55–0.64	84–98	9–10
Strength	3200	0.73–0.77	112–119	14–15

*Values assume a resting energy expenditure equivalent to 40 Kcal per kilogram (18 Kcal/lb) of body weight per day; a male runner who runs 10 miles per day at a pace of 6 minutes per mile with an energy expenditure while running of 0.11 Kcal per minute per pound of body weight; and an additional cost of 2.7 Kcal per pound body weight per day for heavy resistance training.

[†]Data are from Campbell, B., R. Kreider, T. Ziegenfuss, P. La Bounty, M. Roberts, D. Burke, J. Landis, H. Lopez, and J. Antonio. International Society of Sports Nutrition position stand: Protein and exercise. *Journal of International Society of Sports Nutrition* 26(4):1–7, 2007.

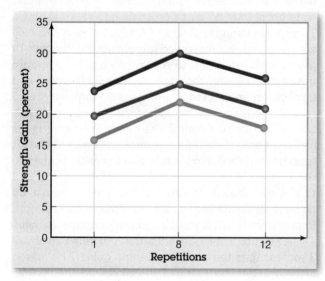

Key

- 1 Set
- 2 Sets
- 3 Sets

FIGURE 4.8
Strength gains from a resistance-training program consisting of various sets and repetitions. All programs were performed 3 days a week for 12 weeks. Note that in this program, the greatest strength gains (+30% improvement) were obtained using 3 sets of 8 reps per set.

gains, most studies suggest that performing 4 or more sets results in overtraining and decreased benefits.

To improve muscular endurance, 4 to 6 sets of 18 to 20 reps for each exercise are recommended. Note that you can improve endurance either by increasing the number of reps progressively while maintaining the same load, or by increasing the amount of weight while maintaining the same number of reps. The advantage of the latter program is that it would also improve muscular strength.

Most research suggests that 2 to 3 days of exercise per week is optimal for strength gains (5). However, studies have also shown that once the desired level of strength has been achieved, one high-intensity training session per week is sufficient to maintain the new level of strength. Finally, although limited research exists regarding the optimal frequency of training to improve muscular endurance, 3 to 5 days per week appear adequate (13).

MAKE SURE YOU KNOW...

- Progressively overloading a muscle can be accomplished by changing the frequency, intensity, and/or duration of the activity. Increasing the weight lifted will increase the intensity of the exercise. Increasing repetitions will increase the duration of the exercise.

- Exercising 2 to 3 days per week is optimal for strength gains; one high-intensity session per week is sufficient to maintain new strength levels; and exercising 3 to 5 days per week is adequate to improve muscular endurance.

Starting and Maintaining a Weight-Training Program

As with any plan for behavior change, you should begin your weight-training program with both short- and long-term goals. Be sure to establish realistic short-term goals that you can reach in the first several weeks of training. Reaching these goals will help motivate you to continue training.

Developing an Individualized Exercise Prescription

An exercise prescription for strength training has three stages: the starter phase, the slow progression phase, and the maintenance phase.

The primary objective of the **starter phase** is to build strength gradually without developing undue muscular soreness or injury. You can accomplish this by starting your weight-training program slowly—beginning with light weights, a high number of repetitions, and only 1 set per exercise, gradually working up to 2 sets per exercise. The recommended frequency of training during this phase is twice per week. The duration of this phase varies from 1 to 3 weeks, depending on your initial strength fitness level. A sedentary person might spend 3 weeks in the starter phase, whereas a moderately trained person may spend only 1 to 2 weeks.

The **slow progression phase** may last 4 to 20 weeks, depending on your initial strength level and your long-term strength goal. The transition from the starter phase to the slow progression phase involves three changes in the exercise prescription: increasing the frequency of training from 2 to 3 days per week; increasing the amount of weight lifted (and decreasing the number of repetitions); and increasing the number of sets performed from 2 to 3. The objective of the slow progression phase is to gradually increase muscular strength until you reach your desired level.

After reaching your strength goal, your long-term objective is to maintain this level of strength; this is the **maintenance phase** of the strength-training exercise prescription. Maintaining strength will require a lifelong weight-training effort. You will lose strength if you do not continue to exercise. The good news is that the effort required to maintain muscular strength is less than the initial effort needed to gain strength: Research has shown that as little as one workout per week is required to maintain strength (16).

COACHING corner

Muscular strength and endurance result from consistency, proper weight selection, and good form. If your motivation begins to wane, then consistency and attention to form may also go. Consider the following ideas for adding variety, accountability, and critical review for your training program.

- Hire a qualified trainer to consult with you on your lifting program.
- Read a supplemental text or attend an exercise-training seminar related to strength training.
- Identify exercises that mimic daily activities to enhance your functionality.
- Develop workouts with a partner and take turns leading the workouts.
- Try a strength-training or conditioning style group fitness class.

Meet trainer at 3 PM

See the sample programs on pages 90–92 to develop your exercise prescription for weight training.

MAKE SURE YOU **KNOW**...

- As you develop your strength-training program, divide it into three phases: a starter phase, a slow progression phase, and a maintenance phase.

starter phase The beginning phase of an exercise program. The goal of this phase is to build a base for further physical conditioning.

slow progression phase The second phase of an exercise program. The goal of this phase is to increase muscle strength beyond the starter phase.

maintenance phase The third phase of an exercise program. The goal of this phase is to maintain the increase in strength obtained during the first two phases.

Strength Training for Older Adults

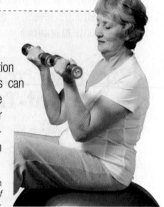

According to the Centers for Disease Control and Prevention (CDC), about 1.9 million people aged 65 and older were treated in emergency rooms for injuries due to falls in 2004. Almost 15,000 people over age 65 died as a result of injuries sustained in falls. In an effort to combat the number and minimize the severity of the falls, the American Academy of Orthopedic Surgeons (AAOS) and the National Athletic Trainers Association (NATA) are teaming up to help older Americans avoid falls and reduce the severity of injuries when falls do occur. The two organizations have established guidelines that call for older adults to keep muscles and bones strong by strength training with weight-bearing and resistance exercise.

Weight-bearing exercises increase bone density and help prevent osteoporosis. Research has shown that resistance training can enhance muscle mass and function even in 90-year-old subjects. Seniors can increase their lean muscle mass, improve dynamic balance, and increase their strength by participating in a well-designed strength-training program 2 or 3 days a week.

Sources: Centers for Disease Control and Prevention and The Merck Company Foundation. *The State of Aging and Health in America 2007.* Whitehouse Station, NJ: The Merck Company Foundation, 2007; Kim, S., and T. Lockhart. Effects of 8 weeks of balance or weight training for the independently living elderly on the outcomes of induced slips. *International Journal of Rehabilitation Research* 33(1):49–55, 2011; MacIntosh, B., P. Gardiner, and A. McComas. *Skeletal Muscle: Form and Function,* 2nd ed. Champaign, IL: Human Kinetics, 2006.

Motivation to Maintain Strength Fitness

The problems associated with starting and maintaining weight-training programs are similar to those associated with cardiorespiratory training. You must find time to train regularly, so good time management is critical.

Another key feature of any successful exercise program is that training must be fun. You can make weight training fun in a variety of ways. First, find an enjoyable place to work out. Locate a facility that contains the type of weights you want to use and in which you feel comfortable and motivated. Second, develop a realistic weight-training routine. Designing a training routine that is too hard may be good for improving strength but will not increase your desire to train. Therefore, design a program that is challenging but fun. Weight training is often more enjoyable with a partner. When looking for a workout buddy, ask a friend who is highly motivated to exercise and has strength abilities similar to yours.

Although the benefits of weight training are numerous, recent studies have shown that improved appearance, elevated self-esteem, and the overall feeling of well-being that result from regular weight training are the most important factors in motivating people to continue to train regularly. Looking your best and feeling good about yourself are excellent reasons to maintain a regular weight-training program. In addition, your elevated resting metabolic rate can help you burn calories more efficiently throughout the day, so even if you put on a few extra pounds of muscle mass, your clothes will fit better, and you will look better.

Sample Exercise Prescriptions for Weight Training

Scan to plan your individualized program for weight training. ▶

As with training to improve cardiorespiratory fitness, the exercise prescription for improving muscular strength must be tailored to the individual. Before starting a program, review the guidelines and precautions listed in Figure 4.9 (page 91).

The sample programs below illustrate the stages of a suggested strength-training exercise prescription. When you reach the strength goals of the program, the maintenance phase begins. You will use the same routine as you used during the progression phase, but you'll need to perform the routine only once per week.

The isotonic strength-training program contains exercises that are designed to provide a whole-body workout. Although you can perform some exercises using either machines or free weights, keep in mind that safety and proper lifting techniques are especially important when using free weights.

Follow the exercise routines described and illustrated on pages 93–99, and develop your program using the guidelines provided. This selection of exercises is designed to provide a comprehensive strength-training program that focuses on the major muscle groups. You can also use Table 4.2 to help you plan a program that works the total body. To avoid overtraining any one muscle group, be aware of which muscle groups are involved in an exercise. Note that it is not necessary to perform all exercises in one workout session; you can perform half of the exercises on one day and the remaining exercises on another day.

1. Warm up before beginning a workout. This involves 5 to 10 minutes of movement (calisthenics) using all major muscle groups.

2. Start slowly. The first several training sessions should involve limited exercises and light weight!

3. Use the proper lifting technique, as shown in the isotonic strength-training exercises in this chapter. Improper technique can lead to injury.

4. Follow all safety rules.

5. Always lift through the full range of motion. This not only develops strength throughout the full range of motion but also helps you maintain flexibility.

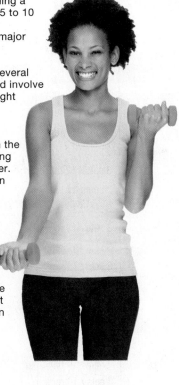

FIGURE 4.9
Follow these guidelines and precautions prior to beginning a strength-training program.

TABLE 4.2	Total-Body Resistance-Training Program		
Target Area	**Muscles**	**Without Weights**	**With Weights**
Arms	Biceps	Pull-up	Biceps curl
	Triceps	Push-up	Triceps extension
Chest	Pectoralis major	Push-up, dip	Fly, chest press, bench press
Upper back	Trapezius, rhomboids	Push-up	Upright row
Abdomen	Rectus abdominis, obliques	Curl-up, plank	Abdominal curl
Lower back	Latissimus dorsi	Pull-up	Lateral pulldown, back extension
Legs	Gluteus maximus	Lunge	Leg press
	Quadriceps	Lunge	Leg extension, leg press
	Hamstrings	Lunge	Hamstring curl
	Gastrocnemius, soleus	Heel raise	Calf raise

Beginner Isotonic Strength-Training Program

Choose exercises from Table 4.2 and on pages 93–99.
Weight = RM for the number of reps (e.g., 15 reps will be done with a 15 RM weight, etc.)

	Monday	Tuesday	Wednesday	Thursday	Friday	Saturday	Sunday
Week 1		1 set / 15 reps			1 set / 15 reps		
Week 2		2 sets / 15 reps			2 sets / 15 reps		
Week 3		2 sets / 15 reps			2 sets / 15 reps		

Intermediate Isotonic Strength-Training Program

Choose exercises from Table 4.2 and on pages 93–99.
Weight = RM for the number of reps (e.g., 12 reps will be done with a 12 RM weight, etc.)

	Monday	Tuesday	Wednesday	Thursday	Friday	Saturday	Sunday
Week 4	2 sets / 12 reps		2 sets / 12 reps		2 sets / 12 reps		
Week 5	2 sets / 12 reps		2 sets / 12 reps		2 sets / 12 reps		
Week 6	3 sets / 12 reps		3 sets / 12 reps		3 sets / 12 reps		
Week 7	3 sets / 12 reps		3 sets / 12 reps		3 sets / 12 reps		
Week 8	3 sets / 12 reps		3 sets / 12 reps		3 sets / 12 reps		
Week 9	3 sets / 12 reps		3 sets / 12 reps		3 sets / 12 reps		
Week 10	3 sets / 12 reps		3 sets / 12 reps		3 sets / 12 reps		
Week 11	3 sets / 12 reps		3 sets / 12 reps		3 sets / 12 reps		
Week 12	3 sets / 12 reps		3 sets / 12 reps		3 sets / 12 reps		
Week 13	3 sets / 12 reps		3 sets / 12 reps		3 sets / 12 reps		
Week 14	3 sets / 10 reps		3 sets / 10 reps		3 sets / 10 reps		
Week 15	3 sets / 10 reps		3 sets / 10 reps		3 sets / 10 reps		
Week 16	3 sets / 10 reps		3 sets / 10 reps		3 sets / 10 reps		
Week 17	3 sets / 10 reps		3 sets / 10 reps		3 sets / 10 reps		
Week 18	3 sets / 10 reps		3 sets / 10 reps		3 sets / 10 reps		
Week 19	3 sets / 10 reps		3 sets / 10 reps		3 sets / 10 reps		
Week 20	3 sets / 10 reps		3 sets / 10 reps		3 sets / 10 reps		

Advanced Isotonic Strength-Training Program

Choose exercises from Table 4.2 and on pages 93–99.
Weight = RM for the number of reps (e.g., 8 reps will be done with a 8 RM weight, etc.)

	Monday	Tuesday	Wednesday	Thursday	Friday	Saturday	Sunday
Week 21	3 sets / 8 reps		3 sets / 8 reps		3 sets / 8 reps		
Week 22	3 sets / 8 reps		3 sets / 8 reps		3 sets / 8 reps		
Week 23	3 sets / 8 reps		3 sets / 8 reps		3 sets / 8 reps		
Week 24	3 sets / 8 reps		3 sets / 8 reps		3 sets / 8 reps		
Week 25	3 sets / 8 reps		3 sets / 8 reps		3 sets / 8 reps		
Week 26	3 sets / 8 reps		3 sets / 8 reps		3 sets / 8 reps		
Week 27	3 sets / 8 reps		3 sets / 8 reps		3 sets / 8 reps		
Week 28	3 sets / 8 reps		3 sets / 8 reps		3 sets / 8 reps		
Week 29	3 sets / 8 reps		3 sets / 8 reps		3 sets / 8 reps		
Week 30	3 sets / 8 reps		3 sets / 8 reps		3 sets / 8 reps		
Week 31	3 sets / 6 reps		3 sets / 6 reps		3 sets / 6 reps		
Week 32	3 sets / 6 reps		3 sets / 6 reps		3 sets / 6 reps		
Week 33	3 sets / 6 reps		3 sets / 6 reps		3 sets / 6 reps		
Week 34	3 sets / 6 reps		3 sets / 6 reps		3 sets / 6 reps		
Week 35	3 sets / 6 reps		3 sets / 6 reps		3 sets / 6 reps		
Week 36	3 sets / 6 reps		3 sets / 6 reps		3 sets / 6 reps		
Maintain	3 sets / 6 reps		3 sets / 6 reps		3 sets / 6 reps		

EXERCISE 4.1 BICEPS CURL

PURPOSE: To strengthen the **elbow flexor muscles** (biceps, brachialis, brachioradialis)

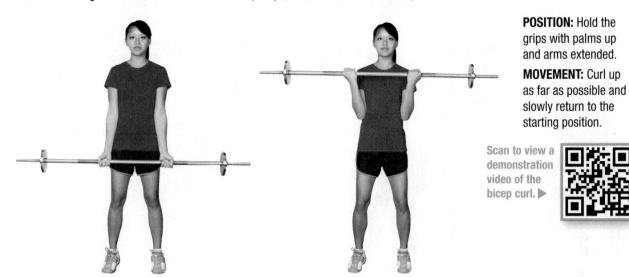

POSITION: Hold the grips with palms up and arms extended.

MOVEMENT: Curl up as far as possible and slowly return to the starting position.

Scan to view a demonstration video of the bicep curl. ▶

EXERCISE 4.2 TRICEPS EXTENSION

PURPOSE: To strengthen the muscles on the **back of the upper arm** (triceps)

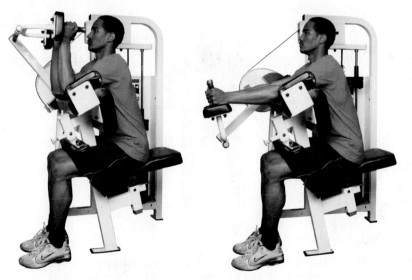

POSITION: Sit upright with elbows bent.

MOVEMENT: With the little-finger side of the hand against the pad, fully extend the arms and then slowly return to the original position.

Scan to view a demonstration video of the triceps extension. ▶

EXERCISE 4.3 DUMBBELL FLY

PURPOSE: To strengthen the muscles of the **chest** (pectoralis major) and **shoulder** (anterior deltoid)

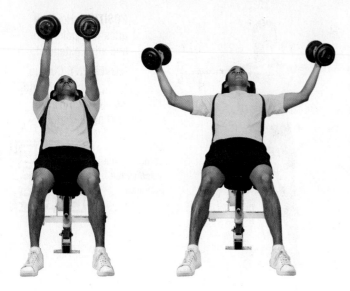

POSITION: Lie on an incline bench set at an angle between 45 and 60 degrees. Hold the dumbbells in front of your body with arms slightly flexed at the elbows.

MOVEMENT: Inhale, then lower the dumbbell until your elbows are at shoulder height. Raise the dumbbell while exhaling.

Scan to view a demonstration video of the dumbbell fly. ▶

EXERCISE 4.4 UPRIGHT ROW

PURPOSE: To strengthen the muscles of the **upper back** (rhomboids, middle trapezius, posterior deltoid, latissimus dorsi)

Scan to view a demonstration video of the upright row. ▶

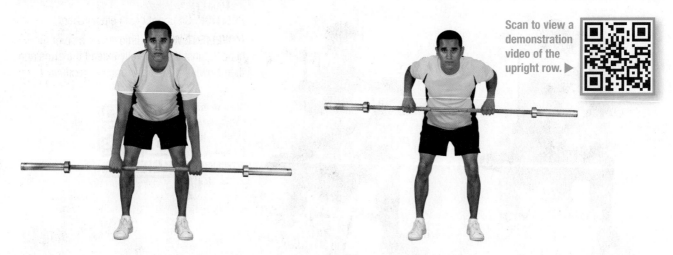

POSITION: Stand with your weight equally distributed on both feet and bend legs slightly. Bend forward at the waist to a 45-degree angle with head up, looking straight ahead. Grasp the bar with an overhand grip and keep hands shoulder width apart.

MOVEMENT: Pull the bar to the chest on the count of 2. Lower the bar to the starting position on the count of 4.

CAUTION: Beginners and people with lower back problems should use very light weight or a dumbbell at first.

EXERCISE 4.5 LUNGE

PURPOSE: To strengthen the muscles of the **hip** (gluteus maximus, hamstrings), **knee** (quadriceps), and **lower back** (erector spinae)

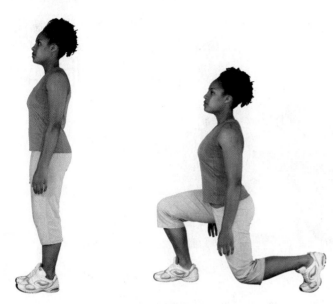

POSITION: Stand with your feet hip-width apart.

MOVEMENT: Lunge forward, putting all of the weight on your leading leg. Do not let the knee of your leading leg move in front of toes. Keep your knee in line with your ankle. Vary the stride length by taking a simple step forward to involve the quadriceps, or a large step forward to place more stress on the hamstrings and gluteals while stretching the quadriceps and hip flexors.

Scan to view a demonstration video of the lunge. ▶

EXERCISE 4.6 LEG EXTENSION

PURPOSE: To strengthen the muscles in the **front of the upper leg** (quadriceps [rectus femoris, vastus lateralis, vastus intermedius, vastus medialis])

Scan to view a demonstration video of the leg extension. ▶

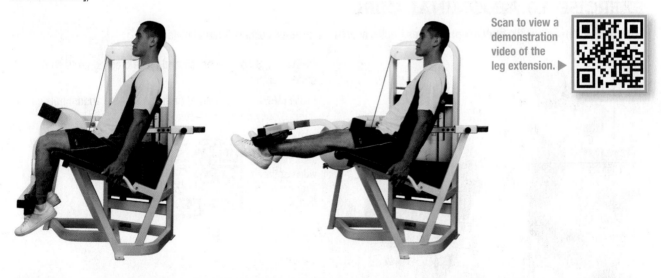

POSITION: Sit in a nearly upright position and grasp the handles on the side of the machine. Position your legs so the pads of the machine are against the lower shin.

MOVEMENT: Extend the legs until they are completely straight and then slowly return to the starting position.

EXERCISE 4.7 HAMSTRING CURL

PURPOSE: To strengthen the muscles on the **back of the upper leg** and **buttocks** (hamstrings [biceps femoris, semimembranosus, semitendinosis])

Scan to view a demonstration video of the hamstring curl. ▶

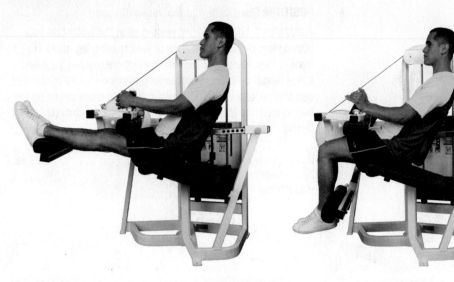

POSITION: In a seated position, extend legs so the pads of the machine are just below the calf muscles.

MOVEMENT: Curl the legs by pushing down on the pads to at least a 90-degree angle and then slowly return to the original position.

EXERCISE 4.8 ABDOMINAL CURL

PURPOSE: To strengthen the **abdominal muscles** (rectus abdominis, external oblique, internal oblique)

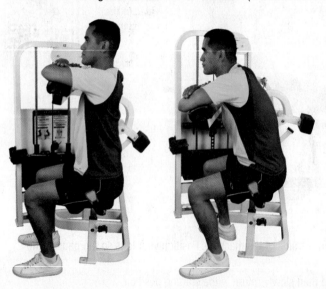

POSITION: Sit on the bench and place crossed arms on the padded armrest.

MOVEMENT: Bend forward until you feel the abdominals engage. Slowly return to starting position.

Scan to view a demonstration video of the abdominal curl. ▶

EXERCISE 4.9 BACK EXTENSION

PURPOSE: To strengthen the muscles of the **lower back** (erector spinae, quadratus lumborum)

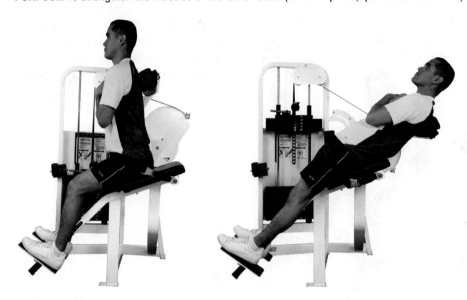

POSITION: Sit with your upper back positioned against the back pads, and your feet flat on the platform. Push back against the pads until the spine is straight. Cross your arms over your chest and straighten your spine.

MOVEMENT: Press backward against the back pad and slowly extend at the hip, keeping your spine straight. Slowly return to the starting position, keeping the spine straight.

EXERCISE 4.10 BENCH PRESS

PURPOSE: To strengthen the muscles in the **chest**, the **front of the shoulders** (pectoralis major, anterior deltoid), and the **back of the upper arm** (triceps)

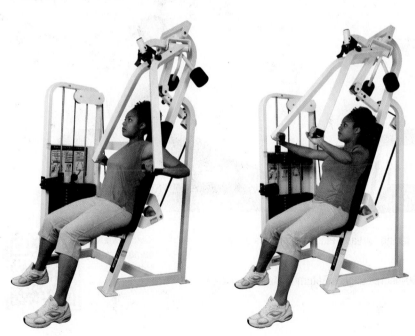

POSITION: Sit on the bench with the bench press hand grips level with your chest and your feet flat on the floor.

MOVEMENT: Grasp the bar handles and press outward until your arms are completely extended. Return slowly to the original position.

CAUTION: Do not arch your back while performing this exercise.

Scan to view a demonstration video of the bench press. ▶

EXERCISE 4.11 PULLOVER

PURPOSE: To strengthen the muscles of the **chest** (pectoralis major) and **shoulder** (triceps, latissimus dorsi, teres major)

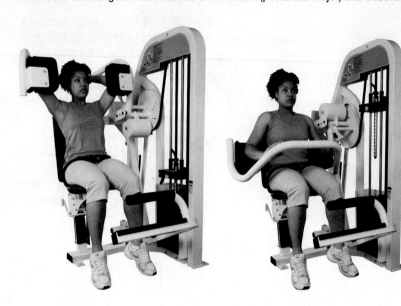

POSITION: Sit with your elbows against the padded ends of the movement arm and grasp the bar behind your head.

MOVEMENT: Press forward and down with your arms, pulling the bar overhead and down to your abdomen. Slowly return to the original position.

EXERCISE 4.12 DIP

PURPOSE: To strengthen the muscles of the **upper back**, **chest** (pectoralis major), and **shoulder** (triceps, deltoid)

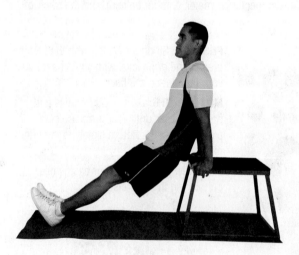 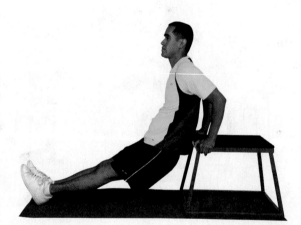

POSITION: Stand in front of a platform or a box, facing forward. Place both hands on the platform behind you.

MOVEMENT: Dip down until the elbows are at 90-degree angles. Return to starting position.

Scan to view a demonstration video of the dip. ▶

EXERCISE 4.13 TOE RAISE

PURPOSE: To strengthen the **calf muscles** (gastrocnemius, soleus).

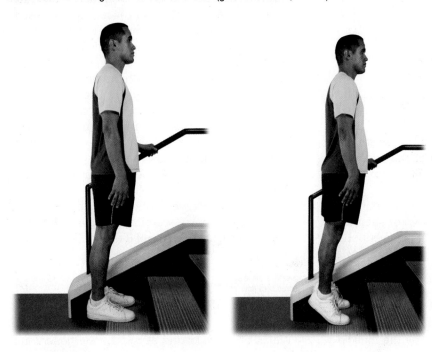

POSITION: Stand with your feet flat on the floor, or on the edge of a step.

MOVEMENT: Raise yourself up using the ankle joint only, and lower yourself back to starting position.

Scan to view a demonstration video of the toe raise. ▶

SUMMARY

Listen and see chapter review videos at **www.pearsonhighered.com/powers.**

HEAR IT! STUDY REVIEW

1. Strength training can reduce low back pain, reduce the incidence of exercise-related injuries, decrease the incidence of osteoporosis, and help maintain functional capacity, which normally decreases with age.

2. Muscular strength is the ability of a muscle to generate maximal force. In simple terms, this refers to the amount of weight that an individual can lift during one maximal effort. Muscular endurance is the ability of a muscle to generate force over and over again. In general, increasing muscular strength by exercise training will also increase muscular endurance. In contrast, training to improve muscular endurance does not always result in improved muscular strength.

3. Skeletal muscle is composed of a collection of long thin cells (fibers). Muscles are attached to bone by thick connective tissue (tendons). Muscle actions result in the tendons pulling on bone, causing movement.

4. Muscle action is regulated by signals coming from motor nerves, which originate in the spinal cord and branch out to individual muscles throughout the body. The motor nerve plus all of the muscle fibers it controls make up a motor unit.

5. Isotonic exercises result in movement of a body part. Isometric exercises involve developing tension within the muscle but result in no movement of body parts. Concentric muscle actions (positive work) involve muscle shortening. In contrast, eccentric muscle actions (negative contractions) involve muscle lengthening.

6. Human skeletal muscle can be classified into three major fiber types: slow-twitch, fast-twitch, and intermediate fibers. Slow-twitch fibers shorten slowly but are highly fatigue resistant. Fast-twitch fibers shorten rapidly but fatigue rapidly. Intermediate fibers combine the characteristics of fast- and slow-twitch fibers.

7. The process of involving more muscle fibers to produce increased muscular force is called fiber recruitment.

8. The percentages of slow-twitch, intermediate, and fast-twitch fibers vary among individuals. There is a relationship between predominant muscle fiber type and success in athletics. For example,

champion endurance athletes (e.g., marathon runners) have a high percentage of slow-twitch fibers.

9. Two primary physiological factors determine the amount of force that can be generated by a muscle: the size of the muscle and the number of fibers recruited.

10. Muscle size is increased primarily because of an increase in fiber size (hypertrophy).

11. The overload principle states that a muscle will increase in strength and/or endurance only when it works against a workload that is greater than normal. The concept of progressive resistance exercise (PRE) is the application of the overload principle to strength and endurance exercise programs.

12. A weight-training program using low repetitions and high resistance results in the greatest strength gains, whereas a program using high repetitions and low resistance results in the greatest improvement in muscular endurance.

13. Isotonic exercise involves contracting a muscle against a movable load (usually a free weight or weights on a weight machine). An isometric strength-training program is based on the concept of contracting a muscle at a fixed angle against an immovable object (using isometric muscle action). Isokinetic exercises require the use of machines that govern the speed of movement during muscle contraction throughout the range of motion.

14. To begin a strength-training program, divide the program into three phases: starter phase—2 to 3 weeks, with 2 workouts per week using 2 sets of 8 reps; slow progression phase—20 weeks, with 2 to 3 workouts per week using 3 sets of 6 reps; and maintenance phase—continues for life with 1 workout per week using 3 sets of 6 reps.

STUDY QUESTIONS

Find more review questions online at
www.pearsonhighered.com/powers.

REVIEW IT!
QUIZZES

1. What type of muscle action occurs as the muscle lengthens and controls the movement with resistance and/or gravity?
   a. concentric action
   b. eccentric action
   c. isometric action

2. A slow-twitch muscle fiber
   a. contracts slowly and produces small amounts of force.
   b. contracts rapidly and generates great amounts of force.
   c. contracts rapidly, produces great force, and fatigues rapidly.
   d. fatigues rapidly and is ideal for short bursts of activity.

3. Muscular strength is defined as
   a. the ability of a muscle to generate force over and over again.
   b. the ability of a muscle to generate maximal force.
   c. the ability of a muscle to shorten as it moves a resistance.
   d. the ability of a muscle to increase in size.

4. Which of the following is a benefit of a regular strength training program?
   a. reduces the incidence of a back pain
   b. increases $\dot{V}O_{2\,max}$
   c. reduces the incidence of colds
   d. increases endurance exercise capacity

5. Which of the following should be the general rule to follow to increase strength in a weight-training program?
   a. high resistance—high repetitions
   b. low resistance—low repetitions
   c. low resistance—high repetitions
   d. high resistance—low repetitions

6. Define the following terms:
   hypertrophy
   hyperplasia
   isotonic exercise
   isometric exercise
   isokinetic exercise
   motor unit
   progressive resistance exercise
   static contraction
   Valsalva maneuver

7. List at least three reasons why training for strength and endurance is important.

8. List and discuss the characteristics of slow-twitch, fast-twitch, and intermediate skeletal muscle fibers.

9. Discuss the pattern of muscle fiber recruitment with increasing intensities of contraction.

10. Discuss the relationship of muscle fiber type to success in various types of athletic events.

11. What factors determine muscle strength?

12. What physiological changes result from strength training?

13. Describe the concept of progressive resistance exercise.

14. Discuss the concept of specificity of training.

15. Compare and contrast the differences in training to increase strength versus training to increase endurance.

16. Define the concept of 1 RM.

17. List the phases of strength- and endurance-training programs, and discuss how they differ.

18. Distinguish isometric, concentric, and eccentric muscle actions.

19. Describe each of the following types of exercise: isokinetic, isometric, and isotonic.

For links to the organizations and websites listed, visit **www.pearsonhighered.com/powers.**

DO IT!
WEBLINKS

HELPFUL WEBLINKS

American College of Sports Medicine
Comprehensive website that provides equipment recommendations, how-to articles, book recommendations, and position statements about all aspects of health and fitness. www.acsm.org

Muscle Physiology
Includes in-depth discussions of how muscle works, as well as recent research articles from a world-renowned muscle physiology lab. www.muscle.ucsd.edu

WebMD
General information about exercise, fitness, wellness. Great articles, instructional information, and updates. www.webmd.com

Name _____   Date _____

Evaluating Muscular Strength: The 1 RM Test

The 1 RM test is used to measure muscular strength. You can use the following procedure to determine your 1 RM:

1. Begin with a 5- to 10-minute warm-up using the muscles to be tested.

2. For each muscle group, select an initial weight that you can lift without undue stress.

3. Gradually add weight until you reach the maximum weight that you can lift at one time. If you can lift the weight more than once, add additional weight until you reach a level of resistance such that you can perform only one repetition. Remember that a true 1 RM is the maximum amount of weight that you can lift one time.

The seated chest press and the leg press are two common methods for the 1 RM test. The seated chest press measures upper-body muscular strength, and the leg press measures muscular strength in the lower body.

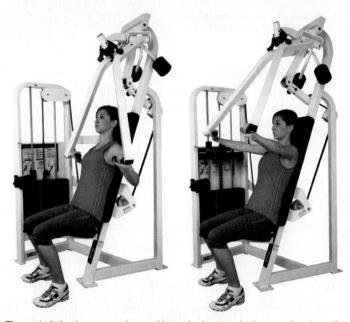

Scan to view a demonstration video of the chest press. ▶

The seated chest press can be used to evaluate upper-body muscular strength.

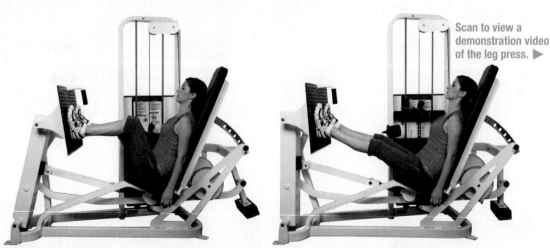

Scan to view a demonstration video of the leg press. ▶

A leg press can be used to evaluate lower-body muscular strength.

Your muscle strength score is the percentage of your body weight lifted in each exercise. To compute your strength score, divide your 1 RM weight in pounds by your body weight in pounds, and then multiply by 100. For example, suppose a 150-pound man has a bench press 1 RM of 180 pounds. This individual's muscle strength score for the bench press is computed as

$$\frac{1 \text{ RM weight}}{\text{body weight}} \times 100 = \text{muscle strength score}$$

Therefore,

$$\text{muscle strength score} = \frac{180 \text{ pounds}}{150 \text{ pounds}} \times 100 = 120$$

Table 4.3 and Table 4.4 on page 104 list strength score norms for college-aged men and women for the seated chest press and leg press, respectively. According to Table 4.3, a muscle strength score of 120 on the seated chess press places a college-aged man in the "good" category.

In the spaces below, record your muscular strength score and fitness category for the 1 RM tests for the leg press and seated chess press.

Age: _____   **Body weight:** _____ **lb**

Date: _____

Exercise	1 RM (lb)	Muscular Strength	Fitness Category
Seated chest press			
Leg press			

GOAL SETTING

1. Based on your results, write a goal to maintain or improve your current fitness level. For example, if you scored "fair" on this test, your goal might be to improve your fitness level to a "good" rating. If your fitness level indicated a score of "excellent," your goal might be to maintain your current fitness status.

   Goal: _____

2. Write three strategies for how you intend to achieve the goal you wrote. For example, one strategy for improving your current fitness status might be to perform 1 set of 10 repetitions at 50% of your 1 RM, 3 times a week. To progressively overload the muscles, increase the number of sets, and increase the weight load by 5–10 lb.

   1. _____

   _____

   2. _____

   _____

   3. _____

   _____

Muscle Strength Score Calculation is based on: Roitman, J. (Ed.). *ACSM's Resource Manual for Guidelines for Exercise Testing and Prescription.* Philadelphia: Lippincott, Williams, & Wilkins, 2001.

TABLE 4.3 **Strength Score Norms for the Seated Chest Press**
Locate your fitness level for upper-body muscular strength using your seated chest press score.

Men	Superior	Excellent	Good	Average	Poor	Very Poor
20–29 yrs	>148	130–147	114–129	99–113	89–98	<89
30–39 yrs	>124	110–123	98–109	88–97	79–87	<79
40–49 yrs	>110	98–109	88–97	80–87	73–79	<73
50–59 yrs	>97	88–96	79–87	71–78	64–70	<64
60+ yrs	>89	80–87	72–79	66–71	58–65	<58
Women	Superior	Excellent	Good	Average	Poor	Very Poor
20–29 yrs	>90	80–90	70–79	59–69	52–58	<52
30–39 yrs	>76	70–76	60–69	53–59	48–52	<48
40–49 yrs	>71	62–71	54–61	50–53	44–49	<44
50–59 yrs	>61	55–61	48–54	44–47	40–43	<40
60+ yrs	>64	54–64	47–53	43–46	39–42	<39

1 RM seated bench press with bench press weight ratio = weight pushed ÷ body weight × 100.

TABLE 4.4 **Strength Score Norms for the Leg Press**
Locate your fitness level for lower-body muscular strength using your seated leg press score.

Men	Superior	Excellent	Good	Average	Poor	Very Poor
20–29 yrs	>227	213–227	197–212	183–196	164–182	<164
30–39 yrs	>207	193–207	177–192	165–176	153–164	<153
40–49 yrs	>191	182–191	168–181	157–167	145–156	<145
50–59 yrs	>179	171–179	158–170	146–157	133–145	<133
60+ yrs	>172	162–172	149–161	138–148	126–137	<126
Women	Superior	Excellent	Good	Average	Poor	Very Poor
20–29 yrs	>181	168–181	150–167	137–149	123–136	<123
30–39 yrs	>160	147–160	133–146	121–132	110–120	<110
40–49 yrs	>147	137–147	123–136	113–122	103–112	<103
50–59 yrs	>136	125–136	110–124	99–109	89–98	<89
60+ yrs	>131	118–131	104–117	93–103	86–92	<86

1 RM seated leg press with leg press weight ratio = weight pushed ÷ body weight × 100.

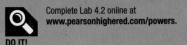
Name _____   **Date** _____

Evaluating Muscular Strength: The Estimated 1 RM Test

You can use the following procedure to determine your estimated 1 RM for any particular lift (e.g., chest press):

1. First, perform a set of 10 repetitions using a light weight.

2. Next, add 5 lb. and perform up to 10 repetitions.

3. Repeat this process until you reach a weight that you can lift 2–10 times. This is called your repetitions maximum (RM) for that weight. For example, if you can bench press 100 lb. only 6 times, then 100 lb. is your 6 RM weight.

Be sure to have an experienced instructor supervise the process so that your 10 RM weight can be discovered in fewer than five trials. Rest about 5 minutes after each trial to recover.

After determining your 2–10 RM, you can use Table 4.5 on page 106 to estimate your 1 RM. For example, if your RM for 100 lb. is 6, then the estimate for the 1 RM would be about 116 lb.

Remember, strength is largely determined by your body size. Thus, to determine your "standardized" muscle strength from the estimated 1 RM, use the same formula that you used in Lab 4.1:

$$\text{muscle strength score} = \frac{1 \text{ RM weight}}{\text{body weight}} \times 100$$

Record your muscular strength scores below, and use Table 4.3 or Table 4.4 in Laboratory 4.1 to determine your fitness category.

Age: _____   **Body weight:** _____ **lb**

Date: _____

Exercise	1 RM (lb)	Muscular Strength	Fitness Category
Seated chest press			
Leg press			

GOAL SETTING

1. Based on your results, write a goal to maintain or improve your current fitness level. For example, if your score was "fair" on this test, your goal might be to improve your fitness level to a "good" rating. If your fitness level indicated a score of "excellent," your goal might be to maintain your current fitness status.

    Goal: _____

2. Write three strategies for how you intend to achieve the goal you wrote. For example, one strategy for improving your current fitness status could be to perform 1 set of 10 repetitions at 50% of your 1 RM, 3 times a week. To progressively overload the muscles, increase the number of sets, and increase the weight load by 5–10 lb.

    1. _____

    _____

    2. _____

    _____

    3. _____

    _____

Muscle Strength Score Calculation is based on: Roitman, J. (Ed.). *ACSM's Resource Manual for Guidelines for Exercise Testing and Prescription.* Philadelphia: Lippincott, Williams, & Wilkins, 2001.

TABLE 4.5 1 RM Prediction Table

Wt (lb)	Repetitions									
	1	2	3	4	5	6	7	8	9	10
10	10	10	11	11	11	12	12	12	13	13
15	15	15	16	16	17	17	18	19	19	20
20	20	21	21	22	23	23	24	25	26	27
25	25	26	26	27	28	29	30	31	32	33
30	30	31	32	33	34	35	36	37	39	40
35	35	36	37	38	39	41	42	43	45	47
40	40	41	42	44	45	46	48	50	51	53
45	45	46	48	49	51	52	54	56	58	60
50	50	51	53	55	56	58	60	62	64	67
55	55	57	58	60	62	64	66	68	71	73
60	60	62	64	65	68	70	72	74	77	80
65	65	67	69	71	73	75	78	81	84	87
70	70	72	74	76	79	81	84	87	90	93
75	75	77	79	82	84	87	90	93	96	100
80	80	82	85	87	90	93	96	99	103	107
80	80	82	85	87	90	93	96	99	103	107
85	85	87	90	93	96	99	102	106	109	113
90	90	93	95	98	101	105	108	112	116	120
95	95	98	101	104	107	110	114	118	122	127
100	100	103	106	109	113	116	120	124	129	133
105	105	108	111	115	118	122	126	130	135	140
110	110	113	116	120	124	128	132	137	141	147
115	115	118	122	125	129	134	138	143	148	153
120	120	123	127	131	135	139	144	149	154	160
125	125	129	132	136	141	145	150	155	161	167
130	130	134	138	142	146	151	156	161	167	173
135	135	139	143	147	152	157	162	168	174	180
140	140	144	148	153	158	163	168	174	180	187
145	145	149	154	158	163	168	174	180	186	193
150	150	154	159	164	169	174	180	186	193	200
155	155	159	164	169	174	180	186	192	199	207
160	160	165	169	175	180	186	192	199	206	213
165	165	170	175	180	186	192	198	205	212	220
170	170	175	180	185	191	197	204	211	219	227
175	175	180	185	191	197	203	210	217	225	233
180	180	185	191	196	203	209	216	223	231	240
185	185	190	196	202	208	215	222	230	238	247
190	190	195	201	207	214	221	228	236	244	253
195	195	201	206	213	219	226	234	242	251	260
200	200	206	212	218	225	232	240	248	257	267
205	205	211	217	224	231	238	246	255	264	273

Wt (lb)	Repetitions									
	1	2	3	4	5	6	7	8	9	10
210	210	216	222	229	236	244	252	261	270	280
215	215	221	228	235	242	250	258	267	276	287
220	220	226	233	240	248	256	264	273	283	293
225	225	231	238	245	253	261	270	279	289	300
230	230	237	244	251	259	267	276	286	296	307
235	235	242	249	256	264	273	282	292	302	313
240	240	247	254	262	270	279	288	298	309	320
245	245	252	259	267	276	285	294	304	315	327
250	250	257	265	273	281	290	300	310	322	333

Source: Adapted from M. Brzycki, "Strength Testing: Predicting a One-Rep Max from a Reps-to-Fatigue." Reprinted with permission from the January 1993 *Journal of Physical Education, Recreation, and Dance.*

LABORATORY 4.3

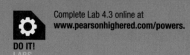

Complete Lab 4.3 online at
www.pearsonhighered.com/powers.

DO IT!
LABS

Name _____ Date _____

Tracking Your Progress

Use the log below to chart your strength-training progress. Record the date, number of sets, reps, and the weight for each of the exercises listed in the left column.

Date				
Exercise	St/Rp/Wt	St/Rp/Wt	St/Rp/Wt	St/Rp/Wt
Biceps curl (see Exercise 4.1)				
Triceps extension (see Exercise 4.2)				
Dumbbell fly (see Exercise 4.3)				
Upright rows (see Exercise 4.4)				
Lunges (with or without weights) (see Exercise 4.5)				
Abdominal curl (see Exercise 4.8)				
Quadriceps extension (see Exercise 4.6)				
Hamstring curl (see Exercise 4.7)				
Bench press or chest press (see Exercise 4.10)				

St/Rp/Wt = Sets/Reps/Weight *Example:* 2/6/80=2 sets of 6 reps each with 80 lb.

Name _____ **Date** _____

Measuring Muscular Endurance: The Push-Up and Curl-Up Tests

THE STANDARD PUSH-UP TEST

Scan to view a demonstration video of the push-up test. ▶

Perform the standard push-up test as follows:

1. Position yourself on the ground in push-up position (Figure a). (Note that you can instead use the modified push-up position shown in Figures c and d.) Place your hands about shoulder-width apart, and extend your leg in a straight line with your weight on your toes.

2. Lower your body until your chest is within 1 to 2 inches off the ground (Figure b), and raise yourself back to the up position. Be sure to keep your back straight and to lower your entire body as a unit.

3. Select a partner to count your push-ups and time your test (test duration is 60 seconds). Warm up with a few push-ups, and rest for 2 to 3 minutes after the warm-up to prepare for the test.

4. When your partner says "Go," start performing push-ups. Have your partner count your push-ups aloud, and ask him or her to let you know periodically how much time remains.

5. Record your score and fitness classification (from Table 4.6 on page 110) in the chart on page 111.

THE STANDARD PUSH-UP

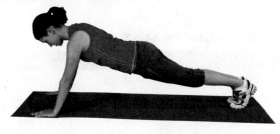

(a)

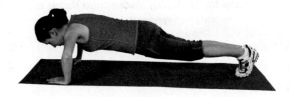

(b)

Scan to view a demonstration video of the standard push-up. ▶

THE MODIFIED PUSH-UP

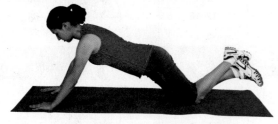

(c)

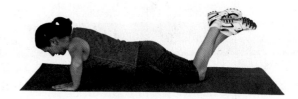

(d)

Scan to view a demonstration video of the modified push-up. ▶

109

THE CURL-UP TEST

Scan to view a demonstration video of the curl-up test. ▶

You can perform the curl-up test as follows:

1. Lie on your back with your legs shoulder-width apart, your knees bent 90 degrees, your arms straight at your sides, and your palms flat on the mat (Figure a).

2. Extend your arms so that your fingertips touch a strip of tape perpendicular to your body. A second strip of tape is located toward the feet and parallel to the first (10 centimeters apart).

3. Use the cadence provided on a metronome set to 50 beats per minute. Slowly curl up your upper spine until your fingers touch the second strip of tape. Then slowly return to the lying position with your head and shoulder blades touching the mat and your fingertips touching the first strip of tape. Breathe normally throughout, exhaling during the curling up stage.

4. Have your partner count the number of consecutive curl-ups you do in 1 minute, maintaining the metronome cadence and without pausing, to a maximum of 25. Record your score and fitness classification (from Table 4.7) in the chart on page 111.

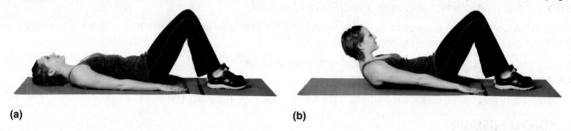

(a)   (b)

TABLE 4.6 **Norms for Muscular Endurance Using the Push-Up and Modified Push-Up Tests**

Men	Superior	Excellent	Good	Fair	Poor	Very Poor
20–29 yrs	≥62	47–61	37–46	29–36	22–28	≤21
30–39 yrs	≥51	39–51	30–38	24–29	17–23	≤16
40–49 yrs	≥39	30–39	24–29	18–23	11–17	≤10
50–59 yrs	≥38	25–38	19–24	13–18	9–12	≤8
60+ yrs	≥27	23–27	18–22	10–17	6–9	≤5
Women (modified push-up)	Superior	Excellent	Good	Fair	Poor	Very Poor
20–29 yrs	≥45	36–44	30–35	23–29	17–22	≤16
30–39 yrs	≥39	31–38	24–30	19–23	11–18	≤10
40–49 yrs	≥33	24–32	18–23	13–17	6–12	≤5
50–59 yrs	≥28	21–27	17–20	12–16	6–11	≤5
60+ yrs	≥20	15–19	12–14	5–11	2–4	≤1
Women (full push-up)	Superior	Excellent	Good	Fair	Poor	Very Poor
20–29 yrs	≥42	28–41	21–27	15–20	10–14	≤9
30–39 yrs	≥39	23–38	15–22	11–14	8–10	≤7
40–49 yrs	≥20	15–19	13–14	9–12	6–8	≤5
50–59 yrs	—	—	—	—	—	—
60+ yrs	—	—	—	—	—	—

— indicates data not available.

Source: Reprinted with permission from The Cooper Institute®, Dallas, Texas from a book called *Physical Fitness Assessments and Norms for Adults and Law Enforcement.* Available online at www.CooperInstitute.org.

TABLE 4.7 Norms for Muscular Endurance Using the Curl-Up Test

Men	Excellent	Very Good	Good	Fair	Needs Improvement
15–19 yrs	25	23–24	21–22	16–20	≤15
20–29 yrs	25	21–24	16–20	11–15	≤10
30–39 yrs	25	18–24	15–17	11–14	≤10
40–49 yrs	25	18–24	13–17	6–12	≤5
50–59 yrs	25	17–24	11–16	8–10	≤7
60–69 yrs	25	16–24	11–15	6–10	≤5
Women	Excellent	Very Good	Good	Fair	Needs Improvement
15–19 yrs	25	22–24	17–21	12–16	≤11
20–29 yrs	25	18–24	14–17	5–13	≤4
30–39 yrs	25	19–24	10–18	6–9	≤5
40–49 yrs	25	19–24	11–18	4–10	≤3
50–59 yrs	25	19–24	10–18	6–9	≤5
60–69 yrs	25	17–24	8–16	3–7	≤2

Source: Canadian Physical Activity, Fitness & Lifestyle Approach: CSEP-Health & Fitness Program's Appraisal and Counselling Strategy, 3rd edition, © 2003. Reprinted with permission from the Canadian Society for Exercise Physiology.

Age: _____

Date: _____

Number	Fitness Category
Push-ups (1 min):	
Curl-ups (1 min):	

GOAL SETTING

1. Based on your results, write a goal to maintain or improve your current fitness level. For example, if your score was "fair" on this test, your goal might be to improve your fitness level to a "good" rating. If your fitness level indicated a score of "excellent," your goal might be to maintain your current fitness status.

    Goal: _____

2. Write three strategies for how you intend to achieve your goal. For example, a strategy for improving your current fitness status might be to perform 1 set of 10 push-ups (or curl-ups), 3 times a week. To progressively overload the muscles, increase the number of sets to 2 and then 3.

    1. _____

    _____

    2. _____

    _____

    3. _____

    _____

Source: Curl-up test from *Canadian Physical Activity, Fitness & Lifestyle Approach: CSEP-Health & Fitness Program's Appraisal and Counselling Strategy*, 3rd edition, © 2003. Reprinted with permission from the Canadian Society for Exercise Physiology.

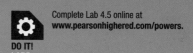
Name _____ **Date** _____

Measuring Core Strength and Stability

Position a watch on the ground where you can easily see it.

1. Assume the basic press up position, with your elbows on the ground (see the figure below). Hold this position for 60 seconds.

2. Lift your right arm off the ground. Hold this position for 15 seconds.

3. Return your right arm to the ground, and lift your left arm off the ground. Hold this position for 15 seconds.

4. Return your left arm to the ground, and lift your right leg off the ground. Hold this position for 15 seconds.

5. Return your right leg to the ground, and lift your left leg off the ground. Hold this position for 15 seconds.

6. Lift your left leg and right arm off the ground. Hold this position for 15 seconds.

7. Return your left leg and right arm to the ground, and lift your right leg and left arm off the ground. Hold this position for 15 seconds.

8. Return to the basic press up position (elbows on the ground). Hold this position for 30 seconds.

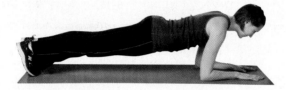

Basic press-up position

Scan to view a
demonstration video
of the basic
press-up. ▶

ANALYSIS

Analysis of the result involves comparing it with the results of previous tests. It is expected that, with appropriate training between each test, the analysis would indicate an improvement.

If you were able to complete this test, you have good core strength. If you were unable to complete the test, then repeat the routine 3 or 4 times a week until you can.

Source: Modified from the Core Muscle Strength Test by Brian Mackenzie, www.brianmac.co.uk/coretest.htm.

GOAL SETTING

1. Based on your results, write a goal to maintain or improve your current core strength and stability. For example, if you were able to hold the position for 60 seconds in step 1 but were unable to lift your right arm off the ground (step 2), your goal might be to work on completing step 2 and step 3. If you completed all steps, your goal could be to maintain your current core strength and stability.

    Goal: _____

2. Write three strategies for how you intend to achieve your goal. For example, an objective for improving your current fitness status might be to perform steps 3 and 4 three times a week. To progressively overload the muscles, increase to steps 5 and 6.

    1. _____

    _____

    2. _____

    _____

    3. _____

    _____

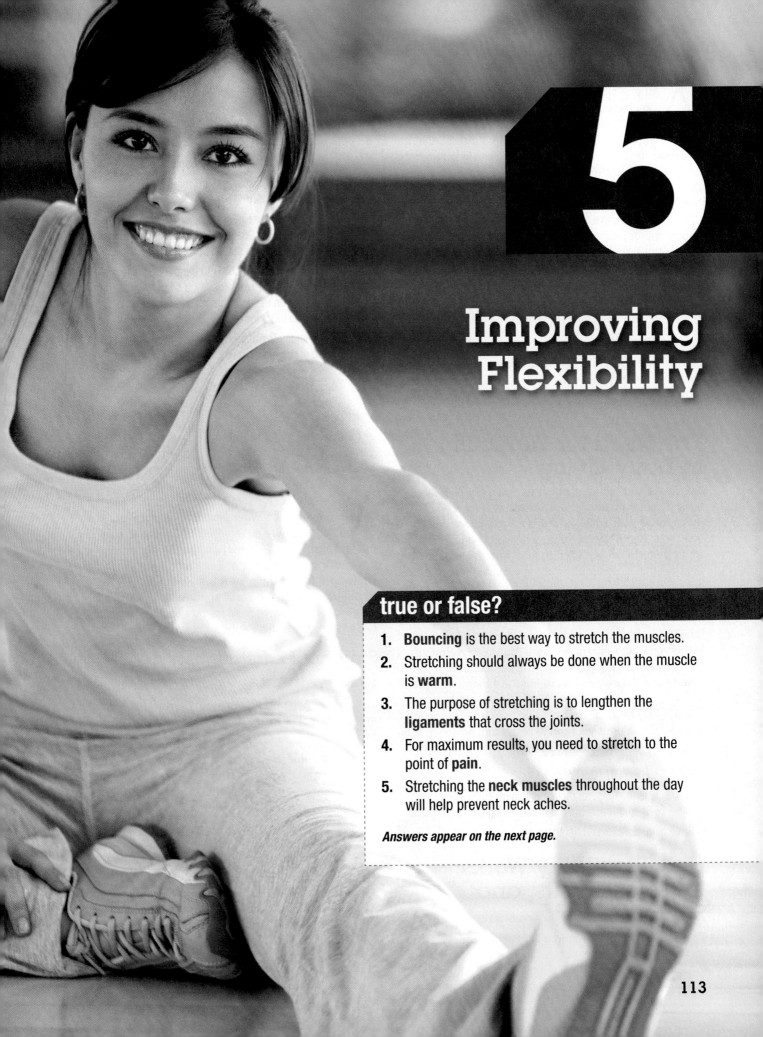

5

Improving Flexibility

true or false?

1. **Bouncing** is the best way to stretch the muscles.
2. Stretching should always be done when the muscle is **warm**.
3. The purpose of stretching is to lengthen the **ligaments** that cross the joints.
4. For maximum results, you need to stretch to the point of **pain**.
5. Stretching the **neck muscles** throughout the day will help prevent neck aches.

Answers appear on the next page.

Abby is a 22-year-old college junior whose biology major requires a lot of paper writing. She finds herself at the library at least four nights a week, conducting hours of research about cell behavior and gene function. Often, by the time she looks up from her textbook, her eyes are blurry, and her neck aches. Abby's fitness instructor advised her to take periodic breaks during her study time and to stretch her neck muscles to alleviate the kink in her neck. Although she knows this is probably good advice, she hasn't tried it yet because she's not sure how to properly stretch her neck muscles, and she forgets to look it up when she has a chance. Hence, the stiffness in her neck continues.

What do you think is causing Abby's stiff neck? Do you think her instructor's advice to stretch her neck will help alleviate the problem? Do you know how to properly stretch your neck muscles? In this chapter we'll discuss what causes muscle tightness and how stretching can improve flexibility. We'll also discuss the proper way to do various stretches and to target specific areas of the body for improved flexibility.

The Need for Flexibility in Daily Living

Gymnasts and ice skaters are not the only people who need to maintain adequate **flexibility**. When you bend down to tie your shoes or reach up to pull a sweatshirt over your head, you're relying on your body's flexibility to perform these tasks. In fact, any movement that requires you to stretch, reach, or twist your body without pain or stiffness is possible because you enjoy a range of motion around your joints. Unfortunately, you may not appreciate the importance of flexibility as a fitness component until you experience an injury that keeps you from performing these routine movements.

People vary in their degrees of flexibility because of differences in body structure, and the range of motion of most joints can decline with disuse. Tightness of the muscle, tendon, and connective tissue surrounding a joint can limit your range of motion; however, this restriction can be eliminated through proper stretching.

MAKE SURE YOU KNOW...
- Flexibility is the range of motion of a joint; it allows you to bend, twist, and reach without experiencing pain or stiffness.
- Stretching can alleviate tightness at a joint.

How Flexibility Works: Muscles, Joints, and Stretching

The range of motion around a joint is determined partly by the shapes and positions of the bones that make up the joint and partly by the composition and arrangement

answers

1. **FALSE** Bouncing can lead to a strained or torn muscle. For most people, slow static stretching will allow muscles to lengthen gradually.

2. **TRUE** A "cold" muscle is more reluctant to stretch than a warm muscle.

3. **FALSE** The purpose of stretching is to stretch muscles and tendons. Stretching the ligaments will cause injury and affect the stability of the joint.

4. **FALSE** Although stretching to the point of discomfort will help improve flexibility, a sharp pain during stretching can indicate that a ligament, muscle, or tendon has been torn.

5. **TRUE** Holding a muscle in one position for a long period of time, such as by staring at a computer screen for several hours, can result in muscle stiffness. Stretching can help alleviate this.

of muscles, tendons, and connective tissue around the joint (1, 2). Although the structure of the bones cannot be altered, the soft tissues can be lengthened to allow for greater range of motion. Remember, moderate tension to the muscles being stretched can make a significant improvement in your flexibility over time.

Of course, there are some movements that you will not be able to do, no matter how much you stretch, without causing yourself harm. You can't bend your fingers backward, for example, or rotate your arm 360 degrees at the elbow. The reason is that you are limited in the range of motion at your joints by your body's anatomy. Let's take a closer look at how this works.

Structural Limitations to Movement

There are five primary anatomical factors that limit movement (see **Figure 5.1** on page 115):

1. *The shape of the bones* determines the amount of movement possible at each joint. For example, because of the way they are structured, ball and socket joints, such as the shoulder and hip, have greater range of motion than hinge joints, such as the elbow and knee.

2. *A stiff muscle* will limit the range of motion at a joint; likewise, a warmed-up muscle will be flexible and allow a greater range of motion.

3. *The connective tissue* within the joint capsule provides stability at the joint. **Ligaments**, for example, are positioned around the joint to prevent the bone ends from coming apart, as in a dislocation injury. They prevent movements that a normal, healthy joint is not supposed to make. **Cartilage** covers

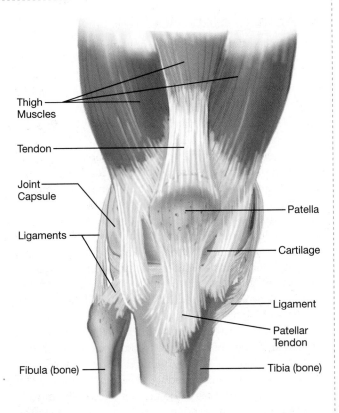

Before we examine specific stretching exercises, let's see how stretching works.

Stretching and the Stretch Reflex

When a doctor taps you on the knee with a rubber hammer, your knee extends. This is a **stretch reflex** caused by the rapid stretching of the **muscle spindles** within the quadriceps muscles that move the knee joint. Activating the stretch reflex is counterproductive to flexibility, because during the stretch the muscle shortens rather than lengthens. (Remember that the goal of stretching is to lengthen the muscle.) Fortunately, you can avoid the stretch reflex if you stretch the muscles and tendons very slowly. In fact, if you hold a muscle stretch for several seconds, the muscle spindles allow the muscle being stretched to further relax and permit an even greater stretch (2, 3). Therefore, stretching exercises are most effective when they avoid promoting a stretch reflex.

Muscle spindles are one type of **proprioceptor**, specialized receptors in muscles and tendons that provide feedback to the brain about the position of the body parts. When you were learning to catch a ball, you had to look at the position of your arms and hands to make sure they were in line with the path of the ball. As your catching skills improved, you no longer had to look at the arm position to know that it was lined up with the ball. The proprioceptors in your muscles and tendons provided feedback to your brain about where the arm was positioned. The proprioceptors within the muscles are muscle spindles, and the proprioceptors within the tendons are **Golgi tendon organs**.

FIGURE 5.1
A view of the knee joint and the anatomical structures that influence movement.

Source: Adapted from Johnson, Michael D., *Human Biology: Concepts and Current Issues, 4th Ed.,* © 2008. Reprinted and Electronically reproduced by permission of Pearson Education, Inc., Upper Saddle River, New Jersey.

the ends of the bones and creates a better fit between the bones, which helps eliminate unnecessary movements.

4. *Tendons,* which connect muscle to bones and to connective tissue surrounding joints, are extensions of the muscle tissue. If the muscle is tight, the tendon will also be tight.

5. *Tight skin* can limit the range of motion at a joint.

Exercise aimed at improving flexibility does not change the structure of bone, but it alters the soft tissues (muscle, joint connective tissue, and tendons) that contribute to flexibility. The resistance of the various soft tissues to total joint flexibility are: joint capsule (47%), muscle (41%), tendon (10%), skin (2%). Note that the structures associated with the joint capsule, muscles, and tendons provide most of the body's resistance to movement. Therefore, flexibility exercises must alter the resistance of one of these three to increase the range of motion around a joint. Stretching the muscle and tendon is desirable because these soft tissues can lengthen over time and thus improve flexibility. Stretching the ligaments in the joint capsule, in contrast, is undesirable because it can lead to a loose joint that would be highly susceptible to injury.

flexibility The ability to move joints freely through their full range of motion.

ligaments Connective tissues within the joint capsule that hold bones together.

cartilage A tough connective tissue that forms a pad on the end of long bones such as the femur, tibia, and humerus. Cartilage acts as a shock absorber to cushion the weight of one bone on another and to provide protection from the friction due to joint movement.

stretch reflex Involuntary contraction of a muscle due to rapid stretching of that muscle.

muscle spindles The type of proprioceptor found within muscle.

proprioceptor Specialized receptor in muscle or tendon that provides feedback to the brain about the position of body parts.

Golgi tendon organs The type of proprioceptor found within tendons.

MAKE SURE YOU KNOW...

- The structural and physiological limits to flexibility are due to the characteristics of bone; muscle; connective tissue within the joint capsule, such as ligaments and cartilage; the tendons, which connect muscle to bones and to connective tissue surrounding joints; and skin.

- If muscle spindles are stretched suddenly, they initiate a stretch reflex that causes the muscle to contract and shorten. However, if muscles are stretched slowly, the stretch reflex can be avoided.

- The proprioceptors (muscle spindles and Golgi tendon organs) monitor the muscles and tendons and report their positions to the brain.

Benefits of Flexibility

Although increased flexibility provides numerous benefits, including increased joint mobility, efficient body movement, and good posture (1, 3, 4), there is no research evidence to support the idea that it reduces the incidence of muscle injury during exercise. In fact, one critical review article suggests that stretching may contribute to injury (5). However, most studies suggest that stretching offers protection from muscle injury when combined with a general warm-up, and improved flexibility does help keep your joints healthy and can prevent lower back pain. Let's look at these benefits more closely.

Keeping Joints Healthy

Joints will suffer from lack of movement if you do not regularly engage them. If a joint is not moved enough, or has a limited range of motion, scar tissue can form that further restricts the joint motion and can be painful to the point that you may not be able to move the joint. The shoulder joint is particularly susceptible to such scar tissue formation. Mild stretching on a daily basis can prevent a joint from becoming immobile.

Joint mobility is also important for keeping the joint lubricated. Joints contain synovial fluid, which is needed to reduce friction and decrease wear and tear. Moving the joint helps circulate the synovial fluid, which in turn reduces the friction on the cartilage between the bones. Too much friction can damage cartilage, setting the stage for arthritis. Mild stretching can improve the mobility of the joint and promote normal wear on the cartilage covering the ends of the bones.

Stretching also directly affects the joints by reducing tension within the fibers of a muscle. When a muscle is stretched, these fibers are free to slide past one another, and the tension is literally worked out of the muscle. Reduced muscle tension reduces the tension exerted by the tendon as it crosses the joint. The force of the muscle exerted through the tendon on the bone can cause the bone ends in the joint to be pulled closer together, thus limiting the joint's range of motion. In essence, stretching can have the same effects on muscle tension as a manual muscle massage, at a much lower cost.

COACHING Corner

Tempted to skip your stretching routine? Skipping stretches may "seem" like a time saver, but the return on your time invested in stretching is significant. Consider allowing yourself the "gift of stretching" the next time you consider skipping it.

- Try achieving a mind–body connection through stretching and breath work. Inhale deeply as you feel your muscles lengthen and exhale deeply as you relax out of your stretch. Repeat 2–3 times and move to the next stretch.

- Be intentional about your stretch routine. Measure your range of motion at major joints and work to increase or improve that range of motion over a realistic time period.

- Allow your stretches to be enjoyable. Initiate the stretch only to a point of mild discomfort and then gradually ease out of the stretch.

- Work to enhance your experience by listening to your favorite music while you stretch.

- Attempt to clear your mind or concentrate on an affirming mantra while you slide into your stretches.

- Notice if you have different ranges of motion in the major joints. For example, compare the flexibility of your right shoulder to your left shoulder. Are there imbalances?

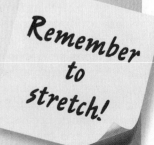

Remember to stretch!

Preventing Lower Back Pain

Another benefit of improved flexibility is that it can help prevent low back problems. Lower back pain (LBP) is sometimes called a **hypokinetic disease**, that is, a disease associated with a lack of exercise. The weak abdominal muscles commonly seen in sedentary individuals and the lack of flexibility in the hip flexor muscles are two common causes of LBP.

The abdominal muscles play a significant role in keeping the pelvic girdle in a neutral alignment with the spine (Figure 5.2). When the abdominal muscles are weak, the pelvis tilts forward and creates an increased hyperextension (forward curve), called *lordosis*, in the lower back. The muscles that flex the hip can affect the pelvis in the same way; however, they pull the pelvis forward when they are tight. Stretching these muscles and strengthening the abdominal muscles are important to keep the pelvis in a neutral alignment.

In addition to the abdominal muscles and the hip flexor muscles, the hamstrings and the lower back muscles also attach to the posterior side of the pelvis and can affect its alignment. The hamstring muscles exert a downward pull on the pelvis, whereas the lower back muscles exert an upward pull. Keeping all four muscle groups in balance helps keep the pelvis in a neutral alignment with the lumbar region of the spine and thus diminishes the likelihood for LBP.

Up to 80% of people will experience LBP, and approximately 15% of Americans will be disabled by LBP in their lifetime (6). Men and women are affected equally by back pain, usually between the ages of 25 and 60. Most pain in the lower back goes away in a few days or weeks. Lower back pain that lasts for longer than 6 months is considered chronic.

People who regularly carry heavy backpacks are at increased risk of lower back problems. In one study (7), curvature of the spine significantly increased as subjects carried weight high on the back rather than on the lower back. Although this study did not examine resulting back problems from the chronic wearing of a backpack, the findings certainly suggest that long-term backpack use can result in misalignment in the lower back.

The psychological, social, and physical costs of lower back pain are high, as are the economic costs. The medical, insurance, and business/industry costs are generally considered to be in the billions of dollars per year. Developing and maintaining healthy low back function requires a balance of flexibility, strength, and endurance. Table 5.1 outlines the top contributors to lower back pain, and the stretching you can do to help maintain a healthy back.

MAKE SURE YOU KNOW...

- Improved flexibility increases joint mobility and joint health, increases resistance to muscle injury, helps prevent low back problems, allows for efficient body movement, and improves posture and personal appearance.

- Flexibility of the hamstrings and lower back and strong abdominal muscles are important for a healthy back.

 Yoga is a great way to exercise your body and mind. Watch *Twist to Get Fit* at www.pearsonhighered.com/powers.

SEE IT! VIDEOS

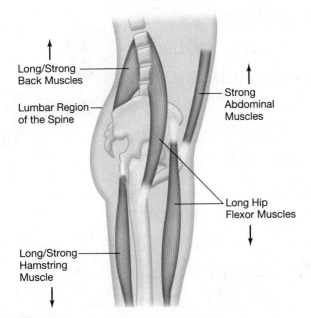

FIGURE 5.2
Strong abdominal and hip flexor muscles, balanced with strong back and hamstring muscles, help keep the spine and pelvis in neutral alignment, thereby lowering the risk of LBP.

Long/Strong Back Muscles
Lumbar Region of the Spine
Long/Strong Hamstring Muscle
Strong Abdominal Muscles
Long Hip Flexor Muscles

TABLE 5.1	Top Potential Contributors to Lower Back Pain and Sample Exercises to Maintain a Healthy Back
Contributor to LBP	**Exercise**
Poor low back lumbar flexibility	Modified hurdler's stretch (Exercise 5.5) Lower back stretch (Exercise 5.8)
Poor hamstring flexibility	Leg stretch (Exercise 5.4) Modified hurdler's stretch (Exercise 5.5)
Poor gluteal flexibility	Hip and gluteal stretch (Exercise 5.7)
Poor strength of the anterior and lateral abdominals	Curl-ups (page 133)
Poor flexibility of the back extensor muscles	Lower back stretch (Exercise 5.8)

hypokinetic disease Disease associated with a lack of exercise.

Preventing Poor Posture

Posture is the position of your joints that you hold while standing or sitting. Good posture is the result of holding positions that place the least amount of strain on the supporting muscles and ligaments around your joints. By routinely holding your body in good posture, you are maintaining the proper balance between the length and tension of all of the muscles around the joints.

Bad posture occurs when you hold positions that stretch muscles on one side of a joint, while shortening them on the other side. This can place undue strain on muscles, ligaments, and joints that will, over time, cause misalignment, pain, and possible damage to joints. Thus, bad posture leads to worse posture!

By incorporating strength and flexibility exercises into your daily routine, you can help correct any imbalances that you may have in your posture and prevent problems from occurring in the future. Here are some benefits of good posture:

- Minimizes any abnormal wear on joint surfaces that could result in arthritis.
- Reduces the stress on the ligaments holding the joints of the spine together.
- Prevents the spine from becoming fixed in abnormal positions, which may help prevent nerve stress and associated pains.
- Prevents fatigue because muscles are being used more efficiently.
- Prevents strain or overuse problems.
- Prevents backache and muscular pain.
- Contributes to a good appearance.

Use Laboratory 5.1 to evaluate your posture and then determine how your flexibility (determined in the next section) might be affecting your posture. Then make sure to include in your exercise routine those flexibility exercises that can help with correcting imbalances around joints.

MAKE SURE YOU KNOW...

- Posture refers to the position of your joints that you hold while standing or sitting.
- Strength and flexibility exercises can help you correct imbalances in your posture.

Evaluating Flexibility

Flexibility is joint specific. That is, you might be flexible in one joint but lack flexibility in another. You may also notice that you are more flexible on one side of your body than the other. This disparity is often due to greater usage of the dominant side of the body.

Although no single test is representative of total body flexibility, measurements of trunk and shoulder flexibility are commonly evaluated. The **sit-and-reach test** measures the ability to flex the trunk, which means stretching the lower back muscles and the muscles in the back of the thigh (hamstrings). In Laboratory 5.2, the first figure illustrates the sit-and-reach test using a sit-and-reach box.

The **shoulder flexibility test** evaluates the range of motion at the shoulder. See Laboratory 5.2 at the end of the chapter for a walk-through of the sit-and-reach test and shoulder flexibility tests.

Once you complete the sit-and-reach test and the shoulder flexibility test, you will better understand how flexible or inflexible you are. Both active and inactive individuals are often classified as average or below average for trunk and shoulder flexibility. In fact, only individuals who regularly perform stretching exercises are likely to possess flexibility levels that exceed the average. Regardless of your current flexibility classification, your flexibility goal should be to reach a classification of above average (i.e., good, excellent, or superior).

MAKE SURE YOU KNOW...

- Flexibility measurements are joint specific.
- Two popular tests to evaluate flexibility are the sit-and-reach test and the shoulder flexibility test.

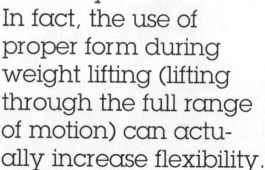

consider this!

Contrary to popular belief, weight lifting does not decrease flexibility. In fact, the use of proper form during weight lifting (lifting through the full range of motion) can actually increase flexibility.

A CLOSER LOOK

Pilates—More Than Stretching?

Pilates (pronounced Puh-**lah**-teez) is a widely used form of exercise among professional dancers, gymnasts, recreational exercisers, and rehabilitation specialists. It involves gentle, subtle stretching and contracting of muscles to produce very fluid, controlled movements that emphasize a mind–body interaction.

This body-conditioning routine improves flexibility, strength, endurance, and coordination without increasing muscle bulk. There are two forms of exercise in Pilates. The first form focuses on mat exercises that use your body weight as the resistance force. The other form involves using specialized machines to tone and strengthen the body. One piece of Pilates equipment, called the Reformer, consists of a moving carriage on a horizontal frame. There is a series of up to 100 exercises that can be performed on it without stopping.

Pilates emphasizes the following basic principles:

- *Concentration*—The mind–body connection. This stresses that conscious control of movement enhances body awareness.

- *Control/precision*—It's not about intensity or multiple "reps"; it's more about proper form.

- *Centering*—A mental focus within the body calms the spirit; a particular focus on the torso develops a strong core and enables the rest of the body to function efficiently. All action initiates from the trunk and flows outward to the extremities.

- *Stabilizing*—Before you move, you have to be still. This helps provide a safe starting place for mobility.

- *Breathing*—Deep, coordinated, conscious diaphragmatic patterns of inhaling and exhaling initiate movement, help activate deep muscles, and keep you focused.

- *Alignment*—Proper alignment is key to good posture. You'll be aware of the position of your head and neck on the spine and pelvis, right down through the legs and toes.

- *Fluidity*—Smooth, continuous motion rather than jarring repetitions.

- *Integration*—Several different muscle groups are engaged simultaneously to control and support movement. All principles come together, making for a holistic mind–body workout.

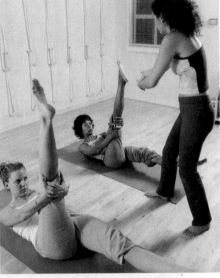

Designing a Flexibility Training Program

Because flexibility training is a key part of any fitness program, you'll want to include stretching exercises in your fitness routine. As with designing programs for the other fitness components, your first step will be to set short- and long-term goals. Do you want to become more flexible in the shoulders, or is your aim more to improve your hamstring and low back flexibility? No matter what your goal, you will want to think about how you will get there before you begin your new flexibility training routine. Also consider keeping a record of your workouts and improvements to follow your progress and plan your future training schedule.

Once you've set your goals, you can consider the types of stretches to include in your program. Three kinds of stretching techniques are commonly used to increase flexibility: **dynamic stretching**, **ballistic stretching**, and **static stretching**. A fourth type of stretching called

sit-and-reach test A fitness test that measures the ability to flex the trunk.

shoulder flexibility test A fitness test that measures the ability of the shoulder muscles to move through their full range of motion.

dynamic stretching Stretching that involves moving the joints through the full range of motion to mimic a movement used in a sport or exercise.

ballistic stretching A type of stretch that involves sudden and forceful bouncing to stretch the muscles.

static stretching Stretching that slowly lengthens a muscle to a point where further movement is limited.

STEPS FOR BEHAVIOR CHANGE

Are you too stiff?

Answer the following questions to help determine whether you would benefit from increased flexibility.

Y N

☐ ☐ Do you often feel as though you have a stiff neck?

☐ ☐ Is your mobility impaired when you turn your head to the left or right?

☐ ☐ Do you have difficulty washing your own back?

☐ ☐ Does your lower back feel stiff when you sit at your desk for prolonged periods of time?

☐ ☐ Do your ankles and feet feel stiff when you get out of bed in the morning?

If you answered yes to more than one question, check out the following tips.

TIPS TO IMPROVE FLEXIBILITY

Tomorrow, you will:

☑ Sit on the edge of your bed when you wake up and make 10 small and 10 large circles to the right and then to the left with your right foot. Repeat with your left foot.

☑ Use the shower as an opportunity to incorporate stretching. Let the warm water hit the back of your neck, shoulders, and upper back. Perform 10 shoulder rolls forward, 10 backward, and 10 neck tilts to the left and right while the shower spray is aimed at your neck and shoulders.

☑ Stretch if your neck feels stiff when you are working at your desk. Perform 5 minutes of gentle neck stretches and shoulder rolls at the top of every hour.

Within the next 2 weeks, you will:

☑ Try to increase the flexibility in your shoulders by holding a washcloth in your right hand as you reach behind your head. Try to grasp the washcloth with your left hand as you reach behind your back. By the end of the first 2 weeks, you should be able to reach it. Try pulling the washcloth up and down as you grasp it in both hands, increasing your range of motion with each up-and-down movement.

By the end of the semester, you will:

☑ Find a physioball for prolonged sitting. If your lower back is stiff after sitting for prolonged periods of time, try sitting on a physioball instead of a desk chair. The smaller muscles of the spine will be exercised as you balance on the physioball.

---

proprioceptive neuromuscular facilitation (PNF) is often used in rehabilitation settings (2, 8).

Dynamic stretching is equally effective for exercise programs and sports training. The fluid, exaggerated movements in dynamic stretches mimic the movements of many exercises. Ballistic stretching, in contrast, involves rapid and forceful bouncing movements to stretch the muscles. The movements of ballistic stretching are more likely to cause injury, so exercises to warm up the muscles prior to stretching are helpful. Ballistic stretches may be most beneficial to athletes involved in quick, explosive movements. With ballistic stretching, the athlete trains the nervous system and the muscles to adapt to the movements that she routinely performs. However, for the average fitness enthusiast seeking to increase flexibility, ballistic movements may activate the stretch reflex, injuring muscles and tendons. For this reason, ballistic stretching techniques are not usually incorporated into a nonathlete's fitness program.

Most people will benefit from incorporating dynamic, static, and PNF techniques into their fitness program. We'll discuss static and PNF stretching techniques next.

Static Stretching

Static stretching is extremely effective for improving flexibility (2, 4). Static stretching involves slowly lengthening a muscle to a point at which further movement is limited (slight discomfort is felt) and holding this position for a fixed period of time, normally 20 to 30 seconds, and repeating it 3 to 4 times, to improve flexibility (4). Compared with ballistic stretching, the risk of injury to the muscle or tendon is minimal with static stretching. When performed during the cool-down period, static stretching may reduce the muscle stiffness associated with some exercise routines (2, 4).

You can perform static stretches at home, and you don't need any special equipment to do them. You can

A CLOSER LOOK

A CLOSER LOOK

When Muscles Cramp

A muscle cramp is one of the most common problems encountered in sports and exercise. For many years, the primary causes of muscle cramps were thought to be dehydration and/or electrolyte imbalances. Accordingly, drinking enough fluids and ensuring that the diet contains sufficient amounts of sodium (from table salt, for example) and potassium (e.g., from bananas) have long been encouraged as preventive measures. When muscles cramp, stretching and/or massage have been used to relieve the cramping until electrolyte balance can be restored.

More recent research, however, suggests that cramping may be due to abnormal spinal control of motor neuron activity, especially when a muscle contracts while shortened (8). For example, the cramping that often occurs in the calf muscles of recreational swimmers when their toes are pointed may occur because those calf muscles are contracting while they are shortened.

The most prevalent risk factors for cramps during exercise are muscle fatigue and poor stretching habits (failure to stretch regularly and long enough during each session). Other risk factors include older age, higher body mass index, and a family history of muscle cramps.

If cramping occurs, you should do the following:

- Passively stretch the muscle. Such stretching induces receptors that sense the stretch to initiate nerve impulses that inhibit muscle stimulation.

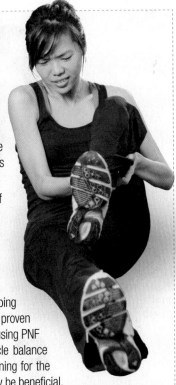

- Drink plenty of water to avoid dehydration or electrolyte imbalances. Sports drinks can help replenish glucose and electrolytes, but do not use salt tablets or drink fluids containing caffeine.

- Seek medical attention if multiple muscle groups are involved, because this could be a sign of more serious problems.

Although no strategies for preventing muscle cramping during exercise have been proven effective, regular stretching using PNF techniques, correcting muscle balance and posture, and proper training for the exercise activity involved may be beneficial.

COACHING Corner

Stretching is a nonnegotiable part of a comprehensive fitness plan. Make the most of your stretch time with these time-saving tips.

- Perform stretches that involve more than one joint at a time.

- Stretch only to a point of mild discomfort, take several breaths, and then release.

- Stretching is essential and more productive at the end of a workout than at the beginning. Save time by stretching when it matters most!

- Add variety to your flexibility training while enhancing your strength and range of motion through classes like yoga.

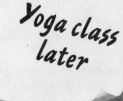

Yoga class later

even do them while watching television or sitting at your computer. See Exercises 5.1 through 5.12 for examples of static stretches.

Proprioceptive Neuromuscular Facilitation

Proprioceptive neuromuscular facilitation (PNF) combines stretching with alternately contracting and relaxing muscles. There are two common types of PNF stretching: *contract–relax (CR) stretching* and *contract–relax/antagonist contract (CRAC) stretching.* The CR stretch technique calls for first contracting the muscle to be stretched. Then, after the muscle is relaxed, it is slowly stretched. The CRAC method calls for the same contract–relax routine but adds the contraction of the **antagonist** muscle, the muscle on the opposite side of the joint. The purpose of contracting the antagonist muscle is to promote a reflex relaxation of the muscle to be stretched.

proprioceptive neuromuscular facilitation (PNF) A series of movements combining stretching with alternating contraction and relaxation of muscles.

antagonist The muscle on the opposite side of a joint.

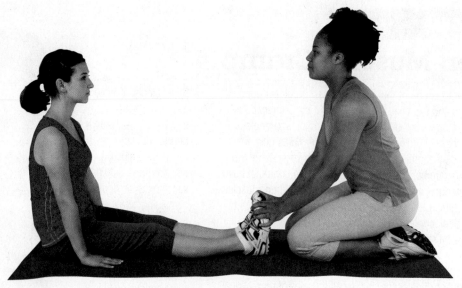

FIGURE 5.3
An example of a partner-assisted CRAC procedure for stretching the calf muscles. The exerciser contracts the calf muscles against resistance provided by the assistant. Then, unassisted, the exerciser contracts the shin (antagonist) muscles, thereby relaxing the calf muscles. Finally, while the exerciser continues contracting the shin muscles, the assistant stretches the calf muscles.

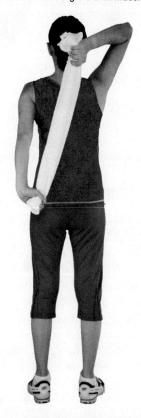

FIGURE 5.4
You can use a towel to do some PNF stretches without a partner.

How do PNF techniques compare with ballistic and static stretching? First, PNF has been shown to be safer and more effective in promoting flexibility than ballistic stretching (8). Further, studies have shown PNF programs to be equal to, or in some cases superior to, static stretching for improving flexibility (9).

Passive and Active Stretching

Some PNF stretches cannot be done alone—that is, they require a partner. The partner supplies resistance to the body part during the contraction of the antagonist muscles, thus preventing the body part from moving. This sequence of movements allows the muscle to relax more than in a static stretch, and greater range of motion can be achieved. The only drawback to this type of stretch is that the partner must provide resistance, which can be very tiring over a short period of time.

The following steps illustrate how a CRAC procedure can be done with a partner (**Figure 5.3**):

1. After the assistant moves the limb in the direction necessary to stretch the desired muscles to the point of tightness (where mild discomfort is felt), the exerciser isometrically contracts the muscle being stretched for 3 to 5 seconds and then relaxes it.

2. The exerciser then moves the limb in the opposite direction of the stretch by isometrically contracting the antagonist muscles. The exerciser holds this isometric contraction for approximately 5 seconds, during which time the muscles to be stretched relax. While the desired muscles are relaxed, the assistant may increase the stretch of the desired muscles.

3. The exerciser then isometrically contracts the antagonist muscles for another 5 seconds, which relaxes the desired muscles, and the assistant again stretches the desired muscles to the point of mild discomfort.

This cycle of three steps is repeated 3 to 5 times.

Some PNF stretches can also be done without a partner (**Figure 5.4**). Using a towel or other object to provide resistance can achieve the same benefits without fatiguing an assistant.

MAKE SURE YOU KNOW...

- Ballistic stretching involves sudden, forceful bouncing.
- Dynamic stretching involves moving the joints through a range of motion that is specific to a sport or activity.
- Static stretches involve stretching a muscle to the limit of movement and holding the stretch for an extended period of time.
- Proprioceptive neuromuscular facilitation (PNF) combines stretching with alternating contraction and relaxation of muscles to improve flexibility.
- Stretching exercises should be performed 2 to 5 days per week for 10 to 30 minutes each day.
- The intensity of a stretch is considered to be maximal when "mild discomfort" is felt.
- You can minimize your risk of injury during stretches by avoiding hazardous exercises and making sure to perform stretches correctly.

Motivation to Maintain Flexibility

Maintaining flexibility requires a commitment to performing regular stretching. Just as in other types of fitness training, good time management is critical if you are going to succeed. Set aside time for 3 to 5 stretching periods per week, and stick to your schedule. Remember that you can stretch almost anywhere, because you don't need special equipment. So take advantage of "windows" of free time in your day and plan stretching workouts.

You are not likely to maintain a lifetime stretching program if you do not enjoy your workouts. One suggestion for making stretching more fun is to perform workouts while listening to music or during a television program you enjoy.

Sample Exercise Prescriptions for Flexibility

Scan to plan your individualized program for flexibility. ▶

So what are the best frequency, intensity, time (duration), and type for your stretching routine (the FITT principle)? The answers vary according to your present level of flexibility, among other factors, but a good rule of thumb is that the first week, or starter phase, of a stretching regimen should include one stretching session. During the next 4 weeks, the slow progression phase of the program, one stretching session should be added per week. Initially, the duration of each training session should be approximately 5 minutes and should increase gradually to 20 to 30 minutes after 6 to 12 weeks of stretching during the slow progression phase.

The physiological rationale for increasing the duration of stretching is that each stretch position is held for progressively longer durations as the program continues. For example, begin by holding each stretched position for 15 seconds, then add 5 seconds each week, up to 30 seconds. Start by performing each of the exercises once (1 rep), and progress to 4 reps. The frequency and duration of a stretching exercise prescription should be 2 to 5 days per week for 10 to 30 minutes each day.

What about the intensity of stretching? In general, a limb should not be stretched beyond a position of mild discomfort. The intensity of stretching is increased by extending the stretch to the limits of your range of motion. Your range of motion will gradually increase as your flexibility improves during the training program.

To improve overall flexibility, all major muscle groups should be stretched. Just because you have good flexibility in the shoulders does not mean your flexibility will be good in the hamstrings. Exercises 5.1 through 5.12 illustrate the proper methods of performing 12 different stretching exercises. Integrate these exercises into the programs outlined on page 125.

In considering the type of exercises to be performed, these exercises are designed to be used in a regular program of stretching to increase flexibility. For safety reasons, all flexibility programs should consist of either PNF or static stretching exercises. The exercises presented involve the joints and major muscle groups for which range of motion tends to decrease with age and disuse. The exercises include both static and PNF movements and may require a partner. To avoid injury, be sure to follow the guidelines in Figure 5.5.

Some stretches that were once thought to improve flexibility are now known to be potentially damaging to the musculoskeletal system. The photos starting on page 132 show some common exercises that may cause injury, and provide substitute exercises that help accomplish the same goals.

1. Don't hold your breath. Try to breathe as normally as possible during the exercise.

2. Do not fully extend the knee, neck, or back.

3. Do not stretch muscles that are already stretched.

4. Do not stretch to the point that joint pain occurs.

5. Avoid stretching when having someone help you with passive stretches. Make sure you communicate about the end of the range of motion.

6. Avoid forceful extension and flexion of the spine.

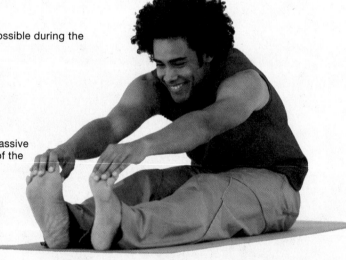

FIGURE 5.5
Follow these guidelines to avoid injury during stretches.

Beginner Flexibility Training Program

	Monday	Tuesday	Wednesday	Thursday	Friday	Saturday	Sunday
Week 1	1 rep / 15 sec			1 rep / 15 sec			
Week 2	1 rep / 15 sec			1 rep / 15 sec			
Week 3	2 reps / 15 sec each			2 reps / 15 sec each			

Intermediate Flexibility Training Program

	Monday	Tuesday	Wednesday	Thursday	Friday	Saturday	Sunday
Week 4		2 reps / 20 sec each		2 reps / 20 sec each			2 reps / 20 sec each
Week 5		2 reps / 20 sec each		2 reps / 20 sec each			2 reps / 20 sec each
Week 6		2 reps / 20 sec each		2 reps / 20 sec each			2 reps / 20 sec each
Week 7		2 reps / 20 sec each		2 reps / 20 sec each			2 reps / 20 sec each
Week 8		3 reps / 25 sec each		3 reps / 25 sec each			3 reps / 25 sec each
Week 9		3 reps / 25 sec each		3 reps / 25 sec each			3 reps / 25 sec each
Week 10		3 reps / 25 sec each		3 reps / 25 sec each			3 reps / 25 sec each
Week 11		3 reps / 25 sec each		3 reps / 25 sec each			3 reps / 25 sec each

Advanced Flexibility Training Program

	Monday	Tuesday	Wednesday	Thursday	Friday	Saturday	Sunday
Week 12		4 reps / 30 sec each		4 reps / 30 sec each	4 reps / 30 sec each		4 reps / 30 sec each
Week 13		4 reps / 30 sec each		4 reps / 30 sec each	4 reps / 30 sec each		4 reps / 30 sec each
Week 14		4 reps / 30 sec each		4 reps / 30 sec each	4 reps / 30 sec each		4 reps / 30 sec each
Week 15		4 reps / 30 sec each		4 reps / 30 sec each	4 reps / 30 sec each		4 reps / 30 sec each
Week 16		4 reps / 30 sec each		4 reps / 30 sec each	4 reps / 30 sec each		4 reps / 30 sec each
Maintain		4 reps / 30 sec each		4 reps / 30 sec each	4 reps / 30 sec each		4 reps / 30 sec each

EXERCISE 5.1 LOWER LEG STRETCH

PURPOSE: To stretch the **calf** muscles (gastrocnemius, soleus) and the **Achilles' tendon**.

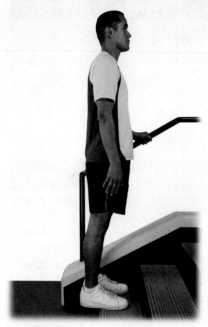 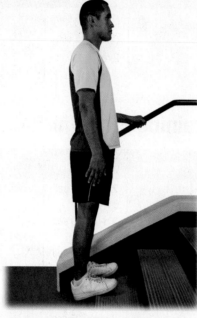

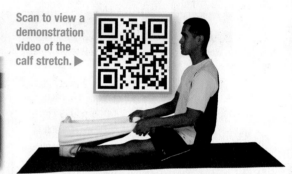

Scan to view a demonstration video of the calf stretch. ▶

POSITION: Stand on the edge of a surface that is high enough to allow your heel to drop lower than your toes. Have a support nearby to hold for balance.

MOVEMENT: Rise up on your toes as far as possible for several seconds, then lower your heels as far as possible. Shift your body weight from one leg to the other for added stretch of the muscles.

VARIATION: Sit on the floor with leg outstretched, loop a towel under the ball of your foot, and gently pull your foot upward so that the top of the foot moves closer to your shin. Another variation (not pictured) is to sit on the floor with one leg outstretched and the other leg flexed, with the sole of your foot along the knee of your other leg. Reach down, grasp the toes of the outstretched leg, and gently pull the foot upward so that the top of the foot moves closer to the shin.

EXERCISE 5.2 SHIN STRETCH

PURPOSE: To stretch the muscles of the **shin** (tibialis anterior, extensor digitorum longus, extensor hallucis longus).

Scan to view a demonstration video of the shin stretch. ▶

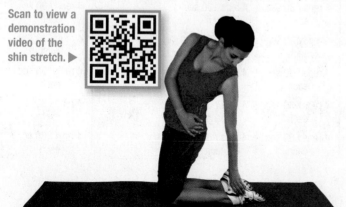

POSITION: Kneel on both knees, with your trunk rotated to one side and the hand on that side pressing down on your ankle.

MOVEMENT: While pressing down on your ankle, move your pelvis forward; hold for several seconds. Repeat on the other side.

EXERCISE 5.3 THIGH STRETCH

PURPOSE: To stretch the muscles in the front of the **thigh** (quadriceps) of the extended (rear) leg.

Scan to view a demonstration video of the thigh stretch. ▶

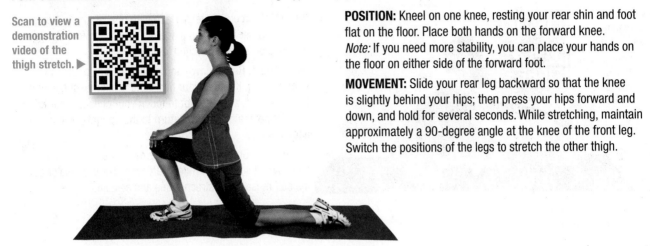

POSITION: Kneel on one knee, resting your rear shin and foot flat on the floor. Place both hands on the forward knee.
Note: If you need more stability, you can place your hands on the floor on either side of the forward foot.

MOVEMENT: Slide your rear leg backward so that the knee is slightly behind your hips; then press your hips forward and down, and hold for several seconds. While stretching, maintain approximately a 90-degree angle at the knee of the front leg. Switch the positions of the legs to stretch the other thigh.

EXERCISE 5.4 LEG STRETCH

PURPOSE: To stretch the muscles on the **back of the hip** (gluteus maximus), the **back of the thigh** (hamstrings), and the **calf** (gastrocnemius and soleus).

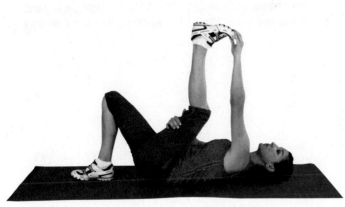

POSITION: Lying on your back, bring one knee toward your chest, and grasp your toes with the hand on the same side. Place the opposite hand on the back of the leg just below the knee.

MOVEMENT: Pull your knee toward your chest while pushing your heel toward the ceiling and pulling your toes toward your shin. Straighten your knee until you feel sufficient stretch in the muscles of the back of the leg, and hold for several seconds. Repeat for the other leg.

EXERCISE 5.5 MODIFIED HURDLER'S STRETCH

PURPOSE: To stretch the **lower back muscles** (erector spinae) and muscles in the **back of the thigh** (hamstrings).

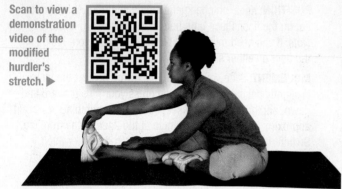

Scan to view a demonstration video of the modified hurdler's stretch. ▶

POSITION: Sit on a level surface with one leg out in front, bend the other knee, and place the sole of the foot alongside the knee of the outstretched leg.

MOVEMENT: Reach down and grab the ankle of the outstretched leg. Keeping your head and trunk straight, lean your trunk forward, and attempt to touch your chest to your knee. Hold for several seconds. Return to the upright position, and alternate legs.

VARIATION: Grasp the toes of the extended leg, and pull your toes toward your shin while stretching. This will also stretch the calf muscles (gastrocnemius and soleus).

EXERCISE 5.6 INSIDE LEG STRETCH

PURPOSE: To stretch the muscles on the **inside of the thighs** (adductors and internal rotators).

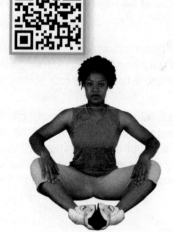

Scan to view a demonstration video of the inner thigh stretch. ▶

POSITION: Sit with the bottoms of your feet together and place your hands just below your knees.

MOVEMENT: Try to raise your knees while pushing down with your hands and forearms. Then relax, and, using your hands, press your knees toward the floor; hold for several seconds.

EXERCISE 5.7 HIP AND GLUTEAL STRETCH

PURPOSE: To stretch the muscles at the **hip** (gluteals, tensor fasciae latae).

Scan to view a demonstration video of the hip and gluteal stretch. ▶

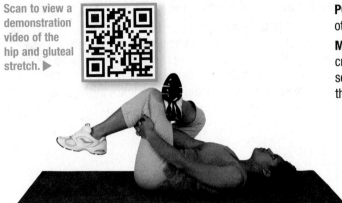

POSITION: Lie on your back, with one leg crossed over the other and both shoulders and both arms on the floor.

MOVEMENT: Grasp behind the knee of the leg that is not crossed over, and pull the thigh toward your chest. Hold for several seconds. Reverse the positions of the legs, and repeat the stretch.

EXERCISE 5.8 LOWER BACK STRETCH

PURPOSE: To stretch the muscles of the **lower back** (erector spinae) and **buttocks** (gluteals).

Scan to view a demonstration video of the lower back stretch. ▶

POSITION: Lie on your back with your hips and knees bent, your feet flat on the floor, and your arms positioned along your sides.

MOVEMENT: First, arch your back and lift your hips off the floor; hold for several seconds. Then relax and return to starting position. Place your hands behind your knees, and pull the knees to your chest. Hold for several seconds.

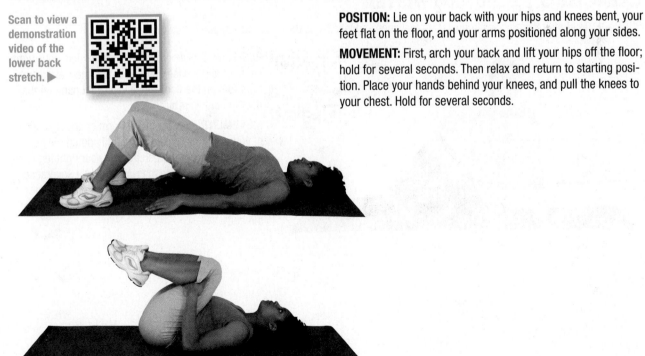

EXERCISE 5.9 SIDE STRETCH

PURPOSE: To stretch the muscles of the **upper arm** (triceps) and **side of the trunk** (latissimus dorsi).

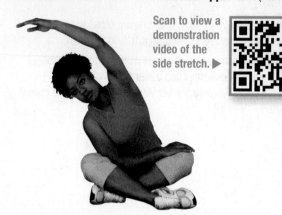

Scan to view a demonstration video of the side stretch. ▶

POSITION: Sit on the floor with your legs crossed.

MOVEMENT: Stretch one arm over your head while bending at your waist in the same direction. With the opposite arm, reach across your chest as far as possible; hold for several seconds. Do not rotate your trunk; try to stretch the muscle on the same side of the trunk as the overhead arm. Alternate arms to stretch the other side of the trunk.

EXERCISE 5.10 TRUNK TWISTER

PURPOSE: To stretch the muscles of the **trunk** (obliques and latissimus dorsi) and **hip** (gluteus maximus).

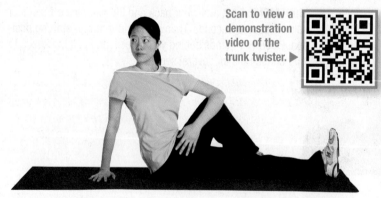

Scan to view a demonstration video of the trunk twister. ▶

POSITION: Sit with your left leg extended, your right leg bent and crossed over your left knee, and your right foot on the floor. Place your right hand on the floor behind your buttocks.

MOVEMENT: Placing your left arm on the right side of your right thigh and your right hand on the floor, use your left arm to push against your right leg while twisting your trunk to the right; hold for several seconds. Then assume the starting position with your right leg extended, and stretch the opposite side of the body.

EXERCISE 5.11 CHEST STRETCH

PURPOSE: To stretch the muscles across the **chest** (pectoralis major) and **shoulder** (anterior deltoid and biceps).

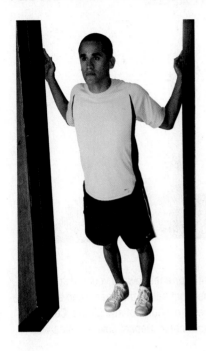

POSITION: Stand in a doorway, and grasp the frame of the doorway at shoulder height.

MOVEMENT: Press forward on the frame for 5 seconds. Then relax and shift your weight forward until you feel the stretch of muscles across your chest; hold for several seconds.

Scan to view a demonstration video of the chest stretch. ▶

EXERCISE 5.12 NECK STRETCH

PURPOSE: To stretch the muscles that rotate the **head** (sternocleidomastoid).

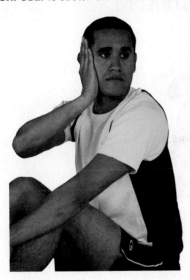

Scan to view a demonstration video of the neck stretch. ▶

POSITION: After turning your head to one side, place your hand against your cheek with your fingers toward the ear and your elbow pointing forward.

MOVEMENT: Try to turn your head and neck against the resistance of your hand; hold for a few seconds. Remove your hand and relax, then turn your head as far as possible in the same direction. Repeat the stretch, turning in the other direction.

PURPOSE: To stretch the **lower back** and **buttocks.**

MAY CAUSE INJURY:

KNEE PULL

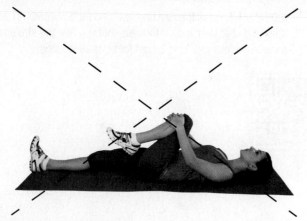

This position places undue stress on the knee joint.

TRY THIS INSTEAD:

LEG PULL

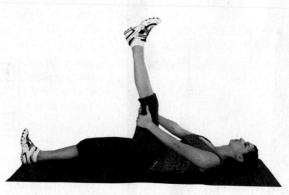

Lie on your back and pull your knee toward your chest by pulling on the back of your leg just below the knee. Then extend the knee joint and point the sole of your foot straight up. Continue to pull your leg toward your chest. Repeat several times with each leg.

PURPOSE: To strengthen the **upper leg** and stretch the **lower leg.**

MAY CAUSE INJURY:

DEEP KNEE BEND

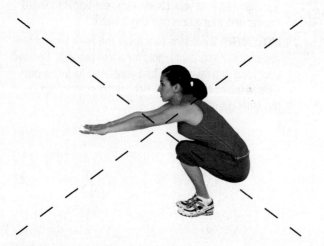

This movement hyperflexes the knee and "opens" the joint while stretching the ligaments.

TRY THIS INSTEAD:

LUNGE

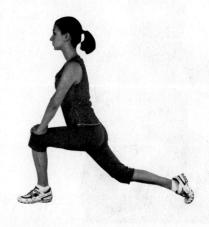

From a standing position, step forward with either foot and touch the opposite knee to the ground. Repeat with the opposite leg.

132

PURPOSE: To stretch the **lower back**, **buttocks**, and **hamstrings**.

MAY CAUSE INJURY:

STANDING TOE TOUCH

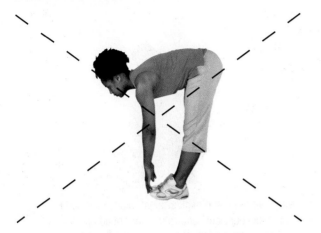

This movement could damage the lower back.

TRY THIS INSTEAD:

SITTING HAMSTRING STRETCH

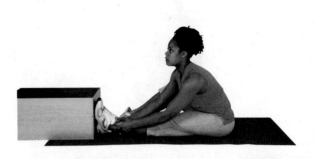

Sit at leg-length from a wall. With your foot on the wall and the other knee bent with the foot between the wall and your buttocks, bend forward, keeping your lower back straight. The bent knee can fall to the side.

Scan to view a demonstration video of the sitting hamstring stretch. ▶

PURPOSE: To strengthen the **abdominal muscles**.

MAY CAUSE INJURY:

SIT-UP (HANDS BEHIND HEAD)

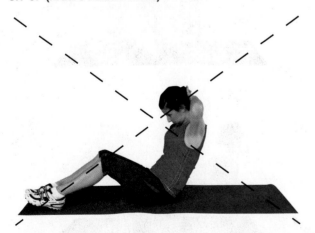

This movement could cause hyperflexion of the neck and strain the neck muscles.

TRY THIS INSTEAD:

CURL-UP

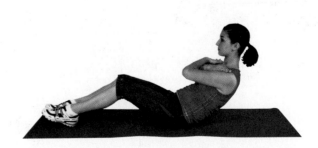

Lie on your back with your knees bent, and cross your arms over your chest. Using your abdominal muscles, curl up until the upper half of your back is off the floor, and then return to the starting position.

PURPOSE: To stretch the **neck muscles**.

May Cause Injury:

NECK CIRCLES

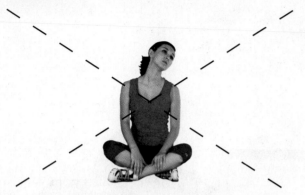

This movement hyperextends the neck, which can pinch arteries and nerves as well as damage disks in the spine.

TRY THIS INSTEAD:

NECK STRETCHES

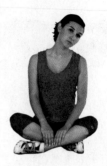

Sit with your head and neck straight. Move your head down to flex your neck, and return your head upright. Then slowly turn your head from side to side as far as possible; attempt to point your chin at each shoulder.

PURPOSE: To stretch and strengthen the **buttocks**.

May Cause Injury:

DONKEY KICK

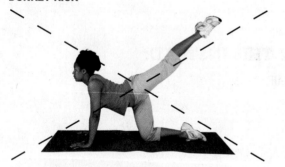

When kicking the leg back, most people hyperextend the neck and/or back.

TRY THIS INSTEAD:

KNEE-TO-NOSE TOUCH

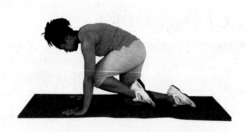

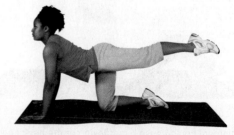

While on your hands and knees, lift one knee toward your nose and then extend that leg to the horizontal position. Alternate legs. Do not lift your leg higher than your hips, and keep your neck in line with your back.

SUMMARY

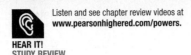

Listen and see chapter review videos at
www.pearsonhighered.com/powers.

HEAR IT!
STUDY REVIEW

1. Flexibility is the range of motion of a joint.
2. Improved flexibility results in the following bene-fits: increased joint mobility, prevention of low back problems, efficient body movement, and improved-posture and personal appearance.
3. The five structural and physiological limits to flex-ibility are the shape of bone; muscle; connective tissue within the joint capsule; the tendons, which connect muscle to bones and to connective tissue that surrounds joints; and skin.
4. Proprioceptors are constantly monitoring the ten-sion of the muscles and tendons and providing feedback to the brain. If muscle spindles are sud-denly stretched, they respond by initiating a stretch reflex that causes the muscle to contract. However, if the muscles and tendons are stretched slowly, the stretch reflex can be avoided.
5. Designing your flexibility program involves set-ting short-term and long-term goals and selecting stretches that will help you meet your goals. Static stretches involve stretching a muscle to the limit of movement and holding the stretch for an extend-ed period of time. Dynamic stretches involve fluid, exaggerated movements designed to mimic the movements of a given sport or activity.
6. Proprioceptive neuromuscular facilitation (PNF) combines stretching with alternating contraction and relaxation of muscles to improve flexibility. Bal-listic stretches may be appropriate for some ath-letes but are not safe for the general public.
7. Flexibility exercises are important in maintaining good posture and preventing misalignment and de-bilitating changes in the musculoskeletal system.

STUDY QUESTIONS

Find more review questions online at
www.pearsonhighered.com/powers.

REVIEW IT!
QUIZZES

1. Which of the following is not an anatomical factor that can limit movement at a joint?
   a. shape of the bones
   b. tight skin
   c. tight tendons
   d. length of the bone
2. Proprioceptors include which of the following?
   a. motor units
   b. Golgi organs
   c. muscle spindles
   d. both b and c
3. Static stretching is not advisable for nonathletes.
   a. true
   b. false
4. To avoid injury, most stretching should be done
   a. only at night.
   b. after the muscles have been warmed up.
   c. while watching television.
   d. to the point of pain.
5. Lower back pain is the result of
   a. weak abdominal muscles.
   b. weak hamstring muscles.
   c. hyperextension of the lower back.
   d. all of the above.

6. Define the following terms:
   flexibility   range of motion   cartilage
   ligament   tendon   antagonist
   proprioceptive neuromuscular facilitation
7. Describe the difference in function between liga-ments and tendons.
8. Compare static and ballistic stretching.
9. List three primary reasons why maintaining flexibil-ity is important.
10. List the factors that limit flexibility. Which factors place the greatest limitations on flexibility?
11. Briefly outline the exercise prescription to improve flexibility.
12. Describe why the stretch reflex should be avoided.
13. List four benefits of having good posture.

HELPFUL WEBLINKS

For links to the organizations and websites listed,
visit www.pearsonhighered.com/powers.

DO IT!
WEBLINKS

American College of Sports Medicine
Provides information, articles, and position statements about health and fitness. www.acsm.org

Mayo Clinic
General information about fitness and wellness. Includes flexibility exercises for particular muscle groups, sports, and conditions. www.mayoclinic.org

WebMD
General information about exercise, fitness, wellness. Great articles, instructional information, and updates. www.webmd.com

LABORATORY 5.1

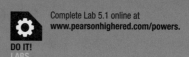
Complete Lab 5.1 online at
www.pearsonhighered.com/powers.

DO IT!
LABS

Name _____ **Date** _____

Assessing Your Posture

Scan to view a demonstration
video of the posture test. ▶

Poor posture is all too common and can lead to severe muscle and joint misalignment, possibly resulting in debilitating musculo-skeletal problems. In fact, poor posture often progresses so slowly that you may notice its symptoms (back and neck pain, stiffness, increased injury, and reduced range of motion) well before you notice a change in your posture.

The first step to improving posture is finding out what your posture looks like. Then you can compare it to "good" posture and determine the kind of exercise that will help you to correct the misalignments.

STEP 1: Take a Photograph to Determine Your Posture

You can determine what your posture looks like by taking a photograph of yourself standing against a wall. Have a friend or relative photograph you standing against a plain, flat surface, from the back and side.

You can compare your body position to a straight plane by placing a string behind you. Attach the string to an object overhead and then tie it to an object to the other end, just above the floor. Center the string between your feet in back view photograph. Center the string on the medial malleolus (bone protrusion on the side of the ankle) in the side view photograph.

STEP 2: Score Your Posture

Once you have the photographs of your posture from the back and side, compare them to the scoring chart on the following page. With each aspect of the posture shown, determine your score from the values shown at the top of the chart.

STEP 3: Review Your Scores

Review each of the posture aspects that you evaluated.

A score of 2 in all the categories indicates that your posture is good. A strength and flexibility exercise program should help you maintain your excellent posture.

If you scored a 1, you might want to find some flexibility exercise that will help you to realign that aspect.

If you scored a 0, begin flexibility exercises now to correct that aspect of your posture. This is important since the misalignment will almost certainly lead to pain and/or permanent alterations to your posture in the future.

Note the date of your assessment in the space provided on the right side of the chart. In 6 weeks, reassess you posture and your scores. Remember: Be conscious of your posture throughout the day. Continue to use both strength and flexibility exercise to help correct any misalignment you detect.

	Good—2	Fair—1	Poor—0	Scores	
Back View				Date 1	Date 2
Head	Head erect, gravity passes directly through center	Head twisted or turned to one side slightly	Head twisted or turned to one side markedly		
Shoulders	Shoulders level horizontally	One shoulder slightly higher	One shoulder markedly higher		
Spine	Spine straight	Spine slightly curved	Spine markedly curved laterally		
Hips	Hips level horizontally	One hip slightly higher	One hip markedly higher		
Knees and Ankles	Feet pointed straight ahead, legs vertical	Feet pointed out, legs deviating outward at the knee	Feet pointed out markedly, legs deviated markedly		
Side View				Date 1	Date 2
Neck and Upper back	Neck erect, head in line with shoulders, rounded upper back	Neck slightly foward, chin out, slightly more rounded upper back	Neck markedly forward, chin markedly out, markedly rounded upper back		
Trunk	Trunk erect	Trunk inclined to rear slightly	Trunk inclined to rear markedly		
Abdomen	Abdomen flat	Abdomen protruding	Abdomen protruding and sagging		
Lower back	Lower back normally curved	Lower back slightly hollow	Lower back markedly hollow		
Legs	Legs straight	Knees slightly hyperextended	Knees markedly hyperextended		

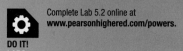
Name _____   Date _____

Assessing Flexibility: Trunk Flexion (Sit-and-Reach) Test and Shoulder Flexibility Test

THE SIT-AND-REACH TEST

Scan to view a
demonstration video of the
sit-and-reach test. ▶

To perform the sit-and-reach test, start by sitting upright with your feet flat against a sit-and-reach box. Keeping your feet flat on the box and your legs straight, extend your hands as far forward as possible, and hold this position for 3 seconds. Repeat this procedure 3 times. Your score on the sit-and-reach test is the distance, measured in inches, between the edge of the sit-and-reach box closest to you and the tips of your fingers during the best of your three stretching efforts.

Note that you should warm up by stretching for a few minutes before you perform the test. To reduce the possibility of injury, avoid rapid or jerky movements during the test. It is often useful to have a partner help by holding your legs straight during the test and by measuring the distance. After completing the test, consult Table 5.2 on page 139 to locate your flexibility fitness category, and record your scores on the same page.

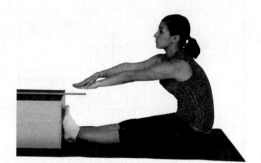

The sit-and-reach test.

THE SHOULDER FLEXIBILITY TEST

Scan to view a demonstration
video of the shoulder
flexibility test. ▶

To perform the shoulder flexibility test, follow these steps: While standing, raise your right arm and reach down your back as far as possible. At the same time, extend your left arm behind your back and reach upward toward your right hand. The objective is to try to overlap your fingers as much as possible. Your score on the shoulder flexibility test is the distance, measured in inches, of finger overlap.

Measure the distance of finger overlap to the nearest inch. For example, an overlap of 3/4 inch would be recorded as 1 inch. If your fingers fail to overlap, record this score as −1. Finally, if your fingertips barely touch, record this score as 0. After completing the test with the right hand up, repeat the test in the opposite direction (left hand up).

As with the sit-and-reach test, you should warm up with a few minutes of stretching prior to performing the shoulder flexibility test. Again, to prevent injury, avoid rapid or jerky movements during the test. After completing the test, consult Table 5.3 on page 139 to locate your shoulder flexibility category, and record your scores on the same page.

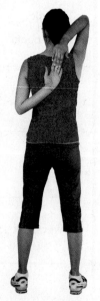

The shoulder flexibility test.

TABLE 5.2 Physical Fitness Norms for Trunk Flexion

BOX Sit-and-Reach Test (centimeters)					
Men	Excellent	Very Good	Good	Fair	Needs Improvement
15–19 yrs	≥39	34–38	29–33	24–28	≤23
20–29 yrs	≥40	34–39	30–33	25–29	≤24
30–39 yrs	≥38	33–37	28–32	23–27	≤22
40–49 yrs	≥35	29–34	24–28	18–23	≤17
50–59 yrs	≥35	28–34	24–27	16–23	≤15
60–69 yrs	≥33	25–32	20–24	15–19	≤14
Women	Excellent	Very Good	Good	Fair	Needs Improvement
15–19 yrs	≥43	38–42	34–37	29–33	≤28
20–29 yrs	≥41	37–40	33–36	28–32	≤27
30–39 yrs	≥41	36–40	32–35	27–31	≤26
40–49 yrs	≥38	34–37	30–33	25–29	≤24
50–59 yrs	≥39	33–38	30–32	25–29	≤24
60–69 yrs	≥35	31–34	27–30	23–26	≤22

Source: Canadian Physical Activity, Fitness & Lifestyle Approach: CSEP-Health & Fitness Program's Appraisal and Counseling Strategy, 3rd edition, © 2003. Reprinted with permission from the Canadian Society for Exercise Physiology.

TABLE 5.3 Physical Fitness Norms for Shoulder Flexibility

Right Hand Up Score	Left Hand Up Score	Fitness Classification
<0	<0	Very poor
0	0	Poor
+1	+1	Average
+2	+2	Good
+3	+3	Excellent
+4	+4	Superior

Note that these norms are for both men and women of all ages. Units for the shoulder flexibility test score are inches and indicate the distance between the fingers of your right and left hands.

Source: Fox, Edward L.; Kirby, Timothy; Fox, Ann Roberts, *Bases of Fitness, 1st Ed.,* © 1987. Reprinted and Electronically reproduced by permission of Pearson Education, Inc., Upper Saddle River, New Jersey.

Date: _____

Sit-and-reach score (centimeters): _____ Fitness category: _____

Shoulder flexibility (inches)

Left side: _____ Fitness category: _____

Right side: _____ Fitness category: _____

GOAL SETTING

1. Based on your results for the flexibility testing, write a goal to either improve or maintain your fitness category.

2. Write three objectives to help you achieve your goal.

1. _____

2. _____

3. _____

LABORATORY 5.3

Complete Lab 5.3 online at
www.pearsonhighered.com/powers.

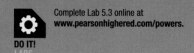

DO IT!
LABS

Name _____ Date _____

Flexibility Progression Log

Use this log to record your progress in increasing flexibility in selected joints. Record the date, hold time, and sets for each of the exercises listed in the left column.

Date							
Exercise	St/Hold	St/Hold	St/Hold	St/Hold	St/Hold	St/Hold	St/Hold
Lower leg stretch (see Exercise 5.1)							
Shin stretch (see Exercise 5.2)							
Thigh stretch (see Exercise 5.3)							
Leg stretch (see Exercise 5.4)							
Modified hurdler's stretch (see Exercise 5.5)							
Inside leg stretch (see Exercise 5.6)							
Hip and gluteal stretch (see Exercise 5.7)							
Lower back stretch (see Exercise 5.8)							
Side stretch (see Exercise 5.9)							
Trunk twister (see Exercise 5.10)							
Chest stretch (see Exercise 5.11)							
Neck stretch (see Exercise 5.12)							

St/Hold = sets and hold time *Example:* 2/30 = 2 sets held for 30 seconds each

Name _____ **Date** _____

Stretching to Prevent or Reduce Lower Back Pain

Stretching exercises are important in maintaining a flexible and healthy back. Our daily activities often result in overuse and tightening of back muscles. Chronic overuse and straining can cause significant back pain and increase your risk of back injury.

In this lab, you will learn exercises to stretch the muscles of your lower back to help in maintaining flexibility. Performing these stretches will help prevent back pain and may help reduce back aches.

BACK EXTENSION—PRONE

Scan to view a demonstration video of the back extension stretch. ▶

1. Lie on your stomach.
2. Prop yourself up on your elbows, extending your back.
3. Start straightening your elbows, further extending your back.
4. Continue straightening your elbows until you feel a gentle stretch.
5. Hold for 15 seconds.
6. Return to the starting position.
7. Repeat 10 more times.

CAT STRETCH

Scan to view a demonstration video of the cat stretch. ▶

1. Get down on the floor on your hands and knees.
2. Push your back up toward the ceiling (like a cat arching its back).
3. Continue arching until you feel a gentle stretch in your back.
4. Hold for 15 seconds.
5. Return to the starting position.
6. Repeat 10 more times.

THE PELVIC TILT

Scan to view a demonstration video of the pelvic tilt. ▶

1. Lie on your back, with your knees bent and feet flat on the floor.
2. Exhale, and press the small of your back against the floor.
3. Hold for 15 seconds.
4. Return to the starting position.
5. Repeat 10 more times.

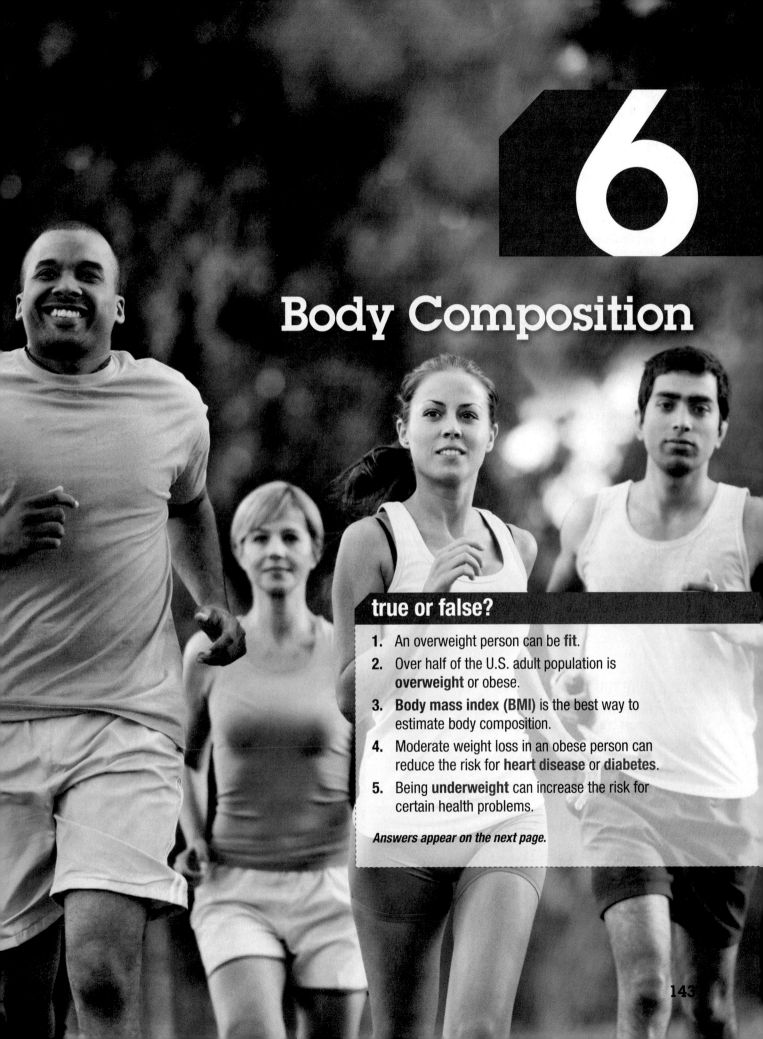

6

Body Composition

true or false?

1. An overweight person can be **fit**.
2. Over half of the U.S. adult population is **overweight** or obese.
3. **Body mass index (BMI)** is the best way to estimate body composition.
4. Moderate weight loss in an obese person can reduce the risk for **heart disease** or **diabetes**.
5. Being **underweight** can increase the risk for certain health problems.

Answers appear on the next page.

143

Many people worry about their body weight. However, how much you weigh is not always a good index of whether your body composition is healthy. In fact, based on height and weight charts, some athletes appear to be 25 pounds overweight but really have very little body fat. How is this possible? Read more in this chapter to find out! We will discuss how to assess your level of body fat, consider how much body fat is healthy for you, and examine the health problems associated with having too much body fat.

What Is Body Composition and What Does It Tell Us?

Body composition refers to the relative amounts of fat and fat-free tissues (e.g., bone, muscle, and internal organs) in the body. Body composition is typically expressed as a percentage of fat in the body. So if a person has 20% body fat, 20% of her body weight is fat mass, and the remaining 80% of her body weight is fat-free or lean body mass. Having a high percentage of body fat is associated with an increased risk of heart disease, diabetes, and other disorders, but having too low a percentage can also be linked to health problems, such as osteoporosis.

Measuring percentage of body fat can help determine whether a person is at a healthy weight, **overweight,** or **obese.** Someone who is "overweight" has a body fat percentage above the level that is considered to be "healthy," based on research examining the relationship between body fatness and rates of disease. A person classified as obese has a very high percentage of body fat, generally over 25% for men and over 35% for women (1–5).

MAKE SURE YOU KNOW...

- Body composition refers to the relative amount of fat and fat-free mass in the body and is generally reported in terms of the percentage of fat in the body.

- Measuring body fat percentage can help determine whether someone is overweight or obese.

How Is Body Composition Related to Health?

Maintaining a healthy body composition is an important goal to achieve a lifetime of wellness. To determine a healthy body weight, you need to consider percentage of body fat. The following sections introduce the types of body fat, as well as the health problems that can ensue from too much body fat.

answers

1. **TRUE** Research has shown that individuals who are overweight, but active or fit, have lower risk for heart disease than both low-active, low-fit overweight individuals and low-active, low-fit normal-weight individuals.

2. **TRUE** It is estimated that approximately 65% of U.S. adults are overweight or obese.

3. **FALSE** BMI can provide information about whether a person is at a healthy weight, and BMI is related to body fat percentage. However, there are limitations for BMI in assessing body fat percentage, because it can overestimate body fat for muscular individuals.

4. **TRUE** A weight loss of as little as 5%–10% can reduce the risk of heart disease and diabetes in overweight and obese individuals.

5. **TRUE** The relationship between weight and health follows what is referred to as a J-shaped curve. Although disease risk is greater for obese individuals, people at the lowest end of the range are also at increased risk for disease.

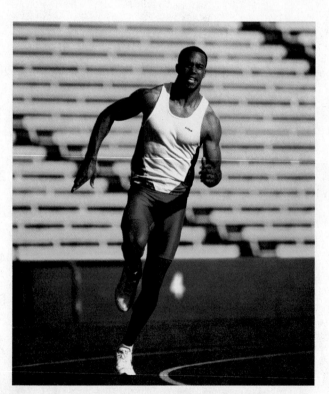

Some muscular athletes can be "overweight" without being over-fat.

The human body contains two major types of fat: (1) essential fat and (2) storage fat. **Essential fat** is necessary for body functions such as facilitating nerve

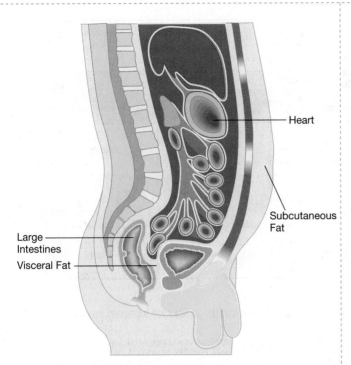

FIGURE 6.1
Storage fat can be visceral or subcutaneous. Visceral fat is stored around the organs; subcutaneous fat is stored between the skin and muscle layers.

impulses. Locations of this fat include nerves and cell membranes. Men have approximately 3% of their body weight as essential fat, and women—who carry more fat in their breasts, uterus, and other sex-specific sites—have approximately 12%.

The second type of body fat is called **storage fat**, which is contained within **adipose tissue** (i.e., fat cells) in the body. This fat may be **visceral fat**, which is located around internal organs, or **subcutaneous fat**, which is located just below the skin **(Figure 6.1)**. Storage fat provides energy for activity, insulates the body to retain heat, and protects against trauma to the body. However, high levels of storage fat, particularly in the visceral region of the body, increase the risk of numerous diseases including cardiovascular disease, diabetes, and cancer. This is why maintaining a healthy body composition is such an important goal.

In general, a healthy percentage of body fat for young men (20–39 years) can range from 8% to 19%, and for young women (20–39 years), from 21% to 32% (1). However, many public health experts recommend levels at the lower end of these ranges for young adults, 12%–15% and 21%–25% for men and women, respectively (1). For most people, a body fat percentage outside these ranges indicates an unhealthy body weight. However, athletes or very active individuals might have lower values. Some athletic men have as little as 5%–13% fat, and athletic women can have as little as 12%–22% (1). Keep in mind that these values are not recommended for the general population and that you can be healthy if your body fat percentage falls within the ranges mentioned. See **Figure 6.2** on page 146 for recommended ranges of percent body fat according to sex and age.

It is not just *how much* body fat a person carries that can greatly affect his risk for several chronic diseases; *where* he carries it also matters. Fat cells are unequally distributed throughout the body, and the distribution of body fat is determined largely by genetics. We inherit specific fat storage traits that determine the regional distribution of fat. For example, many men have a high number of fat cells in the upper body and as a result store more fat within the abdominal area (e.g., around the waist). This is referred to as the **android pattern** of obesity. In contrast, women tend to carry more fat cells in the waist, hips, and thighs of the lower body. This is called the **gynoid pattern** of obesity. People who carry body fat primarily in the abdominal or waist area are at greater risk of developing heart disease and diabetes than are those who store body fat in the hips or lower part of the body (6, 7). The next sections discuss the incidence of overweight people in the U.S. and the importance of maintaining a healthy level of body fat.

body composition The relative amounts of fat and fat-free mass in the body.

overweight A weight above the recommended level for health.

obese An excessive amount of fat in the body, typically above 25% for men and 35% for women.

essential fat Body fat that is necessary for physiological functioning.

storage fat Excess fat reserves stored in the body's adipose tissue.

adipose tissue Tissue where fat is stored in the body.

visceral fat Fat stored in the abdomen and around the organs.

subcutaneous fat Fat stored just beneath the skin.

android pattern A pattern of fat distribution characterized by fat stored in the abdominal region; more common in men.

gynoid pattern A pattern of fat distribution characterized by fat stored in the hips and thighs; more common in women.

Gender	20–39 years		40–59 years		60+ years		Weight Status	Health Risk
	Body Fat	BMI	Body Fat	BMI	Body Fat	BMI		
Men	<8%	<18.5	<11%	<18.5	<13%	<18.5	Underweight	Increased
Women	<21%	<18.5	<23%	<18.5	<24%	<18.5		
Men	8%–19%	18.6–24.9	11%–21%	18.6–24.9	13%–24%	18.6–24.9	Average	Normal
Women	21%–32%	18.6–24.9	23%–33%	18.6–24.9	24%–35%	18.6–24.9		
Men	20%–24%	25.0–29.9	22%–27%	25.0–29.9	25%–39%	25.0–29.9	Overweight	Increased
Women	33%–38%	25.0–29.9	34%–39%	25.0–29.9	36%–41%	25.0–29.9		
Men	>25%	>30	>28%	>30	>30%	>30	Obese	High
Women	>35%	>30	>40%	>30	>42%	>30		

FIGURE 6.2

Health risks associated with varying levels of body fat for men and women according to age. Note that health risks are increased for both underweight individuals and overweight individuals.

Sources: Data from National Institutes of Health. Assessing Your Weight and Health Risk, 2012. http://www.nhlbi.nih.gov/health/public/heart/obesity/lose_wt/risk.htm and Shah, N. R. and E. R. Braverman. Measuring adiposity in patients: The utility of body mass index (BMI), percent body fat, and leptin. *PLoS ONE* 7(4): e33308, 2012.

Overweight and Obesity in the United States

Obesity is often defined as a percentage of body fat greater than 25% for men and greater than 35% for women. Current estimates for the United States suggest that nearly 34% of adults and approximately 17% of children and adolescents (ages 2–19) meet the criteria for obesity (8). Obesity is a major health problem in the United States, and numerous diseases have been linked to being too fat. Because of a strong link between obesity and disease, the National Institutes of Health has estimated that obesity directly contributes to 15%–20% of the deaths in the United States (9).

The burden of obesity has also had a significant effect on health-care costs. Currently, an estimated 10% of all medical costs in the United States are attributed to overweight- and obesity-related health problems. This adds up to the hefty price tag of $147 billion per year in direct medical costs and this number is predicted to rise sharply in the future (10, 11). The World Health Organization reports that the obesity rates in

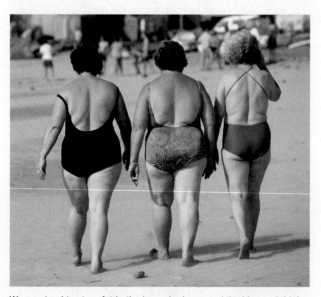

Women tend to store fat in the lower body, around the hips and thighs.

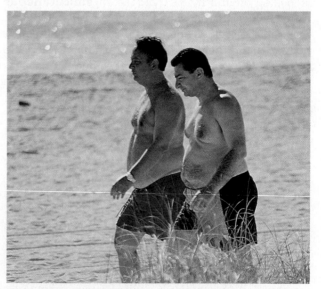

Men tend to store fat in the upper body, around the abdomen.

the United States are the highest in the world and are continuing to climb. The reports are based on studies indicating that the number of obese or overweight people in the United States has increased rapidly during the past 20 years (12). In 2010, no state had a prevalence of obesity less than 20%, 36 states had a prevalence of 25% or more, and 12 states had a prevalence of 30% or more (Figure 6.3). The good news is that the increase in adult obesity in the United States is leveling off. The bad news is that 67% of all Americans are either obese or overweight, and there is no evidence of a decrease in the rate of obesity among children (9, 13). Thus, obesity continues to be a major threat to wellness in the United States.

Why are so many Americans obese? There is no single answer. Obesity is related to both genetic traits and lifestyle (14, 15). (These influences will be discussed

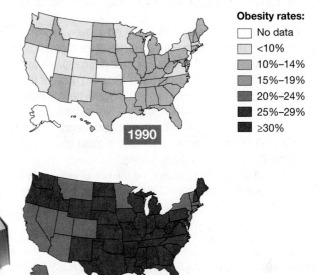

FIGURE 6.3
Obesity rates in the United States have increased rapidly in the 20 years between 1990 and 2010. Note that in 2010 the incidence of obesity was no lower than 20% in any state and that the prevalence of obesity exceeded 30% in 12 states. Where does your home state rank?

Source: Centers for Disease Control and Prevention. U.S. Obesity Trends: 1985–2010, Obesity Trend Maps. www.cdc.gov/nccdphp/dnpa/obesity.

consider this!

On average, college students gain 4–15 pounds during their first year of college.

COACHING corner

The accumulation of fat tissue and the reduction of lean muscle mass have significant long-term consequences. The health risks reach far beyond the more obvious concerns about physical appearance. Consider additional reasons that may be important to you as you begin your journey to change body composition.

- Genetic history may have some predictive power in your long-term health outcomes. Are there people in your family who have developed chronic diseases that are connected to higher levels of fat? Consider interviewing those people to learn if they have experienced high blood pressure, diabetes or reduced insulin sensitivity, fatty liver disease, or enlarged or less efficient heart issues.

- Take a critical look at your food and exercise culture: the assumptions you have come to believe as true as a result of your upbringing. Do you eat or have meal expectations similar to those patterns you had as a kid? In what ways are your exercise habits the same as or different than those of your family members? What changes in your current food and exercise culture might you consider making for your future or that of the family you may develop some day?

Ask Dad about diabetes

The Search for Obesity-Related Genes

Even though obese individuals are found in every segment of the U.S. population, certain subsets of Americans experience the greatest prevalence of obesity. For example, compared to the U.S. population as a whole, the risk of becoming obese is greatest among Mexican American women, African American women, some Native Americans (for example, Pima Indians), and children from low-income families. The high prevalence of obesity in these populations places individuals in those groups at the greatest risk of developing obesity-related diseases.

Research efforts to understand the role of genetics in the high prevalence of obesity in these populations are expanding.

One large investigation, the Heritage Family Study, has been searching for the genes responsible for both obesity and weight loss. This investigation has identified an important gene that is associated with obesity. People with this gene have 1.7 times greater risk of becoming obese compared to people who do not have it (32). Results from this and other genetics studies are expected to provide important information for developing programs that can prevent and treat obesity in high-risk populations.

more in Chapter 9.) Many individuals can experience **creeping obesity,** gradually adding fat over a period of time. This type of slow weight gain is usually attributed to poor diet (including increased food intake) and a gradual decline in physical activity (16). The woman in

Figure 6.4 is gaining one-half pound of fat per month (6 pounds per year); after five years, she will have gained 30 pounds! The weight gain is so gradual that it typically does not become a concern until years later, when the total weight is more noticeable.

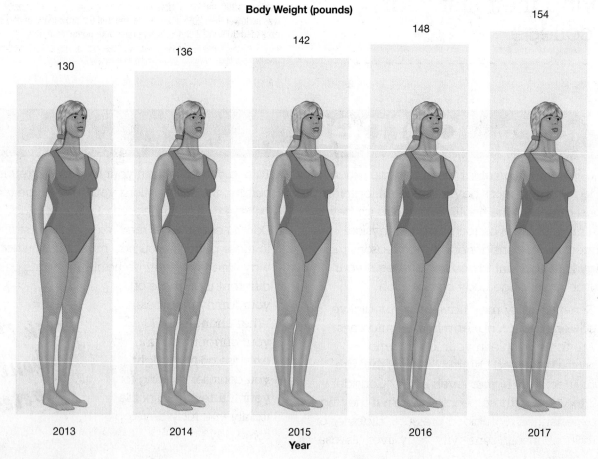

Body Weight (pounds)

| 130 | 136 | 142 | 148 | 154 |
| 2013 | 2014 | 2015 | 2016 | 2017 |

Year

FIGURE 6.4
The concept of creeping obesity.

Chronic Conditions Associated with Overweight and Obesity

Obesity increases the risk of developing at least 26 diseases. Heart disease, colon cancer, hypertension (high blood pressure), kidney disease, arthritis, and diabetes are among the most serious (8, 9, 16).

Heart Disease Heart disease (also called *cardiovascular disease,* or *CVD*) is the leading cause of death in the United States for both men and women. Obesity is considered a major independent risk factor for coronary heart disease, the leading cause of heart attacks. Obesity has been shown to increase the risk of heart attack by 60%–80% (17).

----

consider this!

Sedentary adults are over 2.5 times more likely to experience significant weight gain over 10 years compared to those who report that they exercise vigorously 2 or more times per week.

Hypertension (high blood pressure) is more common among overweight and obese individuals. However, on a positive note, blood pressure is usually reduced with weight loss. Obesity is linked to elevated cholesterol levels and unhealthy blood lipid profiles. As with hypertension, the cholesterol profile typically improves with weight loss. High blood pressure and cholesterol levels are also independent risk factors for coronary heart disease, so the combination of obesity with these risk factors poses a significantly greater risk for a heart attack. (Heart disease will be discussed in much greater detail in Chapter 10.)

Diabetes Diabetes is a metabolic disorder characterized by high blood glucose levels; it affects over 18 million people. Chronic elevation of blood glucose is associated with increased incidence of heart disease,

kidney disease, nerve dysfunction, and eye damage. In fact, diabetes is one of the leading causes of death and disability in the United States, and its incidence is increasing.

There is a strong relationship between the onset of type 2 diabetes and body fat: Over 80% of people with this type of diabetes are obese. Type 2 diabetes has traditionally been referred to as *adult-onset diabetes* because its risk increases after age 45. This type of diabetes is largely associated with behavioral factors, such as poor dietary habits, physical inactivity, and obesity. As obesity among young people has increased, so has the incidence of type 2 diabetes among adolescents and young adults.

Type 2 diabetes is also known as non–insulin-dependent diabetes, because insulin is not always required as treatment. In type 2 diabetes, the body can produce insulin, but there is a reduced ability of insulin to transport glucose from the blood to the cells. This problem, called *decreased insulin sensitivity,* results in elevated blood glucose levels. People can have decreased insulin sensitivity but not have blood glucose levels high enough to be diagnosed with diabetes. In this case, a person has *pre-diabetes,* which is also more common among obese individuals. As with heart disease, weight loss can significantly reduce the risk of diabetes and help manage the disease. In fact, research has indicated that modest weight loss of 5%–10% can reduce the risk of heart disease and type 2 diabetes (18, 19).

How can Harold manage his body weight and prevent diabetes? Listen to the online case study at **www.pearsonhighered.com/powers.**

**HEAR IT!
CASE STUDY**

Other Conditions Obesity is a risk factor for some of the most prevalent types of cancers, including breast, prostate, and colon cancer. Overweight and obese individuals are at higher risk for joint problems and osteoarthritis. Sleep apnea (a condition in which a person stops breathing for brief periods while sleeping) and gallbladder disease are more common among obese individuals. Additionally, obese women are more likely to experience menstrual abnormalities, difficulty conceiving, and complications during pregnancy than women of normal weight.

creeping obesity A slow increase in body weight and percentage of body fat over several years.

diabetes A metabolic disorder characterized by high blood glucose levels that is associated with increased risk for heart disease, kidney disease, nerve dysfunction, and eye damage.

STEPS FOR BEHAVIOR CHANGE

Are you at risk for developing diabetes?

Does your body composition, or other factors, put you at increased risk for developing diabetes? To find out whether you are at increased risk, respond true or false to the following statements.

T F

☐ ☐ I have a BMI that puts me in the overweight or obese category.

☐ ☐ I am under 65 years of age AND I get little or no exercise.

☐ ☐ I have a sister or brother with diabetes.

☐ ☐ I have a parent with diabetes.

☐ ☐ I am a woman who has had a baby weighing more than 9 pounds at birth.

In general, the more "true" answers you have, the higher your risk.

TIPS TO REDUCE YOUR RISK OF DIABETES

Today, you will:

☑ Determine whether you are overweight, and if so, make a plan to lose weight. If you have a BMI above the healthy range, schedule a body composition assessment to determine your level of fat. If your percentage of body fat is above the healthy range, talk to your instructor or a health educator at your campus health center about setting goals and preparing a plan for weight loss.

Within the next 2 weeks, you will:

☑ Get more exercise. Be more active most days of the week. (See Chapter 1 for tips to change your health behavior.)

☑ Incorporate more fresh fruits and vegetables and whole grains into your diet, and cut back on the salt and high-fat foods.

By the end of the semester, you will:

☑ See your health-care provider. A lot of people have diabetes and pre-diabetes without knowing it.

Source: Based on the American Diabetes Association. Diabetes Risk Test. www.diabetes.org.

Mental and Physical Benefits of a Healthy Weight

Maintaining a healthy weight is important for physical health, and it is also associated with certain aspects of mental health. People who are overweight or obese are more likely to have poor body image and low self-esteem compared to people of normal weight. An unhealthy body image and poor self-esteem are associated with poor health behavior choices and increased risk for physical and mental health problems, such as depression and increased anxiety (20, 21). Maintaining a healthy body weight will make physical activity and everyday activities easier. Individuals who maintain a healthy body weight have a lower risk of developing major chronic conditions such as cardiovascular disease, type 2 diabetes, and certain types of cancers. Cardiovascular disease and all-cause death rates are also lower in people at their recommended body weights compared to overweight and obese individuals (22–23).

Health Effects of Too Little Body Fat

Although the current rates of overweight and obesity among U.S. adults indicate there is an obesity epidemic, a small percentage of people in the country suffer from health problems associated with being underweight. As with overweight, underweight can be determined by measuring height, weight, and body fat percentage. However, as with determining overweight and obesity, it is best to use a measure of body composition to determine whether one is underweight. Having close to or below the level of essential body fat is an indicator that an individual might be too thin.

Health problems associated with being underweight are typically related to malnutrition, because the person is likely not eating enough to get all the necessary nutrients. Severe and prolonged malnutrition can result in a loss of muscle mass and strength. Further, underweight individuals are at increased

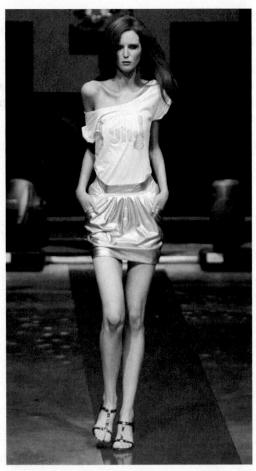

Being underweight can lead to significant health problems.

risk for osteoporosis, and underweight women are at increased risk for menstrual abnormalities that can lead to infertility. People with eating disorders, such as anorexia nervosa and bulimia, can experience many other health problems, including heart problems, digestive disorders, kidney damage, anemia, lethargy, muscle weakness, dry skin, and poor immune function.

Eating disorders are complex conditions that involve much more than just being underweight. (We will discuss these conditions in greater detail in Chapter 9.)

MAKE SURE YOU KNOW...

- Overweight refers to a weight above the recommended level, and obesity refers to a high percentage of body fat.

- A certain amount of fat is needed for normal physiological functioning, but excess storage fat is associated with increased risk for numerous conditions.

- Rates of obesity in the United States are high and contribute significantly to health-care costs.

- The amount and distribution of excess storage fat can lead to increased risk of illness and death associated with heart disease and diabetes.

- Physical and mental health are affected by unhealthy levels of body fat.

- Having too little body fat can lead to significant health problems.

A CLOSER LOOK

Can You Be Fit and Fat?

Although overweight and obesity are associated with numerous unhealthy conditions, and people should always strive for a healthy body weight, it is possible to be fit and overweight. Think about watching your favorite football team. Do all the players look thin and healthy? Probably not. However, because of their intense workouts, even those players with seemingly unhealthy-looking physiques can still be healthy.

Multiple studies have found that overweight individuals can be healthy if they are physically active or fit. The strongest evidence comes from longitudinal studies conducted at the Cooper Clinic in Dallas, Texas. Researchers examined heart disease and death risk and overall death rates in men and women. Death risk was 1.5 times greater for low-fit participants compared to highly fit participants across both normal and overweight BMI classifications. Those with the highest fitness levels and the lowest BMIs had the lowest risk for disease and death. However, overweight but highly fit men and women had lower risk for death than their overweight low-fit counterparts and than low-fit men and women of normal weight. Others have found reduced risk for

heart disease and death in active and fit overweight and obese individuals.

These findings support the fact that efforts to incorporate regular physical activity into one's lifestyle are not in vain, because active overweight individuals do enjoy the benefits of lower risk of heart disease. People who are inactive but at a recommended weight still should consider a regular exercise program to minimize their risk of chronic disease.

Sources: Lohman, T., et al. Body fat measurement goes high-tech: Not all are created equal. *ACSM'S Health and Fitness Journal* 1(1):30–35, 1997; Lee, C. D., S. N. Blair, and A. S. Jackson. Cardiorespiratory fitness, body composition, and all-cause cardiovascular disease mortality in men. *American Journal of Clinical Nutrition* 69:373–380, 1999; Lee, C. D., A. S. Jackson, and S. N. Blair. U.S. weight guidelines: Is it also important to consider cardiorespiratory fitness? *International Journal of Obesity and Related Metabolic Disorders* 22(Suppl. 2):S2–S7, 1998; Church, T., and S. N. Blair. Does physical activity ameliorate the health hazards of obesity? *British Journal of Sports Medicine* 43:80–81, 2009.

Assessing Body Composition

Several field and laboratory methods are available for assessing body composition. Field methods require little equipment and can be easily administered at a fitness center or gym to determine weight status or body composition. The laboratory measures are used more frequently in research or medical settings. Each measure has strengths and limitations.

Field Methods

Several quick and inexpensive field techniques are used to evaluate body composition and the risk for disease (24–26). The procedures discussed in this section have been validated and can provide good estimates of your level of body fat or level of disease risk.

Height/Weight Tables   The application of height/weight tables to determine whether a person is overweight has a long history of use by many groups (e.g., U.S. military, life insurance companies). These tables are designed to determine if an individual is considered to have a body weight greater than normal for a specific height. Although the idea that a simple table can be used to determine if a person is too fat is attractive, there are limits to the usefulness of this approach. The major drawback is that the tables do not reveal how much of the body weight is fat. As mentioned in the chapter introduction, an individual can exceed the ideal body weight on a height/weight chart either by being heavily muscled or by being over-fat. Because of the poor predictive ability of tables in estimating body fat, most experts do not recommend the use of these tables to determine an ideal weight.

Body Mass Index   One of the easiest and most common techniques used to determine whether someone is overweight or obese is the **body mass index (BMI)**. The BMI is computed as the ratio of the body weight (in kilograms; kg) divided by height (in meters squared; m^2):

$$BMI = weight\ (kg) \div height\ (m)^2$$

(*Note*: 1 kg = 2.2 lb and 1 m = 39.37 in.)

For example, for an individual who weighs 64.5 kg and is 1.72 m tall, the BMI would be computed as follows:

$$64.5\ kg/(1.72\ m)^2 = 64.5 \div 2.96 = 21.8\ kg/m^2$$

The concept behind the BMI is that individuals with a low percentage of body fat will have a low BMI. Using **Figure 6.5**, you can estimate your BMI and determine if your BMI indicates that you are underweight, normal, or overweight. For example, men and women with a BMI of less than 25 kg/m^2, respectively, are considered to be at a normal and healthy weight (Figure 6.5). In contrast, men and women with a BMI of greater than 30 kg/m^2 are considered obese. This is important because research has indicated that individuals classified as overweight or obese according to BMI are at increased risk for cardiovascular disease and death.

BMI is a simple and inexpensive method for determining your weight status, but it has limitations. For example, BMI is not a perfect predictor of obesity: In some cases the method can over- or underestimate

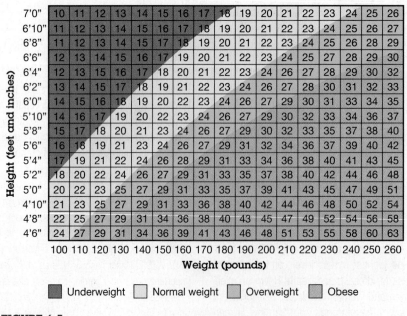

Underweight ■   Normal weight □   Overweight ■   Obese ■

FIGURE 6.5
Estimate your BMI by finding the intersection of your weight and height. For example, if you weigh 150 pounds and your height is 5′8″, your BMI would be estimated to be 23.

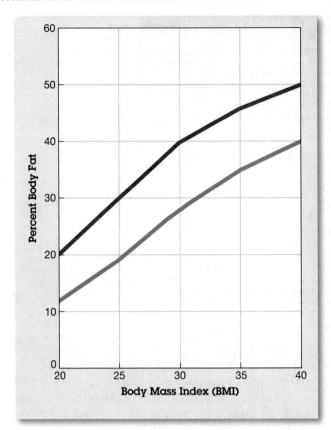

Key

━━━ Women

━━━ Men

FIGURE 6.6

Illustration of the relationship between body mass index (BMI) and % body fat for both men and women (38). Using this figure, you can estimate your % body fat by determining where your BMI intersects with the line representing your gender. For example, if you are female with a BMI of 25, your estimated % body fat is ~30%.

body fatness. For example, an individual with a low percentage of body fat but a high level of muscularity would typically have a relatively high BMI, which would incorrectly suggest a high percentage of body fat.

Additionally, BMI is not a perfect predictor of body fat percentage. **Figure 6.6** illustrates the relationship between BMI and body fat percentage. For example, if you are a male with a BMI of 25, your body fat percentage is estimated to be ~19%. However, your true percentage could be as low as 14% or as high as 24% because several factors (e.g., muscularity) affect the relationship between BMI and body fat percentage.

Regardless of its flaws, BMI has become a widely used method to estimate body composition because BMI is a both a simple and practical predictor of body fat percentage. BMI is best used to obtain an initial estimate of whether one's percentage is at a healthy level. If your BMI suggests that you have too much body fat, you should follow up a calculation with a measure of body fat percentage, especially if you feel you are at a healthy weight and your BMI indicates otherwise.

Skinfold Assessment Because more than 50% of body fat is subcutaneous fat that lies just beneath the skin, a **skinfold test** can be used to estimate a person's overall body fatness (27, 28). In a skinfold test, subcutaneous fat is measured using an instrument called a skinfold caliper. To be accurate, skinfold tests to estimate body fat for both men and women require at least three skinfold measurement sites (16). The anatomical sites to be measured in men (abdominal, chest, thigh skinfolds) and in women (suprailium, triceps, and thigh skinfolds) are illustrated in Laboratory 6.1. Note that for standardization, all measurements should be made on the right side of the body.

Skinfold measurements to determine body fat can be accurate but generally have a $\pm 3\%-4\%$ margin of error (27, 29). Using calibrated metal calipers (instead of plastic) and having a skilled technician do the test are two ways to increase accuracy. Skinfold assessment is an easy measure to obtain and can provide good estimates of body fat when done properly. However, it is not a good measure to assess body composition for obese individuals, because it is often difficult to obtain accurate measures of skinfold thickness. Inaccurate measures of skinfold thickness can be both misleading and discouraging to individuals trying to lose weight and can interfere with setting an appropriate weight goal. Bioelectrical impedance (discussed later in this chapter) may be a preferred method of estimating body fat for some individuals.

Waist Measurement and Waist-to-Hip Ratio Waist measurements and the **waist-to-hip ratio** can be used to estimate the risk of disease associated with high body fat. Note, however, that these techniques do not provide an estimate of body fat percentage. Nonetheless, they are often good indicators of whether body fat distribution is unhealthy.

Waist measurements greater than or equal to 40 inches (102 cm) for men and 35 inches (88 cm) for women are considered health risks and indicate the android pattern of obesity. You can better evaluate your risk according to waist measurement by also considering your BMI

body mass index (BMI) A ratio of body weight (kg) divided by height squared (m²) used to determine whether a person is at a healthy body weight; BMI is related to the percentage of body fat.

skinfold test A field test used to estimate body composition; representative samples of subcutaneous fat are measured using calipers to estimate the overall level of body fat.

waist-to-hip ratio A ratio of the waist and hip circumferences used to determine the risk for disease associated with the android pattern of obesity.

TABLE 6.1 Ranges and Classification for BMI and Waist Circumference

	BMI	Men, ≤102 cm Women, ≤88 cm	Men, >102 cm Women, >88 cm
		Disease Risk* Relative to Normal Weight and Waist Circumference	
Underweight	<18.5	—	—
Normal	18.5–24.9	—	—
Overweight	25.0–29.9	Increased	High
Obesity			
Class I	30.0–34.9	High	Very high
Class II	35.0–39.9	Very high	Very high
Class III	≥40	Extremely high	Extremely high

*Disease risk for type 2 diabetes, hypertension, and cardiovascular disease. Dashes (—) indicate that no additional risk at these levels of BMI was assigned. Increased waist circumference can also be a marker for increased risk even in persons of normal weight.

Source: Data from Gallagher, D., S. B. Heymsfield, M. Heo, S. A. Jebb, P. Murgatroyd, Y. Sakamoto. Healthy percentage body fat ranges: an approach for developing guidelines based on body mass index. *American Journal of Clinical Nutrition* 72(3):694–701, 2000.

(see Table 6.1). A high waist measurement alone might not indicate increased risk. For example, a high waist measurement for someone who is tall might be proportional to his height, and the level of BMI and body fat might be well within the healthy range.

Another way to estimate disease risk according to body fat distribution is the waist-to-hip ratio. An individual with a large fat deposit in the abdominal region would have a high waist-to-hip ratio and would have a higher risk of disease than someone with a lower ratio.

Both waist and hip circumference measurements should be made while the person is standing, using a nonelastic tape. It is important that the person not wear bulky clothing during the measurement, because that could alter the measurements. During measurements, the tape should be placed snugly around the body but should not press into the skin. Record your measurements to the nearest millimeter or sixteenth of an inch. The specific procedure is detailed in Laboratory 6.1.

Laboratory Measures

Body fat measurements performed in a laboratory are considered the gold standard for assessing body composition. However, these techniques require expensive

COACHING **Corner**

Gradual changes in body composition are more desirable than drastic changes that occur quickly. Consider a multi-pronged approach to changing your body composition.

- Beginning or continuing an exercise program while also making dietary adjustments is the best practice for changing body composition.

- Before making a drastic change, consider consulting with a registered dietician about your activity level and your current dietary intake.

- Recognize that fat tissue does not magically morph into muscle and that the reduction of fat tissue requires that you create a deficit in the energy balance equation.

- People who are overweight or obese and who exercise are often more healthy than those of average weight who do not exercise. This means it is not necessary or beneficial to lose weight before beginning an exercise program.

- Being overweight or obese may require adjustments in frequency, intensity, time, and type of exercise to avoid injury.

- Spot reduction through excessive exercising is not practical. Aim for a balanced and diverse exercise program.

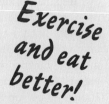
Exercise and eat better!

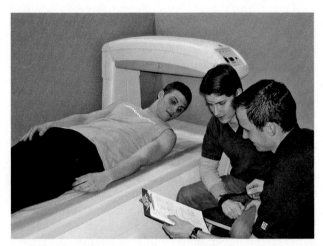

The DXA scan is considered the gold standard for measuring body composition.

specialized equipment and are often not readily available to the general public. The methods are typically used by researchers or clinicians to determine body fat percentage in research participants or patients.

Dual Energy X-Ray Absorptiometry **Dual energy X-ray absorptiometry (DXA)** involves taking a low-radiation X-ray scan (involving considerably less radiation than a typical X-ray scan) of the entire body to obtain estimates of body fat percentage. In this procedure, the person lies still on a table while an X-ray arm passes over the body. The scan typically requires about 15 minutes to complete.

The advantage of using DXA is that it provides a measure of total body fat as well as of regional fat distribution. It can also be used to assess bone density as it relates to osteoporosis and osteoporosis risk. However, the technique is generally not used outside research or clinical settings. The equipment is expensive, and because it uses an X-ray, only trained professionals can perform the scan. Therefore, this technique of determining body composition is not commonly available in fitness and wellness centers.

Hydrostatic Weighing **Hydrostatic weighing,** also called underwater weighing, is a technique that involves weighing the individual both on land and in a tank of water to determine body volume and body density. Lean mass has a higher density than water, whereas fat mass is less dense than water. The more muscular person will weigh more under water. Because fat tends to float, the person with more fat will weigh less under water. After the two weights are obtained, they are used to calculate percentage of body fat.

Underwater weighing is very time consuming and requires expensive equipment. Additionally, this measure typically does not appeal to most individuals, because it involves being completely submerged under water. Thus, this procedure is rarely employed to assess

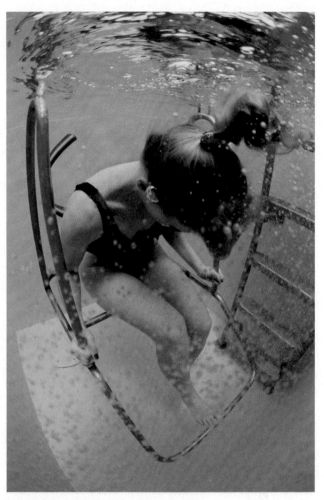

Hydrostatic weighing involves being weighed while submerged in a tank of water.

body composition in fitness centers or in college fitness and wellness courses.

Air Displacement **Air displacement** is another method used to assess body composition; it is similar in principle to hydrostatic weighing, but instead of being submerged in water, the individual is seated in a chamber (the Bod Pod®). Computerized sensors are

dual energy X-ray absorptiometry (DXA) A technique for assessing body composition using a low-radiation X-ray; it is typically used in research or clinical settings and is considered a gold-standard measure.

hydrostatic weighing A method of determining body composition that involves weighing an individual on land and in a tank of water.

air displacement A technique used to assess body composition by estimating body volume based on air displaced when a person sits in a chamber.

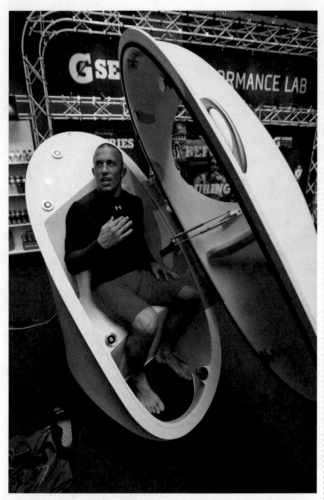

The Bod Pod® uses air displacement to measure body composition.

used to estimate the amount of air that is displaced when the participant is in the chamber. From knowing the amount of air displaced, body volume and then body fat can be calculated. Estimates of body fat percentage from air displacement are similar to measures from hydrostatic weighing.

Air displacement is less time consuming than underwater weighing; however, the equipment is expensive, so this technique is not available in most fitness centers. Air displacement is more commonly used in research settings and has gained wide acceptance as a means of estimating the percentage of body fat in adults.

Bioelectrical Impedance Analysis Bioelectrical impedance analysis (BIA) is a procedure used in fitness centers as well as in research laboratories. With commercially available BIA monitors, the person either stands on sensors of a scale-like piece of equipment or holds sensors between both hands. In the laboratory, the participant lies on a table with surface electrodes placed at the hand and foot. Then a very low level electrical current (too low to be felt) is passed through the body between the electrodes or sensors. Because lean

tissue contains more water, it is a good conductor of the current. Fat tissue, in contrast, contains less water and impedes the flow of the current. Body fat is estimated according to the resistance to the flow of the current.

BIA can be an accurate technique to estimate body fat in many individuals. However, commercially available BIA instruments can vary in quality and the devices do not provide an accurate estimate of percent body fat in all populations (30). For example, the validity of BIA can be influenced by sex, age, and overall level of fatness. Therefore, prior to using this technique, you should determine if the BIA approach has been validated for individuals in your sex and age category (31). For those populations for which BIA has been shown to be valid, the advantages of this technique are numerous, including wide availability of BIA instruments, limited time requirement, and low cost.

A major source of error in the BIA assessment of body fat is a failure to follow precisely the appropriate guidelines in reference to exercise, voiding, eating, and drinking prior to the assessment. Failure to comply with the instructions from the manufacturer can significantly impair the accuracy of this instrument in estimating your percent body fat.

MAKE SURE YOU KNOW...

- There are several laboratory and field methods used to assess body composition and weight status.
- BMI, skinfold, and waist-to-hip ratio are the most common assessments for general use in fitness courses and fitness centers.
- Laboratory assessments such as DXA, hydrostatic weighing, air displacement, and BIA provide very good estimates of body composition, but most are not practical for commercial use because of their cost.

Can you be slim and obese? Watch *Normal Weight Obesity* at **www.pearsonhighered.com/powers.**

**SEE IT!
VIDEOS**

Using Body Composition to Determine Your Ideal Body Weight

The fitness categories presented for body composition differ from those for the other components of health-related physical fitness. Whereas "superior" was the highest fitness level for cardiorespiratory, strength, and muscular endurance fitness, the classification of "optimal" is the highest standard for body composition. Any category other than "optimal" is considered unsatisfactory for health-related fitness. Therefore, your goal should be to reach and maintain an optimal body composition.

Use-At-Home Measurement Devices—Are They Worth the Money?

Did you know that you can buy a bathroom scale that estimates body fat? You can also purchase body composition monitors for $25 to $345. The question is, are such devices worth your money?

The equipment shown in the photo uses the BIA technique, discussed on page 156. The scale assesses body fat in the lower body, and the hand-held device performs an upper body assessment. Because they do not perform total body assessments, the readings from these commercially available monitors are not likely to be as accurate as the laboratory BIA measure or other body composition techniques. Additionally, the partial body readings are influenced by regional fat distribution. Although these devices can provide a general estimate, you are probably better served by getting a skinfold assessment performed by a trained technician.

Research suggests that a range of 8%–19% body fat is an optimal health and fitness goal for men aged 20–39 years, and a range of 21%–32% is optimal for women aged 20–39 years (1). These ranges afford little risk of disease associated with body fatness and permit individual differences in physical activity patterns and diet.

Once you have calculated your body fat percentage and know the optimal range of body fat, how can you determine the desired range of body weight? A typical 20-year-old man who has 30% body fat and weighs 185 pounds can calculate his optimal range of body weight in two simple steps:

Step 1. Compute fat-free weight—that is, the amount of total body weight contained in bones, organs, and muscles:

Total body weight − fat weight = fat-free weight

$$100\% - 30\% = 70\%$$

This means that 70% of total body weight is fat-free weight. Therefore, the fat-free weight for this student is

$$70\% \times 185\ \text{lb} = 129.5\ \text{lb}$$

Step 2. Calculate the optimal weight (which for men is 8%–19% of total body weight): The formula to compute optimum body weight is

Optimum weight
   = fat-free weight ÷ (1 − optimal % fat)

Note that fat percentage should be expressed as a decimal. Thus, for 8% body fat,

Optimum weight = 129.5 ÷ (1 − 0.08)
         = 140.8 pounds

For 19% body fat,

Optimum weight = 129.5 ÷ (1 − 0.19)
         = 159.9 pounds

In making these calculations, we assume that this individual will maintain his lean body mass and lose fat. So his 129.5 pounds of lean mass will be 78%–92% of his new optimal body weight to achieve a healthy body composition. Hence, the optimal body weight for this individual is between 140.8 and 159.9 pounds. Laboratory 6.2 provides an opportunity to compute your optimal body weight using both body fat percentage and body mass index.

MAKE SURE YOU KNOW...

- Healthy body weight should be determined based on the optimal level of body fat for your age, height, and sex.
- Ideal weight can be easily calculated if you know your percentage of body fat.

Behavior Change: Set Goals and Get Regular Assessments

As you attempt to lose or gain weight, it is important to get regular body composition assessments. (You will learn about weight management in Chapter 9.) When we calculated the goal weight based on the optimal level of body fat, we assumed that only fat weight was lost. However, a person experiencing weight loss may also lose water weight and possibly lose lean mass. Incorporating regular aerobic and resistance exercise along with a healthy diet will maximize the amount of fat that is lost and maintain more lean mass.

bioelectrical impedance analysis (BIA) A method of assessing body composition by running a low-level electrical current through the body.

As the body changes with weight loss or gain, the weights that were originally calculated might not correspond exactly with the desired body fat percentage. In the example above, the individual might lose 7 pounds and be in the optimal range if he also increased lean mass. Additionally, regular assessments will help you determine whether the weight you are losing is fat and not lean mass. Therefore, it is important to have regular body composition assessments as you try to reach a new goal weight. Note that it is vital to get the same type of body composition measurement when you get follow-up assessments. If possible, it is also recommended that

the same person perform the assessment. These factors will reduce measurement errors. The frequency of the assessments will depend on your goal.

MAKE SURE YOU KNOW...

- You should have regular body composition assessments when trying to lose or gain weight to ensure the healthiest changes.
- Follow-up assessments should be made with the same procedure as the original assessment.

SUMMARY

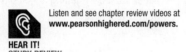

Listen and see chapter review videos at **www.pearsonhighered.com/powers.**

HEAR IT!
STUDY REVIEW

1. Body composition refers to the relative amounts of fat and fat-free tissue in the body. Fat in the body can be essential fat or storage fat. A healthy body weight should be based on the recommended amount of body fat.
2. Body composition is an important component of health-related physical fitness because a high percentage of body fat is associated with an increased risk for numerous diseases. The distribution of fat also affects disease risk associated with overweight and obesity. A very low percentage of body fat is also associated with increased risk for disease.
3. Common field techniques for assessing body fat and healthy weight are skinfold measurements, BMI assessment, and examination of the waist-to-hip ratio.
4. Laboratory techniques for estimating body fat are most commonly used in research and clinical settings. DXA is considered the gold-standard measure for estimating body fat.
5. You can calculate your healthy weight range if you know your desired percentage of body fat or BMI. You should have regular body composition assessments when trying to lose or gain weight.

STUDY QUESTIONS

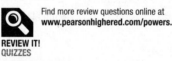

Find more review questions online at **www.pearsonhighered.com/powers.**

REVIEW IT!
QUIZZES

1. How much essential fat does the average man and woman carry?
   a. 25% and 30%
   b. 3% and 12%
   c. 10% and 20%
   d. 5% and 18%
2. Storing excess fat in the hips and thighs puts an individual at greater risk for heart disease and diabetes than storing excess fat in the abdomen.
   a. true
   b. false
3. Which of the following is not a potential health consequence of being overweight or obese?
   a. low self-esteem
   b. gallbladder disease
   c. osteoarthritis
   d. anemia
4. Which is not a potential health consequence of being underweight or having an eating disorder?
   a. malnutrition
   b. menstrual abnormalities
   c. digestive disorders
   d. type 1 diabetes
5. Which technique is used to assess disease risk status associated with regional fat distribution?
   a. waist-to-hip ratio
   b. skinfold test
   c. underwater weighing
   d. bioelectrical impedance analysis
6. For disease risk and health standards, a BMI of _____ kg/m^2 is considered obese.
   a. 27   c. 30
   b. 25   d. 45

7. Which of the following is a common field measure for assessing body composition?
   a. waist measurement
   b. air displacement
   c. hydrostatic weighing
   d. DXA

8. A person classified as normal weight based on a BMI in the healthy range can be overweight.
   a. true
   b. false

9. Discuss the different types of field measurement techniques for assessing body composition. Discuss the strengths and limitations of each.

10. Discuss potential health consequences of not maintaining a healthy body composition.

11. Define overweight and obesity. What is the public health impact of overweight and obesity in the United States?

HELPFUL WEBLINKS

For links to the organizations and websites listed, visit **www.pearsonhighered.com/powers**.

DO IT! WEBLINKS

American College of Sports Medicine
Comprehensive website providing information, articles, and position statements about all aspects of health and fitness. www.acsm.org

American Diabetes Association
Provides diabetes information, including exercise and diet guidelines to reduce your risk. www.diabetes.org

American Heart Association
Contains the latest information about ways to reduce your risk of heart and vascular diseases. Site includes information about exercise, diet, and heart disease. www.heart.org

Centers for Disease Control and Prevention Healthy Weight
Offers information about maintaining a healthy weight and a BMI calculator to assess your weight. www.cdc.gov/healthyweight

LABORATORY 6.1

Complete Lab 6.1 online at
www.pearsonhighered.com/powers.

DO IT!
LABS

Name _____ **Date** _____

Assessing Body Composition

EQUIPMENT

Tape measure, skinfold caliper, scale

DIRECTIONS

Complete the assessments described below as directed by your instructor. Then record your body composition data and weight classifications for skinfold, waist circumference, waist-to-hip ratio, BMI, and/or other measures in the spaces below.

SKINFOLD TEST

Scan to view a demonstration video of the skinfold measurement of percent body fat. ▶

Skinfold Test Sites

Men

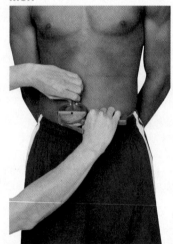

Abdomen

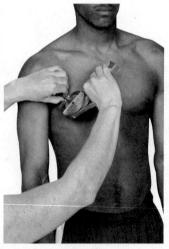

Chest

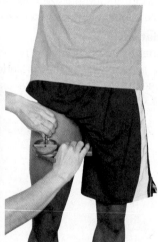

Thigh

Women

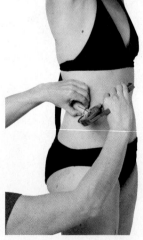

Suprailium

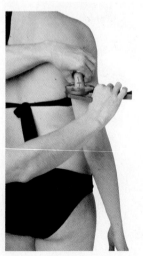

Triceps

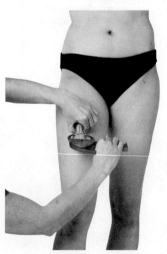

Thigh

To perform skinfold measurements:

- Hold the skinfold between your thumb and index finger.
- Slowly release the tension on the skinfold calipers to pinch the skinfold within ½ inch of your fingers.
- Hold the skinfold, and fully release the tension on the calipers.
- Read the number (the skinfold thickness in millimeters) from the gauge.
- Release the skinfold, and allow the tissue to relax.
- Measure the skinfold thickness at each site.
- Repeat three times, and average the measurements.
- Total the measurements, and use Tables 6.2 and 6.3 on pages 162 and 163 to determine the percent body fat.
- Enter your data in the spaces below.

Sum of 3 skinfolds (mm) _____

Percent body fat _____

Classification:

_____ Underweight

_____ Normal

_____ Overweight

_____ Obese

TABLE 6.2 **Percent Body Fat Estimates for Women (from triceps, suprailiac, and thigh skinfolds)**

Sum of Skinfolds (mm)	Age (years)								
	Under 22	23–27	28–32	33–37	38–42	43–47	48–52	53–57	Over 57
23–25	9.7	9.9	10.2	10.4	10.7	10.9	11.2	11.4	11.7
26–28	11.0	11.2	11.5	11.7	12.0	12.3	12.5	12.7	13.0
29–31	12.3	12.5	12.8	13.0	13.3	13.5	13.8	14.0	14.3
32–34	13.6	13.8	14.0	14.3	14.5	14.8	15.0	15.3	15.5
35–37	14.8	15.0	15.3	15.5	15.8	16.0	16.3	16.5	16.8
38–40	16.0	16.3	16.5	16.7	17.0	17.2	17.5	17.7	18.0
41–43	17.2	17.4	17.7	17.9	18.2	18.4	18.7	18.9	19.2
44–46	18.3	18.6	18.8	19.1	19.3	19.6	19.8	20.1	20.3
47–49	19.5	19.7	20.0	20.2	20.5	20.7	21.0	21.2	21.5
50–52	20.6	20.8	21.1	21.3	21.6	21.8	22.1	22.3	22.6
53–55	21.7	21.9	22.1	22.4	22.6	22.9	23.1	23.4	23.6
56–58	22.7	23.0	23.2	23.4	23.7	23.9	24.2	24.4	24.7
59–61	23.7	24.0	24.2	24.5	24.7	25.0	25.2	25.5	25.7
62–64	24.7	25.0	25.2	25.5	25.7	26.0	26.2	26.4	26.7
65–67	25.7	25.9	26.2	26.4	26.7	26.9	27.2	27.4	27.7
68–70	26.6	26.9	27.1	27.4	27.6	27.9	28.1	28.4	28.6
71–73	27.5	27.8	28.0	28.3	28.5	28.8	29.0	29.3	29.5
74–76	28.4	28.7	28.9	29.2	29.4	29.7	29.9	30.2	30.4
77–79	29.3	29.5	29.8	30.0	30.3	30.5	30.8	31.0	31.3
80–82	30.1	30.4	30.6	30.9	31.1	31.4	31.6	31.9	32.1
83–85	30.9	31.2	31.4	31.7	31.9	32.2	32.4	32.7	32.9
86–88	31.7	32.0	32.2	32.5	32.7	32.9	33.2	33.4	33.7
89–91	32.5	32.7	33.0	33.2	33.5	33.7	33.9	34.2	34.4
92–94	33.2	33.4	33.7	33.9	34.2	34.4	34.7	34.9	35.2
95–97	33.9	34.1	34.4	34.6	34.9	35.1	35.4	35.6	35.9
98–100	34.6	34.8	35.1	35.3	35.5	35.8	36.0	36.3	36.5
101–103	35.3	35.4	35.7	35.9	36.2	36.4	36.7	36.9	37.2
104–106	35.8	36.1	36.3	36.6	36.8	37.1	37.3	37.5	37.8
107–109	36.4	36.7	36.9	37.1	37.4	37.6	37.9	38.1	38.4
110–112	37.0	37.2	37.5	37.7	38.0	38.2	38.5	38.7	38.9
113–115	37.5	37.8	38.0	38.2	38.5	38.7	39	39.2	39.5
116–118	38.0	38.3	38.5	38.8	39.0	39.3	39.5	39.7	40.0
119–121	38.5	38.7	39.0	39.2	39.5	39.7	40.0	40.2	40.5
122–124	39.0	39.2	39.4	39.7	39.9	40.2	40.4	40.7	40.9
125–127	39.4	39.6	39.9	40.1	40.4	40.6	40.9	41.1	41.4
128–130	39.8	40.0	40.3	40.5	40.8	41.0	41.3	41.5	41.8

Source: A. S. Jackson and M. L. Pollock, "Practical Assessment of Body Composition," *The Physician and Sportsmedicine*, Vol. 13, No. 5 (1985): 76–90. Copyright © 1985 JTE Mulitmedia, LLC. Reprinted by permission.

TABLE 6.3 **Percent Body Fat Estimates for Men (from chest, abdomen, and thigh skinfolds)**

Sum of Skinfolds (mm)	Age (years)								
	Under 22	23–27	28–32	33–37	38–42	43–47	48–52	53–57	Over 57
8–10	1.3	1.8	2.3	2.9	3.4	3.9	4.5	5.0	5.5
11–13	2.2	2.8	3.3	3.9	4.4	4.9	5.5	6.0	6.5
14–16	3.2	3.8	4.3	4.8	5.4	5.9	6.4	7.0	7.5
17–19	4.2	4.7	5.3	5.8	6.3	6.9	7.4	8.0	8.5
20–22	5.1	5.7	6.2	6.8	7.3	7.9	8.4	8.9	9.5
23–25	6.1	6.6	7.2	7.7	8.3	8.8	9.4	9.9	10.5
26–28	7.0	7.6	8.1	8.7	9.2	9.8	10.3	10.9	11.4
29–31	8.0	8.5	9.1	9.6	10.2	10.7	11.3	11.8	12.4
32–34	8.9	9.4	10.0	10.5	11.1	11.6	12.2	12.8	13.3
35–37	9.8	10.4	10.9	11.5	12.0	12.6	13.1	13.7	14.3
38–40	10.7	11.3	11.8	12.4	12.9	13.5	14.1	14.6	15.2
41–43	11.6	12.2	12.7	13.3	13.8	14.4	15.0	15.5	16.1
44–46	12.5	13.1	13.6	14.2	14.7	15.3	15.9	16.4	17.0
47–49	13.4	13.9	14.5	15.1	15.6	16.2	16.8	17.3	17.9
50–52	14.3	14.8	15.4	15.9	16.5	17.1	17.6	18.2	18.8
53–55	15.1	15.7	16.2	16.8	17.4	17.9	18.5	19.1	19.7
56–58	16.0	16.5	17.1	17.7	18.2	18.8	19.4	20.0	20.5
59–61	16.9	17.4	17.9	18.5	19.1	19.7	20.2	20.8	21.4
62–64	17.6	18.2	18.8	19.4	19.9	20.5	21.1	21.7	22.2
65–67	18.5	19.0	19.6	20.2	20.8	21.3	21.9	22.5	23.1
68–70	19.3	19.9	20.4	21.0	21.6	22.2	22.7	23.3	23.9
71–73	20.1	20.7	21.2	21.8	22.4	23.0	23.6	24.1	24.7
74–76	20.9	21.5	22.0	22.6	23.2	23.8	24.4	25.0	25.5
77–79	21.7	22.2	22.8	23.4	24.0	24.6	25.2	25.8	26.3
80–82	22.4	23.0	23.6	24.2	24.8	25.4	25.9	26.5	27.1
83–85	23.2	23.8	24.4	25.0	25.5	26.1	26.7	27.3	27.9
86–88	24.0	24.5	25.1	25.7	26.3	26.9	27.5	28.1	28.7
89–91	24.7	25.3	25.9	26.5	27.1	27.6	28.2	28.8	29.4
92–94	25.4	26.0	26.6	27.2	27.8	28.4	29.0	29.6	30.2
95–97	26.1	26.7	27.3	27.9	28.5	29.1	29.7	30.3	30.9
98–100	26.9	27.4	28.0	28.6	29.2	29.8	30.4	31.0	31.6
101–103	27.5	28.1	28.7	29.3	29.9	30.5	31.1	31.7	32.3
104–106	28.2	28.8	29.4	30.0	30.6	31.2	31.8	32.4	33.0
107–109	28.9	29.5	30.1	30.7	31.3	31.9	32.5	33.1	33.7
110–112	29.6	30.2	30.8	31.4	32.0	32.6	33.2	33.8	34.4
113–115	30.2	30.8	31.4	32.0	32.6	33.2	33.8	34.5	35.1
116–118	30.9	31.5	32.1	32.7	33.3	33.9	34.5	35.1	35.7
119–121	31.5	32.1	32.7	33.3	33.9	34.5	35.1	35.7	36.4
122–124	32.1	32.7	33.3	33.9	34.5	35.1	35.8	36.4	37.0
125–127	32.7	33.3	33.9	34.5	35.1	35.8	36.4	37.0	37.6

Source: A. S. Jackson and M. L. Pollock, "Practical Assessment of Body Composition," *The Physician and Sportsmedicine*, Vol. 13, No. 5 (1985): 76–90. Copyright © 1985 JTE Mulitmedia, LLC. Reprinted by permission.

Waist Circumference and Waist-to-Hip Ratio

Scan to view a demonstration video of the waist and hip circumference measurements. ▶

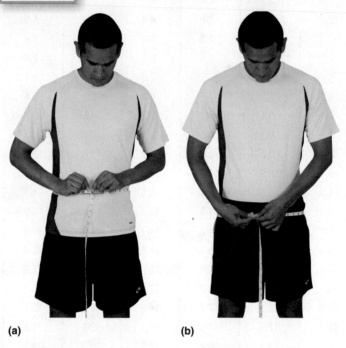

(a)   (b)

To perform waist-to-hip circumference measurements:

• Perform the waist measurement first.

• Place the tape at the level of the navel (a), and make your measurement at the end of a normal breath.

• For the hip measurement, place the tape around the maximum circumference of the buttocks (b).

• Divide the waist circumference by the hip circumference to determine the waist-to-hip ratio.

• Use Table 6.4 on page 165 to determine the waist-to-hip ratio rating.

• Use Table 6.1 on page 154 to determine your waist measurement rating.

• Enter your data in the spaces below.

Waist measurement _____

Hip measurement   _____

Waist-to-hip ratio   _____

Classification:

_____ Low risk

_____ Moderate risk

_____ High risk

_____ Very high risk

TABLE 6.4   Waist-to-Hip Circumference Ratio Standards for Men and Women

Men	Risk			
	Low	Moderate	High	Very High
20–29 yrs	<0.83	0.83–0.88	0.89–0.94	>0.94
30–39 yrs	<0.84	0.84–0.91	0.92–0.96	>0.96
40–49 yrs	<0.88	0.88–0.95	0.96–1.00	>1.00
50–59 yrs	<0.90	0.90–0.96	0.97–1.02	>1.02
60–69 yrs	<0.91	0.91–0.98	0.99–1.03	>1.03

Women	Risk			
	Low	Moderate	High	Very High
20–29 yrs	<0.71	0.71–0.77	0.78–0.82	>0.82
30–39 yrs	<0.72	0.72–0.78	0.79–0.84	>0.84
40–49 yrs	<0.73	0.73–0.79	0.80–0.87	>0.87
50–59 yrs	<0.74	0.74–0.81	0.82–0.88	>0.88
60–69 yrs	<0.76	0.76–0.83	0.84–0.90	>0.90

Source: Data from Bray, G. A., and D. S. Gray. Obesity. Part I–Pathogenesis. *West J Med* 149(4):429–441, 1988.

BMI

Weight (kg) _____

Height (m^2) _____

BMI _____

Classification (see Table 6.1 on page 154):

_____ Underweight

_____ Normal

_____ Overweight

_____ Obese

Other Measure: _____

Percent body fat _____

Classification:

_____ Underweight

_____ Normal

_____ Overweight

_____ Obese

Questions

1.   Are your classifications for each assessment similar? If not, why do you think there are discrepancies?

_____

_____

2.   Which assessment did you feel was most accurate for you, and why?

_____

_____

LABORATORY 6.2

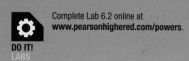

Complete Lab 6.2 online at
www.pearsonhighered.com/powers.

DO IT!
LABS

Name _____ Date _____

Determining a Healthy Body Weight

EQUIPMENT

Results from Laboratory 6.1 and a calculator

DIRECTIONS

If your results from Laboratory 6.1 indicate that you need to lose or gain weight, you should calculate a goal body weight needed to achieve an optimal level of body fat or optimal BMI. Keep in mind that not everyone will need to lose or gain weight. If your weight is within the recommended levels and you are happy with your current body composition, weight maintenance should be your goal.

PART 1

		Example:
Current weight	_____	*Current weight* 176
Current percent fat	_____	*Current percent fat* 38
Current BMI	_____	*Current BMI* 29.3*
Goal percent fat	_____	*Goal percent fat* 25–30†
Goal BMI	_____	*Goal BMI* 20–25 kg/m²

STEP 1: Calculate % of fat-free mass.

1 − _____ (current percent fat‡) = _____ (% fat-free mass)

Example: 1 − (0.38) = 0.62

STEP 2: Calculate fat-free weight.

_____ (% fat-free mass‡) × _____ (current body weight) = _____ (fat-free weight)

Example: 0.62 × 176 = 109.12

STEP 3: Calculate optimal weight, lower and upper ends of the range.

_____ (optimal weight) = _____ (fat-free weight)/(1 − _____ [optimal percent fat‡])

Repeat for the upper end of the range.

Example: 109.12 ÷ (1 − 0.25) = 145.5

109.12 ÷ (1 − 0.30) = 155.9

Example optimal range = 146 to 156 pounds

Your optimal range: _____ to _____

---

*We used a height of 65 inches.

†We selected values within the recommended healthy range. You can use the whole range, or you can use part of the range, as we did. The important thing to remember is that your goal should be within the recommended levels for your age and activity level.

‡Expressed as a decimal.

STEP 4: Calculate BMI based on your optimal weight range.

_____ to _____

Example:

_1m = 39.25 in., 1 lb = 2.2 kg_

_65 in. ÷ 39.25 = 1.65 m_

_146 lb ÷ 2.2 = 66.2 kg_

_66.2 ÷ 1.65² = 24.3 kg/m²_

_156 lb ÷ 2.2 = 70.7 kg_

_70.7 ÷ 165² = 25.9 kg/m²_

BMI: 24.3 to 25.9 kg/m²

PART 2

Repeat the calculations for determining a healthy goal weight, using BMI.

goal weight (kg) = desired BMI × height (m²)

Repeat for the upper end of the range

_____ to _____

Questions

1. Do the BMI values in part 1 of the lab place you in the recommended range? If not, why not?

   _____

   _____

2. Are there any differences between the BMI values from parts 1 and 2? If so, why?

   _____

   _____

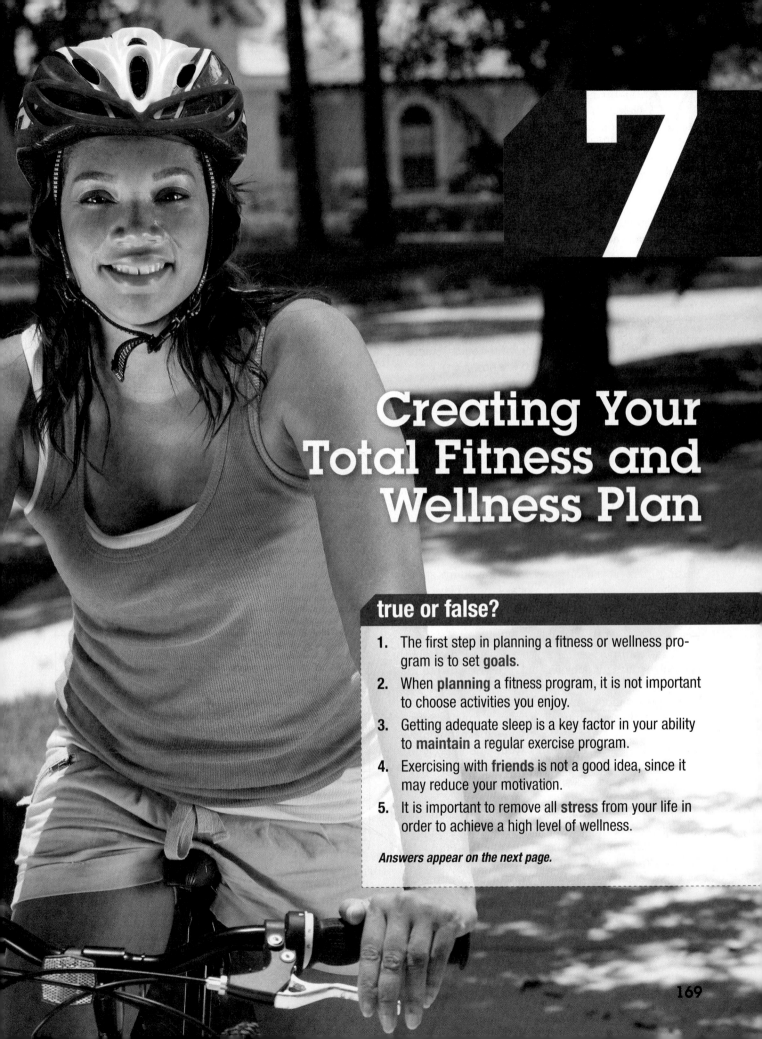

7

Creating Your Total Fitness and Wellness Plan

true or false?

1. The first step in planning a fitness or wellness program is to set **goals**.

2. When **planning** a fitness program, it is not important to choose activities you enjoy.

3. Getting adequate sleep is a key factor in your ability to **maintain** a regular exercise program.

4. Exercising with **friends** is not a good idea, since it may reduce your motivation.

5. It is important to remove all **stress** from your life in order to achieve a high level of wellness.

Answers appear on the next page.

Miguel wants to lose some weight, and Vanessa wants to have more physical strength and endurance. They know that better nutrition and exercise could help, but they don't know how to get started. How can they put together individualized plans to achieve their unique fitness and wellness goals?

In previous chapters, you learned about the general principles and health benefits of wellness and physical fitness (Chapters 1–2) and about exercise programs that can help you achieve fitness in four key areas: cardiorespiratory endurance, muscular strength, muscular endurance, and flexibility (Chapters 3–5). You also read about the importance of body composition (Chapter 6). With this information, you can begin to build an exercise program that promotes all components of health-related physical fitness and a wellness plan for successful behavior change. This chapter offers practical guidelines to help you achieve these goals.

Steps to Develop a Personal Fitness Plan

Now that you understand the benefits and components of physical fitness, it is time to develop an action plan to promote personal fitness. This section presents a four-step procedure for setting up your own fitness program.

Step 1. Set Your Goals

Setting goals is the first and most important step in establishing a successful personal fitness plan. If you don't know what you're working toward, you are not likely to achieve it. Thus, setting goals is a key requirement for any fitness program.

The main purpose of setting goals is to establish clear objectives for achievement. Studies indicate that creating a written list of goals prior to beginning a fitness program increases your chances of maintaining an exercise regime and improving physical fitness. Setting goals helps you focus on what you expect to achieve, and it defines and establishes your priorities. It also reinforces your motivation to succeed. Setting goals is a vital, first step in achieving your fitness objectives.

There are three major types of fitness goals. One type is called a performance goal. This is a specific short-term, intermediate, or long-term target that you set to improve your cardiorespiratory fitness, muscular strength and endurance, or flexibility. For example, a specific short-term performance goal might be to raise your cardiorespiratory fitness rating from poor to average.

Figure 7.1 shows the performance goals set by Susie Jones, who will use fitness testing to determine when she has reached her objectives. The "current status" column shows Susie's fitness ratings based on tests performed prior to starting her exercise program.

answers

1. **TRUE** Setting goals is the first and most important step in establishing a successful personal fitness or wellness plan. Without goals the changes you make are likely to be random, temporary, lack focus, and yield little benefit.

2. **FALSE** Research indicates that performing fitness activities you enjoy is a key element in sustaining a program of regular exercise.

3. **TRUE** Getting an appropriate amount of sleep plays an important role in your ability to maintain a regular exercise program.

4. **FALSE** Exercising with friends can increase your motivation by making exercise more fun and providing positive reinforcement.

5. **FALSE** It is impossible to remove all stress from your life. In order to achieve a high level of wellness, it is important to learn how to cope with the stress in your life.

Name: Susie Jones

Fitness Goals			
Fitness Category	Current Status	Short-term Goal (8 weeks)	Long-term Goal (18 months)
Cardiorespiratory fitness	Poor	Average	Excellent
Muscular strength	Poor	Average	Excellent
Muscular endurance	Very poor	Average	Good
Flexibility	Poor	Average	Good
Body composition	High fat	Moderately high	Optimal

FIGURE 7.1
As you begin thinking about your short-term and long-term goals for each component of physical fitness, fill out a worksheet like this so you can track your progress.

After consulting with her instructor, Susie has set short-term goals that she hopes to achieve within the first 8 weeks of training. She has also set long-term goals that she hopes to reach within the first 18 months. Both short-term and long-term goals are flexible and can be modified to meet changing needs and circumstances.

In addition to performance goals, you can set body composition goals. Progress can be measured by changes in body weight, body mass index (BMI), or other measures of body composition, including how well your clothes fit! Susie's list of fitness goals also shows her body composition objectives (Figure 7.1).

You should also establish adherence goals. That is, you should set a goal to exercise a specific number of days per week. Adherence goals are important because regular exercise is essential to achieve your overall fitness goals.

The following guidelines can help you establish your personal fitness goals:

- *Set realistic short-term goals first.* Short-term goals are typically fitness objectives to be achieved within the first 2 to 6 months of your exercise program. Establishing short-term goals that are realistic is important for two reasons: First, if your goals are too hard to achieve, you may get frustrated and give up. Second, reaching your short-term goals will help motivate you to achieve other goals in the future.

- *Set intermediate and long-term goals.* In addition to short-term goals, it is important to set intermediate and long-term fitness goals. Intermediate goals are typically 6- to 12-month targets, whereas long-term goals can range from 1 to 2 years and beyond.

- *Establish goals that can be measured.* It is also important to make your goals specific and measurable (1). This will help you determine if you have reached them. For example, setting a weight-loss goal of 5 pounds is a measurable goal.

- *Put goals in writing.* Writing your goals down and posting them in a place where you can see them every day will help remind you of your fitness objectives. Keeping your goals in mind is essential to achieving them (2).

- *Establish a reward system for achieving goals.* After you reach each of your specific fitness goals, give yourself a reward! You might do something you enjoy, such as going to a concert or a sporting event. Rewarding achievement is a good way to maintain your motivation and move on to your next goal (2).

Once you begin your fitness program, be prepared for setbacks such as skipping workouts or falling behind in your progress. An occasional setback is normal (3). However, once you realize that you have stopped making progress, you should work to get back on track as soon as possible.

The importance of fitness goals cannot be overemphasized. Goals provide the structure and motivation for a personal fitness program. Complete the laboratories at the end of this chapter to establish your short-term goals (Laboratory 7.1) and your intermediate and long-term goals (Laboratory 7.2).

Step 2. Select Exercises for Your Fitness Program

After establishing your personal fitness goals, the next step is to choose exercises that develop the various components of health-related physical fitness (as described in Chapters 3–6). Remember to target each of the following components.

Cardiorespiratory endurance. Exercises that develop this component involve repetitive movement of large muscle groups, such as the legs. (Details on designing an aerobic exercise program were presented in Chapter 3.) Combining two or more aerobic training techniques, such as cross training and interval training, can make your fitness routine more varied and effective. Just remember that your cardiorespiratory endurance program should be designed to achieve your specific fitness goals (3).

Muscular strength and endurance. Progressive resistance exercise training is the key to increasing muscular strength and endurance. (Use the information presented in Chapter 4 to create a personalized training program that will help you develop this critical fitness component.)

Flexibility. Because flexibility is an important part of any fitness program, you should include stretching exercises in your training routine. (Specifics on how to design a flexibility-training program can be found in Chapter 5.) Again, how you incorporate flexibility training into your weekly exercise routine should be guided by your personal fitness goals.

Body composition. Remember, too, that body composition is an important component of health-related physical fitness (see Chapter 6). Achieving a desirable body composition should be both an intermediate and a long-term goal of your total fitness program.

Step 3. Plan Your Weekly Fitness Routine

The next step is to plan your weekly fitness routine by determining how much time and energy you will devote to each element of your program. This calculation should be based on the FITT principle—frequency, intensity, time, and type (see Chapter 3). **Figure 7.2** on page 172 illustrates how to apply the FITT principle to each component of a health-related physical fitness program. Let's briefly discuss these guidelines.

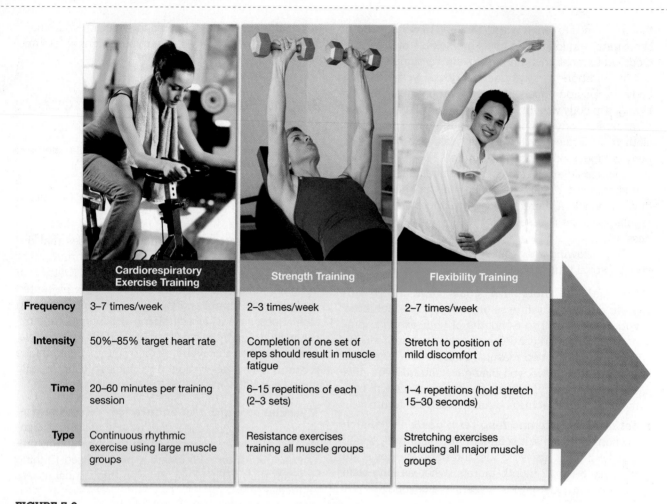

	Cardiorespiratory Exercise Training	Strength Training	Flexibility Training
Frequency	3–7 times/week	2–3 times/week	2–7 times/week
Intensity	50%–85% target heart rate	Completion of one set of reps should result in muscle fatigue	Stretch to position of mild discomfort
Time	20–60 minutes per training session	6–15 repetitions of each (2–3 sets)	1–4 repetitions (hold stretch 15–30 seconds)
Type	Continuous rhythmic exercise using large muscle groups	Resistance exercises training all muscle groups	Stretching exercises including all major muscle groups

FIGURE 7.2
This chart can help you apply the FITT principle to each exercise component of health-related physical fitness.

Training to improve cardiorespiratory fitness. Most cardiorespiratory health benefits occur with 120–150 minutes per week of moderate-intensity aerobic exercise. However, training more than 150 minutes per week can provide even more fitness benefits and help to achieve weight-loss goals. Details of the cardiorespiratory exercise prescription are summarized in Figure 7.2. Examples of different types of aerobic activities and their intensity are listed in Table 7.1.

Training to improve muscular strength and endurance. A training frequency of 2 to 3 days per week—on non-consecutive days—is recommended to improve muscular strength and endurance (4, 5). You should progress until you can perform 2 to 3 sets of each exercise, with 6 to 15 repetitions in each set (Figure 7.2).

Training to improve flexibility. Flexibility exercises should be performed 2 to 7 days per week, with stretches performed on all major muscle groups

(Figure 7.2). One to four repetitions of 15 to 30 seconds each is recommended.

TABLE 7.1 Aerobic Activities and Intensities	
Type of Activity	**Intensity**
Bicycling (level and <10 MPH)	Moderate
Bicycling (>10 MPH)	Vigorous
Race-walking	Moderate to vigorous
Running	Vigorous
Skipping rope	Vigorous
Spinning classes	Moderate to vigorous
Swimming	Vigorous
Tennis (doubles)	Moderate
Tennis (singles)	Vigorous
Walking	Moderate
Water aerobics	Moderate

Weekly Exercise Training Log

Name: Dylan Brown

Week: September 9–15

Activity	Monday	Tuesday	Wednesday	Thursday	Friday	Saturday	Sunday
Aerobics Class	20 min		20 min	20 min	20 min		30 min
Soccer Practice		30 min		20 min		30 min	
Weight Training	2 sets (8 reps) x 8 exercises		2 sets (8 reps) x 8 exercises		2 sets (8 reps) x 8 exercises		
Stretching		15 min		15 min			15 min
Daily Duration (cardiorespiratory endurance exercise)	20 min	30 min	20 min	40 min	20 min	30 min	30 min
Total Weekly Duration (cardiorespiratory endurance exercise)	170 min						

FIGURE 7.3
A weekly exercise training log like this one can help you record your activities and chart your progress.

Step 4. Monitor Your Progress

The final step in designing your fitness plan is to create a training log that records your progress each week. A log that tracks your weekly training activities will give you a sense of accomplishment and help motivate you to continue your program (6). **Figure 7.3** provides an example of a weekly training log. Other types of logs are available on the Internet and as applications on smart phones. You should choose a style that is easy to maintain and that meets your needs. Keeping an exercise log will remind you of your progress and provide an incentive to move forward.

In addition to your log, you might also create charts that show your training progress and fitness improvement in key measurable areas. **Figure 7.4** on page 174 shows a graph that tracks weekly exercise duration. It illustrates the total number of minutes spent per week on cardiorespiratory endurance exercise and compares those figures to the proposed training plan. Remember, too,

that you should monitor your fitness progress in cardiorespiratory endurance and muscular strength by retesting your fitness levels at regularly established intervals—for example, every 3 months—and keeping a record of your improvements.

MAKE SURE YOU KNOW...

- There are four main steps to follow in developing a personal fitness plan: (1) set your goals; (2) select your activities; (3) plan your weekly routine; and (4) monitor your progress.
- It is important to choose fitness activities that target cardiorespiratory fitness, muscular strength and endurance, and flexibility.
- The FITT principle will help you plan your weekly fitness routine.
- A training log is a useful tool to monitor your ongoing progress.

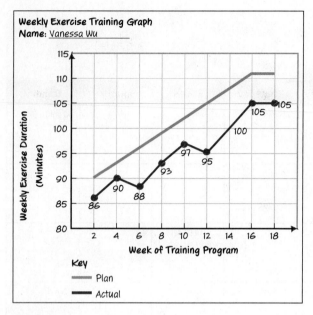

Weekly Exercise Training Graph
Name: _Vanessa Wu_

FIGURE 7.4
A graph like this one—which shows actual and planned time spent per week on cardiorespiratory exercise training—can be a useful tool for monitoring your progress.

Combining Fitness Training Components: Examples and Considerations

Once you have selected activities and created separate exercise programs that target the main components of physical fitness, you are ready to combine these elements in an integrated weekly exercise routine. Sample programs are provided at the end of this chapter on pages 182–183. The first program illustrates a weekly program for a beginner; the second shows a program for someone who has already completed 6 to 20 weeks of exercise training, and the third shows a program for someone who has completed more than 20 weeks of exercise training. To plan and record your own weekly fitness program, you can use the chart in Laboratory 7.3. Consider the following factors when developing your weekly exercise plan:

- **Fun and variety.** You are more likely to achieve success in your fitness program if you choose activities you enjoy. It is also a good idea to add variety to your routine by including different types of activities—such as swimming, tennis, running, and cycling.

- **Current fitness level.** Make sure to construct a fitness program that matches your current fitness level. It is counterproductive to design a training plan that is overly ambitious and impossible to complete. You should create a program that is realistic and achievable.

- **Special health issues.** If you have special health concerns—such as type 1 diabetes or asthma—consult your physician before designing your fitness program. Your doctor should be able to provide information that will help you devise a program to meet your particular needs.

- **Muscle strain.** Keep in mind that muscles need time to rest and recover after weight training. For this reason, you should not schedule weight-training sessions on consecutive days. Note in the sample exercise programs on pages 182–183 that weight training and running are scheduled on alternating days (also see Table 7.2).

- **Flexibility training.** You should perform stretching exercises at least 2 days per week. You should also do them when your muscles are warm—that is, after exercising. Table 7.2 shows a stretching program of 3 days per week. Stretching 5 to 7 days per week is considered ideal, however. As you progress toward your fitness goals, you should add additional stretching days to your exercise program.

MAKE SURE YOU KNOW...

- Your fitness program will be more successful if you include a variety of physical activities you enjoy.
- Your program should be realistic and correspond to your current fitness level.
- If you have special health concerns, consult a doctor when planning your exercise program.
- Strength training should be scheduled on non-consecutive days to allow muscles to recover.
- Stretching exercises should be performed at least 2 days a week, when muscles are warm.

Ever wonder what's the best medication for your muscle soreness? Watch _Understanding Over-the-Counter Painkillers_ at **www.pearsonhighered.com/powers**.

SEE IT! VIDEOS

TABLE 7.2 Weekly Exercise Plan to Promote Overall Fitness							
Activity	**Monday**	**Tuesday**	**Wednesday**	**Thursday**	**Friday**	**Saturday**	**Sunday**
Running	X		X		X		
Cycling		X		X			X
Weight training		X		X		X	
Stretching	X		X		X		

Putting Your Fitness Plan into Action

After setting your goals, planning your fitness routine, and creating a monitoring system to chart your progress, it is time to launch your plan into action and start on the path to improving your personal fitness. Remember that planning a fitness program is often easier than carrying it out. The guidelines below will help you succeed in following your exercise program and achieving your goals.

- **Take a gradual approach.** Begin your exercise program in a careful, measured way. You may cause muscle strain or injury if you push yourself too hard at the start. After adjusting to your routine, you can gradually increase the amount of exercise overload to raise your fitness level. Even small increases in exercise duration and intensity will result in noticeable improvements.

- **Be consistent and methodical.** One key to reaching your fitness goals is to maintain a pattern of regular exercise. If you pick a convenient time and place for your training sessions, you are more likely to stick to your routine.

- **Exercise with friends.** Exercising with friends can make exercise more fun and increase your motivation. Choose a friend with a similar fitness level who shares your exercise goals and is willing to commit to a regular routine. Keep in mind, too, that a canine friend can be a good exercise partner. It has been shown that having a dog will increase your physical activity (7). Dog walking, for example, can be a great way to get daily exercise. So when you are seeking an exercise partner, remember that "man's best friend" may be a good option.

- **Vary your training.** Engaging in a variety of fitness activities will also make your exercise program more enjoyable and productive. Cross training, for example, has many health and fitness benefits (8). Even simple variations such as changing the routes you walk, run, or cycle can help maintain your interest and enthusiasm.

- **Get enough rest.** Getting adequate sleep plays an important role in any fitness program. Good sleep patterns are critical to overall health and well-being (9, 10). Research indicates that irritability, moodiness, and general fatigue are among the first signs of a lack of sleep (11). Most adults need an average of 8 hours of sleep a day, though sleep needs can vary (12). Some people are able to get by on as little as 6 hours of sleep, whereas others can't perform at their peak unless they've slept for 10 hours. You should figure out how much sleep you need to feel revived and refreshed, and then schedule that time into your daily routine.

- **Adapt to changing circumstances.** Don't allow changes in your work or class schedule to disrupt your exercise program. If necessary, adjust your exercise routine so that you continue to pursue your

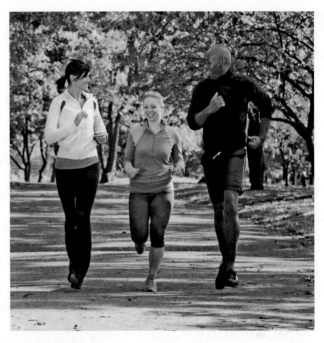

Exercising with friends can increase fun and motivation.

fitness goals. Also, if you are used to exercising outdoors, don't let bad weather or short daylight during winter days interfere with your training. Continue your exercise indoors, either in your own home, a public gym, or a private fitness center.

- **Expect backsliding.** At times you may miss exercise sessions and lose motivation. This may occur because you feel tired or ill, or because other things get in the way. This type of "backsliding" is common and should not discourage you or keep you from getting your fitness program back on track. See the Closer Look box on page 176 for strategies to avoid backsliding.

- **Combine regular exercise with other healthy behaviors.** Although exercise provides major health benefits, it is not a cure-all to achieve good health (13, 14). Other factors, such as following a good diet and avoiding smoking and drug abuse, will improve your chances of remaining healthy. Later in this chapter you will learn more about putting together wellness plans for improved healthy behaviors. (Chapters 8–11 and 15–16 discuss various healthy behaviors that will improve your overall well-being and reduce your risk of disease.)

MAKE SURE YOU KNOW...

- It is important to take a gradual approach to exercise and not overdo it when starting your fitness program.
- It is best to exercise in a regular and consistent pattern.
- Exercising with friends can be very beneficial.
- Varying your training activities can increase motivation.
- Getting enough sleep is critical to the success of your fitness program.

COACHING Corner

Are you losing interest in your strength-training and flexibility programs? It may be time to try a different mode of training! New exercises that include movements involving your body weight can be just as beneficial as lifting in a gym. Here are some additional ideas to keep your workout interesting:

- Try Pilates or yoga.
- Join a group fitness class that emphasizes strength and endurance training.
- Create your own routine that utilizes multi-joint movements that mimic activities of your daily life.
- Create a soundtrack of music that motivates you.
- Consider hiring a certified personal trainer for a different experience.

Try a fitness class!

- It may be necessary to adjust your exercise routine to accommodate changing schedules and circumstances.
- Backsliding in personal fitness is common and should not be a cause for discouragement.
- Exercise should be combined with other healthy behaviors to ensure good health.

Lifetime Adjustments in Your Exercise Prescription

As you age, you will need to adjust your fitness program to adapt to life's changing circumstances. For example, although it is generally safe to exercise when pregnant, pregnancy may require changes in your exercise routine. In addition, aging itself brings various physiological changes that may require adjustments in your exercise program. (Specific details about exercise guidelines during pregnancy and older age are discussed in Chapter 12.)

MAKE SURE YOU KNOW...

- An exercise program should evolve over time. The circumstances of aging and pregnancy, for example, may require changes in the exercise prescription.

Steps to Develop a Wellness Plan

In the first part of this chapter, you learned to design your overall plan for improving your physical fitness. And in Chapter 1 you were introduced to a term that encompasses almost every other aspect of your overall health: wellness. In addition to physical health, wellness includes various aspects of emotional, intellectual, spiritual, social, and environmental health. (In the chapters

A CLOSER LOOK

How to Avoid Backsliding in Your Fitness Program

Reverting to old habits, or backsliding, is common in any behavior change program. Most people who start a new exercise routine have problems maintaining a regular workout schedule. One key to success is to recognize that backsliding is typical. The following tips may help you stay on track and reach your fitness goals:

- If you slip out of your exercise routine, remember that you can get back in just as easily. Focus on your goals for health and fitness and the benefits you hope to gain.
- Try not to become discouraged. A positive attitude is very helpful! Remember that sticking with your program will eventually lead to success.

- If you lose motivation, keep in mind that exercise has a positive impact on physical and mental energy (2, 17). Even if you perform only part of your regular workout, exercise will help lift your mood and make you feel better (6).
- Keeping a training log will also help you stay on track. A log of your accomplishments can help you feel pride in your progress and keep you moving forward to achieve your goals.

that follow, you will go "in-depth" into several aspects of wellness that have a major impact on your health.) If you can combine the fitness concepts discussed previously with the wellness concepts to be presented, you will be well on your way to a lifetime of good health, enhanced quality of life, and a true sense of well-being.

After you have covered the remaining chapters, you will be ready to put together a detailed "Wellness Plan." The 4-step plan outlined below will help you achieve a higher level of wellness.

Step 1. Establish Your Goals

This is the most important step in developing your plan. Without goals, any changes in behavior are likely to be random and temporary, and to lack focus and yield little benefit. Remember in Chapter 1 that we encouraged the use of SMART goals. SMART is an acronym for Specific, Measureable, Action-oriented, Realistic, and Time-stamped. For example, if you decide to reduce the amount of saturated fats in your diet, you would set a goal of, "Beginning tomorrow, I will reduce my intake of saturated fats by 50% (SMRT) by reducing the amount of red meat in my diet (A)."

Putting your goals in writing will help remind you how "specific" the goals are so that you can constantly be looking for new "actions" to help accomplish the goals. By writing down your goals and keeping them easily accessible (such as keeping them on a to-do list in your phone), you can view them often as a reminder of what you are trying to accomplish.

Also, try to reward yourself for accomplishing any of the goals you have listed. This is a great way to reinforce your planning and actions in trying to accomplish the goals. As we discussed earlier, be prepared for setbacks. For example, in reaching your dietary goals, an occasional piece of candy or soda will not undo all of the benefits accomplished. Just look at the jolt in fat/sugar/sodium that you got from it and ask yourself if it was worth it. With that, you are educating yourself as to how and why you are changing your behavior.

Step 2. Select Wellness Concepts to Build Your Wellness Program

While many concepts of wellness play a part in your well-being, we have chosen the ones with the most significant potential impact on your health to discuss here. Thus, the major aspects of wellness that will be discussed in upcoming chapters are dietary considerations, stress management, sexually transmitted infections, and addictions and drug abuse.

Diet.   In the absence of disease, diet and fitness are probably the most significant factors affecting your wellness. Bad dietary habits can lead to a host of ill-health effects such as obesity, cardiovascular disease, diabetes, and many more. Changing dietary habits can lead to significant improvements in health and wellness (as you will see in Chapter 8).

Stress Management.   Everyone has stress in their daily life, and you should strive to reduce it as much as possible. However, it is most important to learn how to cope with stress, as most people will not be able to significantly reduce the stress associated with work, family, and school. (In Chapter 11, you will learn the ill-health effects of high stress levels. In addition, you will examine the sources of stress in your life and the ways by which you can minimize and learn to cope.)

Sexually Transmitted Infections.   Responsible sexual behavior requires asking questions of your potential partner, taking precautions, and educating yourself about the risks associated with sexual activity. (In Chapter 15, you will learn about symptoms and routes of transmission of sexually transmitted infections [STIs]. You will also learn strategies to prevent the unpleasant, sometimes deadly, STIs.)

Addiction and Substance Abuse.   When a person cannot control his actions regarding a certain substance or behavior, we say he is addicted to that substance or action. The addiction may be to alcohol or other drugs, gambling, shopping, or video games. In contrast, substance abuse may or may not involve an addiction. For example, the routine use of anabolic steroids to increase muscle mass is the abuse of a substance, but typically the abuse does not lead to a physical or psychological addiction. (In Chapter 16, you will learn more about addictive behaviors and their causes. Also, you will learn more about what these behaviors are and how you can prevent addictions. You will be able to determine the difference between substance use and abuse.)

Health-Care Choices.   Making good decisions about managing your health care is another very important aspect of wellness, since it is the overarching theme to all aspects of health care. To maintain a high level of wellness, you must be an informed health-care consumer. This includes understanding your health insurance, an especially important topic for those in their early 20s since that is the time that these important decisions are usually made. You should also be informed about choosing a health-care provider. Research your options—there are many available, and learning how to make the best decision can be a challenge. See the Closer Look boxes on pages 178 and 179 for more information about medical specialists and health care.

Do you benefit from healthcare reform? Watch *What Health Care's Passage Means for You* at **www.pearsonhighered.com/powers**.
SEE IT! VIDEOS

Should Eli pay for health care coverage? Listen to the online case study at **www.pearsonhighered.com/powers**.
HEAR IT! CASE STUDY

A CLOSER LOOK

Glossary of Medical Specialists

Everyone, regardless of age, needs a good, reliable health-care provider for common medical problems. A regular provider will be familiar with your medical history, and you are more likely to develop a relationship that will make you more comfortable when discussing your medical issues. Although your health-care provider will likely be a primary care physician, other medical professionals may sometimes address your health-care needs. For example, many women see a nurse practitioner or midwife for annual exams and/or during a pregnancy. Physician's assistants also sometimes conduct routine tests and screenings. These medical professionals can help with many routine and preventive health care needs, but they might need to refer you to a physician for some medical concerns.

Medical specialists are doctors who have received focused training in a specific area of medicine. The following list describes the most common types of medical specialists.

Anesthesiologist Administers anesthesia during surgery and monitors the patient's immediate recovery following surgery.

Cardiologist Diagnoses and treats diseases of the heart and blood vessels.

Dermatologist Specializes in care and treatment of skin diseases.

Emergency room specialist Specializes in the care and treatment of trauma patients and acute illnesses.

Gastroenterologist Diagnoses and treats diseases of the digestive system and liver.

Hematologist Specializes in disorders of the blood.

Internist Specializes in the nonsurgical treatment of adults. Major areas of medical interest may include heart disease, cancer, diabetes, and arthritis.

Neurologist Diagnoses and treats disorders of the brain and nervous system.

Neurosurgeon Specializes in surgical treatment of disorders of the brain and nervous system.

Obstetrician/gynecologist A gynecologist specializes in the treatment of the reproductive systems of women, whereas an obstetrician specializes in the treatment of pregnant women and delivering babies.

Oncologist Specializes in the treatment of cancer.

Otorhinolaryngologist Specializes in diagnosis and treatment of problems in the ear, nose, and throat.

Pediatrician Specializes in the treatment of children.

Physiatrist Specializes in physical medicine and rehabilitation.

Psychiatrist Treats behavioral and mental health disorders using both psychotherapy and medications.

Radiologist Specializes in the use of imaging technology (e.g., X-ray imaging, ultrasound) to diagnose diseases (e.g., cancer) and injuries (e.g., broken bones).

Surgeon Specializes in the use of surgery to diagnose and treat diseases. A general surgeon may perform a wide variety of surgical procedures, whereas other surgeons specialize in a specific area of surgery (e.g., cardiovascular surgery, plastic surgery).

Urologist Diagnoses and treats problems associated with the urinary tract in men and women, and in reproductive disorders in men.

**SEE IT!
VIDEOS** Should conventional doctors incorporate alternative medicine therapies into their treatments? Watch *Holistic Healthcare* at www.pearsonhighered.com/powers.

Step 3. Plan Your Behavior Changes for Wellness

Now that you have learned the importance of setting goals and chosen the specific areas on which you need to focus your effort, let's discuss ways to change your behaviors. To do this, let's use two examples of behavior change that will show you how to begin: quitting smoking and losing weight.

Smoking Cessation. Cigarette smoking increases the risk of cancer and heart disease. Research shows that smoking is the leading cause of preventable death in the United States (15). Although millions of people have quit smoking, the number of smokers has increased since the late 1960s because of an increase in young smokers, particularly young women. Smoking is a difficult behavior to change because it involves an addiction to nicotine, so outside assistance might be necessary to help overcome the addiction.

1. The first step in quitting smoking is having the desire to stop. You may want to quit because you recognize the negative health effects of smoking, or you may have important people in your life who want you to quit.

consider this!

By grade 12, 54% of students have tried cigarette smoking.

2. When you analyze your smoking behavior, pay attention to the times you smoke. Think about the reasons you decide to smoke. Is it automatic after a meal, or when you are with certain friends? Note the times you do not have the desire to smoke or when you choose other behaviors over smoking, and note your barriers for quitting smoking. These are examples of using self-monitoring to change behavior.

3. After you have a good idea of when and why you smoke, it is time to set goals and make a plan. Relapse prevention and substituting behaviors can be very helpful. Mobilize your support network by telling your friends and family what you plan to do—and, specifically, how they can help.

   When you set your goals, make sure they are SMART goals. Also, be sure to set both short-term and long-term goals. Obviously, the long-term goal is to stop permanently, but you should set goals for the things you will do to prepare for and maintain cessation. For example, you might sign a behavioral contract with your roommate and agree to check in after meals to maintain accountability. If you smoke after meals, plan to brush your teeth or chew gum instead of smoking; this is an example of counter conditioning. Relapse prevention might involve eating lunch in a no-smoking restaurant. Planning ahead and having an alternate behavior

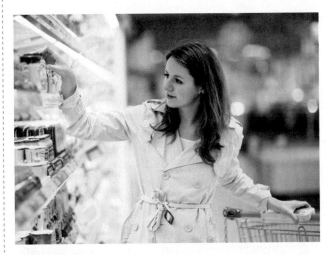

Choosing healthy foods at the grocery store will help you plan healthier meals.

will decrease the likelihood of smoking at your high-risk times.

Quitting smoking "cold turkey" is the most commonly reported method for smoking cessation (15, 16). Continue using behavior modification strategies to move from the action to the maintenance stage. If you smoke even one cigarette during the action stage, you move back into the preparation or possibly the contemplation stage. If you have a setback, reevaluate your decision, try to determine

A CLOSER LOOK

Communicating Effectively with Your Health-Care Provider

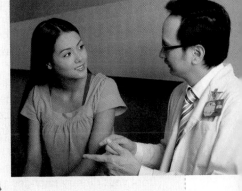

The relationship between patient and health-care provider plays an important role in the quality and effectiveness of medical care. Here are some guidelines for getting the most from your visit to the health-care provider.

- Prepare for your appointment in advance. Studies show that 70% of correct medical diagnoses depend on what you tell your medical professional about your symptoms (13). Prior to your visit, write down a list of your symptoms. Try not to leave anything out of your list, even if you think it seems minor. Something you think is a minor detail might be very important.

- Bring any medications that you are taking to your appointment, including over-the-counter medications, supplements, and herbal treatments, and mention any current medical treatments you are using. You might think they are not important, but they can have side effects and can interact with medications.

- Remember, no question is a dumb question. Write out a list of questions before your appointment, and feel free to ask them. Let your health-care provider know if you do not understand

the answers to your questions or any other information you are given. If you are unclear about any part of your diagnosis and treatment options, ask for another explanation of your problem and the proposed treatment.

- If you want to know more about your condition, ask your doctor to recommend resources where you can find additional information. Finally, prior to leaving the doctor's office, make certain that you understand the next steps for your treatment (i.e., return for another visit, more tests, and/or obtaining a prescription).

SEE IT! VIDEOS

Will you take medical advice from an Internet doctor? Watch *Dr. Web's Credentials* at **www.pearsonhighered.com/powers.**

why you had the lapse, and revise your plan. As you maintain your new healthy behavior of not smoking, be sure to reward yourself for accomplishing your goal.

Weight Loss. Losing weight and keeping it off are difficult for many people. Applying behavior modification principles and using behavior change models are essential. Although no single weight-loss program works for all people, the following are common components of most successful efforts:

1. Make sure that you want to lose weight for yourself. If you want to lose weight to please someone else, your chances for success are not as high.

2. Assess your eating habits, including the kind and amount of food you eat as well as the environmental and social circumstances involved. Also assess your physical activity and exercise patterns.

3. Establish short- and long-term SMART goals. Do not limit your goals to a specific number of pounds to lose. Your action step should include plans for changing your exercise and eating habits as well.

4. Establish your support network and accountability partners. A behavioral contract can be helpful.

5. Develop your specific plan, including dietary and activity changes. Remember to make it very detailed and to include specific steps. For example, a goal to "prepare healthier meals" is not specific enough. Instead, spell out what you will do to prepare healthier meals. Find recipes for dishes that are low in calories and dense in nutrients. Plan meals for an entire week, and make a grocery list for only the foods needed for your menus. Prepare meals according to the plan, and consider portion size. Each step might seem minor, but each takes effort. With this level of detail, you are using shaping, and you can experience success at each level to increase your confidence. (See Chapter 9 for more on weight management.)

6. Relapse prevention and counter conditioning will help plan for situations that might make you slip from your dietary changes and exercise plans. For example, knowing healthy menu options before you get to a restaurant and planning to exercise as soon you get home instead of watching television can help keep you on track.

7. Use your support network and any other outside assistance.

8. Reward yourself for successes along the way (self-reinforcement). Make sure your rewards do not undermine your success. Rewarding yourself with chocolate cake for a week of weight loss is not the best choice, but a dessert once in a while is not unreasonable.

There is a lot of good and bad information out there about ways to lose weight. You need to check information for accuracy when you consider a weight-loss plan. Unsound plans often produce rapid weight loss, but they might leave you missing key nutrients and can cause you to gain more weight later. These plans may also lighten your wallet, but not your body. Stay away from products or services that do not have information about long-term effects. (Refer to Chapter 9 and your instructor to help you evaluate a plan.)

Remember that the key elements in a weight-loss program are the desire to lose weight for oneself, establishing goals, developing a plan, and getting support from your friends and family. As you develop your plan, assess your readiness for change as well as the benefits, barriers, and other factors that will contribute to your success.

Step 4. Monitor Your Progress

As with your fitness plan, you need to begin a weekly log to record your actions aimed toward meeting your goals for behavior change. By doing this, you can see the obstacles you have overcome and accomplishments you have made; these will motivate you to continue! **Figure 7.5** illustrates a way that you can track your behavior change over the course of a week. You may

Weekly Behavior Change Log

Name: Kayla Johnson
Goal: Improve my diet
Week: February 10–16

What did you do this week to work toward your goal?
I determined that the saturated fat in my diet was typically about 200% of what it should be. In the beginning of the week I tried to choose foods that were low in saturated fats.

What obstacles did you encounter as you worked toward your goal? Most foods in my usual diet contained high amounts of saturated fat—red meat, desserts, etc. In trying to make better food choices, I did backslide! On Thursday, I consumed more fat than on Wednesday, but then I resumed my reduction in fat after that.

What supported your efforts this week? I substituted fish and chicken for the red meat in my diet. I like fish and chicken so that made my changes much easier. About 1/2 of the saturated fat was coming from red meat. I eliminated even more fat by eating fruit for dessert instead of sweets.

How will you use this week's experiences to work toward your goal next week? I'll continue to look for foods that are lower in saturated fats to substitute into my diet. If I backslide again, I won't get discouraged, and I'll make an effort to get back on track with my goal.

FIGURE 7.5
This sample log charts progress in a weight loss program.

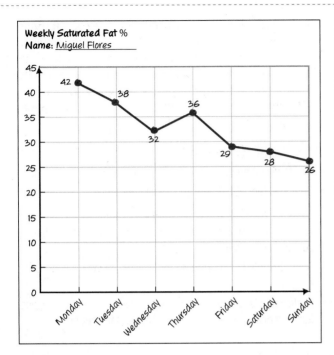

Weekly Saturated Fat %
Name: Miguel Flores

FIGURE 7.6
A progression graph allows you to track improvement and progress toward reaching a goal.

find others on the Internet or download apps for tracking your progress. **Figure 7.6** shows a progression log (graph) that allows you to track how you are improving and how far you need to go to reach your goal. You can use the graph to track such variables as "pounds lost," "calories consumed," "cigarettes smoked," and so on. You can also use such a log to plan rewards for yourself along the way. This would give you short-term goals to provide motivation to reach the long-term goal.

MAKE SURE YOU KNOW...

- Behavior modification can be applied to many health behaviors.
- Choose to modify those aspects of wellness that are most affecting your health.
- Your goals for behavior change should be specific, measurable, action-oriented, realistic, and time-stamped.
- Monitor your progress to identify common obstacles and provide motivation.
- A detailed plan of action is essential for using behavior modification to change your unhealthy behaviors.

Putting Your Wellness Plan into Action

As with your fitness plan, once you have completed the steps outlined above, it is time to put your wellness plan into action! The easy planning part is done; now comes the part where you will perform. The guidelines below will help you to stay on track with the plan.

COACHING **corner**

Every step is necessary in the journey toward reaching your fitness and wellness goals. Sometimes, however, you may find yourself drifting from your original intentions. Consider the following questions as you continue to cement your commitment to a fitness and wellness program. You can discuss your answers with someone who might help hold you accountable for following your plan.

- What are the three most important reasons you have decided to commit to this plan?
- How do you know when your life is in or out of balance?
- On days you do not "feel" like following your plan, what are other options you can use that are "better than nothing at all"?
- Explain your plan and your goals to a close friend. Discuss how that person can best help you when you do not feel like following your plan.

3 reasons for my wellness plan . . .

- **Start slow.** The changes you will be making will take some adjustments by your body. For example, the faster you try to lose weight, the more efficient your body's metabolism will become. Thus, it would take more effort to lose the weight if you lose it fast. Go slow! Losing weight slowly will make it easier for you to develop new habits, will let your body adjust without making drastic changes in metabolism, and will give you longer-lasting results.
- **Be consistent.** Again, your body is trying to adjust to your new behavior. With calorie reduction, spread the deficit over several meals. Don't wait until dinner and take all of your calorie reduction for the day!
- **Form groups with friends.** If you can find friends who are also going through modifications in behavior, it is great to meet and talk with them about their progress. This serves as a motivator and also allows you to exchange new ideas about how plan/reward/ analyze behaviors.
- **Incorporate variety into your plan.** Variety can make changing your behavior easier, and even make it

fun. This will make success even more likely! Using the dieting example again, try to use different combinations of energy expenditure and caloric reduction. For example, how many miles would you need to walk to burn the calories contained in a piece of cake? The use of variety in your planning is extremely useful in helping you to learn about how diet and exercise interact.

- **Adapt to changing schedules.** Make sure your action plan has allowed for some flexibility in your schedule. Look ahead while planning and think about work and/or class schedule changes. How will social outings affect your desire to smoke, drink, or eat? Such considerations are important in getting past those times when you will need lots of willpower to overcome temptations.

- **Expect backsliding.** As discussed in terms of the fitness plan, backsliding is to be expected with the wellness plan. If dieting, an occasional dessert or snack is not going to destroy your plan. Just make

sure not to let it get you away from your plan. If trying to reduce stress in your life, there will be times when it is impossible to remove yourself from a stressful situation. Just use that experience as a learning period to practice the ways that you will cope with stress. The situation may also allow you to learn how to avoid the same situation in the future.

MAKE SURE YOU KNOW...

- Go slowly when you're making changes to improve wellness.
- Be consistent about how you apply your plan.
- Friends can serve as a helpful support system.
- Variation in how you approach and apply your plan will help sustain motivation.
- Being flexible is important to the success of your wellness program.
- Backsliding is expected, and you can use it as a learning opportunity to plan ways to cope with difficulties in your program.

Sample Programs for Fitness

Scan to plan your individualized program for fitness. ▶

The following sample programs will help you plan your weekly exercise routine. Remember to choose a variety of activities you enjoy, and incorporate activities for enhanced cardiorespiratory endurance, muscular strength, and flexibility. Table 7.2 on page 174 shows a sample weekly exercise plan that combines activities in a way that promotes overall fitness. The weekly exercise plans that follow show sample programs for a beginner, someone who has completed 6–20 weeks of training, and someone who has completed over 20 weeks of training. Refer to these weekly samples as you plan your program in Laboratory 7.3.

Beginner Exercise Program (1–5 weeks of training)

This sample exercise program is designed for a beginner who is planning a weekly exercise routine. Before each exercise routine, warm up by performing 5–10 minutes of calisthenics or brisk walking. Cool down by engaging in 5–15 minutes of low-intensity exercise.

For weight training, choose 6–10 exercises designed to target major muscle groups (e.g., arms, chest, abdomen, lower back, and legs).

Activity	Monday	Tuesday	Wednesday	Thursday	Friday	Saturday	Sunday
Cardiorespiratory	10–20 min walking and/or running		10–20 min walking and/or running		10–20 min walking and/or running		
Weight Training		1 set / 15 reps		1 set / 15 reps		1 set / 15 reps	
Stretching	2 reps / 15 sec each		2 reps / 15 sec each		2 reps / 15 sec each		

Intermediate Exercise Program (6–20 weeks of training)

This sample exercise program is designed for someone planning a weekly exercise routine and who has completed 6 to 20 weeks of training. Before each exercise routine, warm up by performing 5–15 minutes of calisthenics or brisk walking. Cool down by engaging in 5–15 minutes of low-intensity exercise.

For weight training, choose 8–10 exercises designed to target major muscle groups (e.g., arms, chest, abdomen, lower back, and legs).

Activity	Monday	Tuesday	Wednesday	Thursday	Friday	Saturday	Sunday
Cardiorespiratory	30–40 min walking and/ or running		30–40 min walking and/ or running		30–40 min walking and/ or running		
Weight Training		2 sets / 6 reps		2 sets / 6 reps		2 sets / 6 reps	
Stretching	2–3 reps / 20 sec each		2–3 reps / 20 sec each		2–3 reps / 20 sec each		

Advanced Exercise Program (20+ weeks of training)

This sample exercise program is designed for someone planning a weekly exercise routine and who has completed over 20 weeks of training. Before each exercise routine, warm up by performing 5–15 minutes of calisthenics or brisk walking. Cool down by engaging in 5–15 minutes of low-intensity exercise.

For weight training, choose 8–10 exercises designed to target major muscle groups (e.g., arms, chest, abdomen, lower back, and legs).

Activity	Monday	Tuesday	Wednesday	Thursday	Friday	Saturday	Sunday
Cardiorespiratory	30–40 min walking and/ or running	20–25 min cycling	30–40 min walking and/or running	20–25 min cycling	30–40 min walking and/or running		30–40 min walking and/or running
Weight Training		3 sets / 6 reps		3 sets / 6 reps		3 sets / 6 reps	
Stretching	3 reps / 30 sec each	3 reps / 30 sec each	3 reps / 30 sec each	3 reps / 30 sec each	3 reps / 30 sec each		

SUMMARY

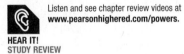

Listen and see chapter review videos at
www.pearsonhighered.com/powers.

HEAR IT!
STUDY REVIEW

1. The four steps in building a personal fitness plan are to (1) establish your goals; (2) select your activities; (3) plan your weekly routine; and (4) monitor your progress.

2. A well-designed fitness program includes activities to improve cardiorespiratory fitness, muscular strength and endurance, and flexibility.

3. The FITT principle provides a useful tool to plan your weekly fitness routine.

4. A training log will help you monitor your progress toward achieving total fitness.

5. Your fitness action plan should take the following guidelines into consideration: Adopt a gradual, consistent approach to exercise; exercise with friends, if possible; vary your training activities and routine; get enough sleep; adapt to changing schedules; anticipate lapses in your training program; and combine exercise with other healthy behaviors.

6. Although exercise provides major health benefits, exercise alone cannot guarantee good health. Choosing a healthy diet and avoiding harmful habits such as smoking and drug abuse can also make a big difference.

7. Aging and other life changes will require adjustments in your fitness program.

8. The term wellness encompasses physical, emotional, intellectual, spiritual, social, and environmental health.

9. When planning goals, make sure your goals are SMART. SMART stands for: Specific, Measureable, Action-oriented, Realistic, and Time-stamped.

10. Prioritize your goals. Choose behaviors to change that are contributing the most to decreasing your level of wellness.

11. Monitor your progress. Record your actions in a Behavior Change Log and plot your progress. This gives you an idea of the obstacles you face and allows you to gain motivation as you see success.

STUDY QUESTIONS

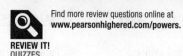

Find more review questions online at
www.pearsonhighered.com/powers.

REVIEW IT!
QUIZZES

1. The first and most important step in establishing a personal fitness plan is
   a. selecting your activities.
   b. creating a training log.
   c. establishing goals.
   d. planning your weekly fitness routine.

2. Most health benefits will occur with _____ minutes of exercise per week.
   a. 50–75   b. 80–100   c. 120–150   d. 200–250

3. Exercise training to improve muscular strength should be performed
   a. 2–3 days per week.
   b. 4–5 days per week.
   c. 5–6 days per week.
   d. 6–7 days per week.

4. At a minimum, stretching should be performed at least
   a. 1 day per week.
   b. 2 days per week.
   c. 3 days per week.
   d. 4 days per week.

5. Which of the following is contained in the concept of wellness?
   a. Consumer health
   b. Disease health
   c. Driving health
   d. Environmental health

6. The first step in development of a wellness plan is to:
   a. monitor your progress.
   b. plan your behavior changes for wellness.
   c. establish your goals.
   d. choose which aspect of wellness you will change.

7. One aspect of being an informed health care consumer is understanding
   a. the medical use of drugs.
   b. your health insurance.
   c. how foods are metabolized in the body.
   d. how to rid your life of stress.

8. A key to weight loss is
   a. use of a support network.
   b. avoidance of rewards.
   c. make sure that one reason you are losing weight is to please others.
   d. develop a plan before establishing your goals.

9. Your wellness action plan should
   a. begin quickly and progress as fast as you can.
   b. not include friends and family.
   c. not incorporate variety in your actions.
   d. adapt to changing schedules.

10. Describe the four steps to developing (a) a fitness plan and (b) a wellness plan.

11. Discuss the three major types of fitness goals, and describe the guidelines which can help you establish your personal fitness goals.

12. What are the components of the FITT principle, and how do these apply to planning your weekly fitness routine?

13. Explain why it is important to take your current fitness level into account when developing your exercise plan.

14. Discuss how keeping a log of your actions will help you reach your wellness goals.

HELPFUL WEBLINKS

For links to the organizations and websites listed, visit
www.pearsonhighered.com/powers.

DO IT!
WEBLINKS

American College of Sports Medicine
This website contains a large volume of contemporary material related to exercise and health. www.acsm.org

Association for Applied Sport Psychology
This site contains a wealth of information about goal-setting and adherence to exercise programs. www.appliedsportpsych.org

Behavior Change/Lifestyle Management Programs
University of California–Riverside provides programs and behavior change direction.
http://wellness.ucr.edu/behavior_change_programs.html

Guide to Behavior Change
National Heart, Lung, and Blood Institute's guide to changing behavior to improve heart health. www.nhlbi.nih.gov/health/public/heart/obesity/lose_wt/behavior.htm

Mayo Clinic
This is a health-related website that contains numerous tips on beginning fitness and wellness programs. www.mayoclinic.org

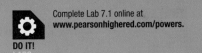
Name _____ **Date** _____

Personal Fitness Program Contract and Short-Term Fitness Goals

I, _____ (signature), am making a commitment to follow my personal fitness plan and achieve my established short-term goals.

My program will begin on _____(date).

My short-term goals:

a.　Performance goals: _____

b.　Body composition goals: _____

c.　Adherence goals: _____

Upon achievement of my goals, I will reward myself as follows:

a.　_____ (goal #1) _____ (date) _____ (reward)

b.　_____ (goal #2) _____ (date) _____ (reward)

c.　_____ (goal #3) _____ (date) _____ (reward)

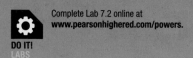
Name _____ **Date** _____

Personal Fitness Program Contract and Intermediate/Long-Term Fitness Goals

I, _____ (signature), am making a commitment to follow my personal fitness plan and achieve my established intermediate and long-term goals.

My intermediate-term goals:

a. Performance goals: _____

b. Body composition goals: _____

c. Adherence goals: _____

My long-term goals:

a. Performance goals: _____

b. Body composition goals: _____

c. Adherence goals: _____

Upon achievement of my goals, I will reward myself as follows:

a. _____ (goal #1) _____ (date) _____ (reward)

b. _____ (goal #2) _____ (date) _____ (reward)

c. _____ (goal #3) _____ (date) _____ (reward)

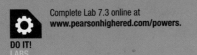
Name _____   **Date** _____

Planning a Personal Fitness Program

Use this lab to plan your personal fitness program. Record the appropriate information in the spaces provided below.

Activity	Intensity*	Duration (min/day)	Monday	Tuesday	Wednesday	Thursday	Friday	Saturday	Sunday
Cardiorespiratory endur-ance exercise									
Muscular strength/ endurance exercise									
Stretching exercises to improve flexibility									

* Establish intensity for your cardiorespiratory endurance exercise using heart rate or RPE (see Chapter 3)

LABORATORY 7.4

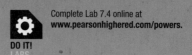
Name _____   **Date** _____

Wellness Profile

In the chapters that follow, you will be introduced to various aspects of wellness and the skills necessary to make significant changes in your behavior. As you prepare to examine the concepts in more detail, you can use this lab to predict what your strengths will be in the six areas of wellness. Refer back to this lab later to reexamine this list, and update it as you evaluate your personal wellness goals and make plans for improving wellness.

Write your top three strengths for each component of wellness below.

PHYSICAL WELLNESS

Maintaining overall physical health and participating in physical activities. Examples of strengths include cardiorespiratory endurance, balance, and flexibility.

1. _____
2. _____
3. _____

EMOTIONAL WELLNESS

Possessing a positive self-concept and dealing appropriately with your feelings. Strengths may include self-confidence, trust, and optimism.

1. _____
2. _____
3. _____

INTELLECTUAL WELLNESS

Retaining knowledge, thinking critically about issues, making sound decisions, and finding solutions to problems. Strengths may include inquisitiveness, curiosity, and dedication.

1. _____
2. _____
3. _____

SOCIAL WELLNESS

Developing lasting relationships with family and friends and contributing to the community. Strengths in this area may include compassion and friendliness.

1. _____
2. _____
3. _____

ENVIRONMENTAL WELLNESS

Protecting yourself from environmental hazards and minimizing your negative impact on the environment. Behaviors such as recycling and carpooling are examples of strengths in this aspect of wellness.

1. _____
2. _____
3. _____

SPIRITUAL WELLNESS

Having a sense of meaning and purpose in life. Behaviors such as prayer, meditation, helping others, and enjoying nature are examples of strengths along this dimension.

1. _____

2. _____

3. _____

Is there an aspect of wellness that you need to develop more fully? If so, which one? What are some specific behaviors you can do now to improve this wellness component in your life?

_____

_____

_____

_____

_____

_____

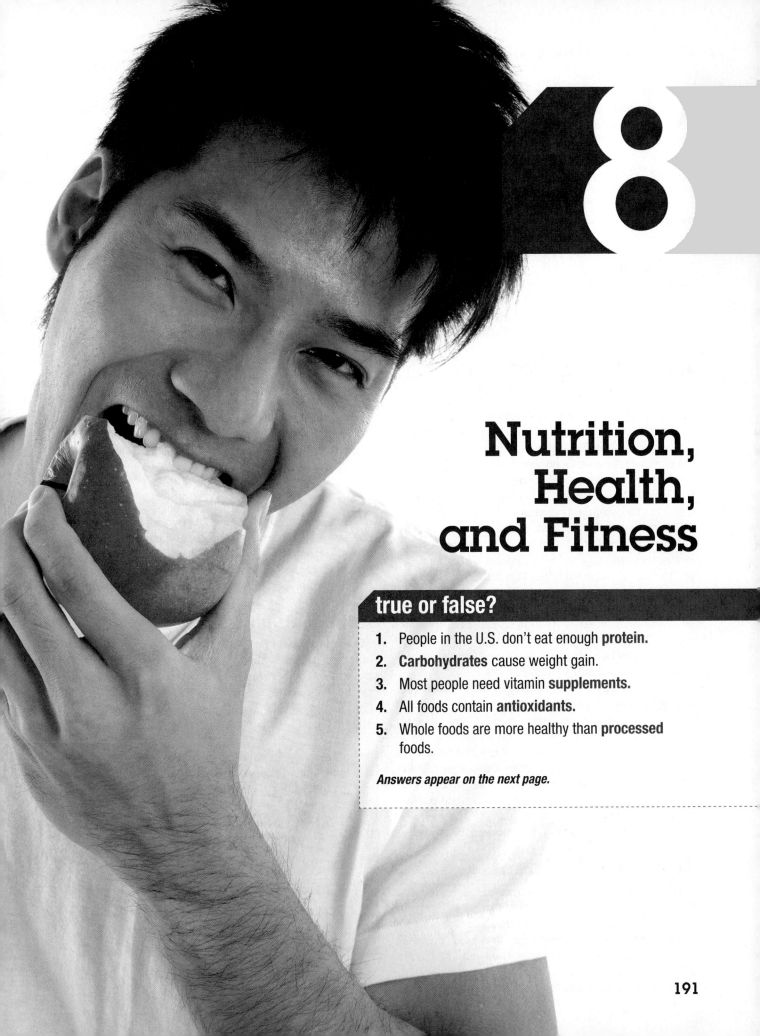

8

Nutrition, Health, and Fitness

true or false?

1. People in the U.S. don't eat enough **protein.**
2. **Carbohydrates** cause weight gain.
3. Most people need vitamin **supplements.**
4. All foods contain **antioxidants.**
5. Whole foods are more healthy than **processed** foods.

Answers appear on the next page.

When you sit down to lunch at your campus cafeteria, do you think to yourself, "Wow, this looks like a great plate of protein, carbohydrate, and phytochemicals"? Or are you more likely to appreciate the hamburger, french fries, and ketchup on your tray? You probably don't often consider the nutrient components of food or how they ultimately drive your body to function, but understanding these nutrients, and the processes that break them down to make them available for use, can help you appreciate their importance to health and help you improve your food choices.

In this chapter, we'll find out how your body uses the food you eat. We'll discuss the classes of nutrients and their functions, the fundamental concepts of good nutrition, and guidelines for a healthy diet. We also explore how exercise training can modify nutritional requirements.

What Is Nutrition and Why Is It Important?

Nutrition is the study of food and the way the body uses it to produce energy and build and repair itself. It involves understanding the relationship between food and health or disease. Good nutrition means a diet that supplies all of the essential nutrients required to maintain a healthy body. Consuming too much or too little of any of the essential nutrients will eventually lead to health problems. In the past, it was dietary deficiencies of nutrients that caused health problems for many people; for example, insufficient intake of vitamin C can lead to scurvy, and insufficient iron intake can lead to a form of anemia—both of which were once prevalent in much of the world's population (and are still common in the developing world). Although these conditions still exist today, excess consumption of calories, and the overweight and obesity that result, are greater causes of health problems in the United States.

Diets that are too high in calories, sugar, fats, and/or sodium have been linked to diseases and conditions such as cardiovascular disease, cancer, obesity, and diabetes, which are the leading killers in the United States (1). According to the U.S. Department of Health and Human Services, over half of all deaths are associated with health problems linked to poor nutrition (2). The good news is that analyzing and modifying your diet can help prevent many of these nutrition-related diseases. A basic understanding of nutrition is therefore important for everyone.

What Are Nutrients?

Nutrients are the basic substances in foods that your body uses to maintain health. They can be divided into two categories: macronutrients and micronutrients. The **macronutrients** (carbohydrates, fats, and proteins) are needed in greater amounts; they primarily build and maintain body tissues and provide energy for daily activities. **Micronutrients** (vitamins and minerals) are

needed in much smaller amounts by your body, but they are essential for numerous processes, including regulating cell functions. The final class of nutrient is water, which is so important for body function that you can't survive more than a few days without it.

Macronutrients

Macronutrients provide the energy, in the form of **kilocalories** (more commonly called *calories*), that your body needs daily to function. Carbohydrates and protein provide 4 calories per gram, and fat provides 9 calories per gram. Under normal conditions, carbohydrates and fats are the primary fuels the body uses to produce

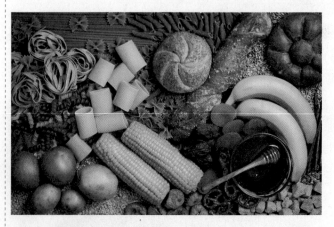

Whole grains, pasta, potatoes, fruits, and vegetables can be excellent sources of carbohydrates.

TABLE 8.1 Food Sources of the Macronutrients		
Carbohydrate (4 calories/gram)	Protein (4 calories/gram)	Fat (9 calories/gram)
Grains	Meats	Butter
Fruits	Fish	Margarine
Vegetables	Poultry	Oils
Concentrated sweets	Eggs	Shortening
Bread	Milk	Cream
Beans/peas	Beans	
	Rice	

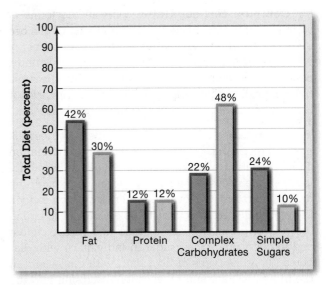

Key

— Typical Diet

— Recommended Diet

FIGURE 8.1

The recommended nutritionally balanced diet compared with the typical U.S. diet. The average American consumes too much fat and simple sugar, and too few complex carbohydrates.

Source: Block, G. Junk foods account for 30% of caloric intake. *Journal of Food Composition and Analysis* 17:439–447, 2004.

energy. The primary role of protein is to build and repair tissues, though when carbohydrate is in short supply or the body is under stress, protein can be used for energy. A well-balanced diet is composed of approximately 58% carbohydrates (including complex carbohydrates and simple sugars), 30% fat, and 12% protein **(Figure 8.1)**.

Table 8.1 lists some major food sources of carbohydrates, proteins, and fats.

Carbohydrates   Whole grains, pasta, fruits, and vegetables are excellent sources of **carbohydrates,** the main source of fuel for your brain. Carbohydrates are especially important during many types of physical activity, because they are a key energy source for muscular contraction. However, not all carbohydrates are created equal—simple carbohydrates (or sugars) are easier for the body to break down and use for energy; complex carbohydrates (starch and fiber) can be used for energy but also serve other purposes.

Types of Carbohydrates   Simple carbohydrates consist of chains of one or two simple sugars. **Glucose** is the most noteworthy of the simple sugars because it is the only sugar molecule that can be used directly by the body. To be used for fuel, all other carbohydrates must first be converted to glucose. The body stores glucose in the form of **glycogen** in skeletal muscles and the liver. Glucose that is not immediately used for energy or stored as glycogen will be stored as fat for future energy use. The central nervous system uses glucose almost exclusively for its energy needs. If you don't consume enough carbohydrates in food, your body has to make glucose from protein. This is undesirable because it results in the breakdown of body protein for use as fuel. Dietary carbohydrates are important not only as a direct fuel source, but also for their protein-sparing effect.

There are several other simple sugars found in foods, including fructose, galactose, lactose, maltose, and sucrose. Fructose is found primarily in fruit, and galactose and lactose are found in milk and dairy products. Maltose is found in some grains, and sucrose, commonly known as table sugar, is the white, granular product used for household baking.

nutrition The study of food and the way the body uses it to produce energy and build or repair body tissues.

nutrients Substances in food that are necessary for good health.

macronutrients Carbohydrates, fats, and proteins, which are necessary for building and maintaining body tissues and providing energy for daily activities.

micronutrients Vitamins and minerals. Micronutrients are involved in many body processes, including regulating cell function.

kilocalorie The unit of measure used to quantify food energy or the energy expended by the body. Technically, a kilocalorie is the amount of energy necessary to raise the temperature of 1 gram of water 1°C. The terms *kilocalorie* and *calorie* are often used interchangeably.

carbohydrate A macronutrient that is a key energy source for muscular contraction.

glucose A simple carbohydrate (sugar) that can be used directly by the body. All other carbohydrates must be converted to glucose before being used for fuel.

glycogen The storage form of glucose in the liver and skeletal muscles.

Complex carbohydrates come in the forms of starch and fiber. **Starches** are long chains of glucose units and are often used for that sudden burst of energy we need during physical activity. **Fiber** is a stringy, nondigestible carbohydrate found in plants. Because fiber is nondigestible, it is not a fuel source. However, it is important in helping prevent some chronic diseases.

The Importance of Fiber Dietary fiber provides bulk in the intestinal tract. This bulk aids in the formation and elimination of food waste products, thus reducing the time necessary for wastes to move through the digestive system and lowering the risk of colon cancer. Dietary fiber is also thought to be a factor in reducing the risk of coronary heart disease and breast cancer and in controlling blood sugar in individuals with diabetes (3). Some types of fiber bind with cholesterol in the digestive tract and prevent its absorption into the blood, thereby reducing blood cholesterol levels.

Fiber can be classified according to its viscosity (its thickness when mixed with digestive juices in the intestines). **Soluble fiber** is more viscous than **insoluble fiber** and is usually found in oats, barley, beans, peas, and citrus fruits. Insoluble fiber is typically concentrated in whole wheat and vegetables. A higher viscosity slows transit in the intestines, allowing nutrients to be absorbed more readily. This helps in regulating glucose levels, appetite, and the reabsorption of bile acids. The primary health benefit of insoluble fiber is its water-binding capacity, which quickens transit time in the large intestine. A faster transit time also helps maintain regularity of bowel movements and reduces the risk of colon cancer (4).

You should eat a minimum of 25 grams of fiber a day; however, be aware that excessive amounts of fiber in the diet can cause intestinal discomfort and decreased absorption of calcium and iron into the blood (3). Your best bet for getting plenty of fiber is to eat adequate amounts of whole grains, legumes, fruits, and vegetables (including the skins) every day. You'll also want to drink plenty of fluid to prevent constipation.

Carbohydrates in Foods Some foods, such as pasta, potatoes, and bread, are famous for containing high amounts of carbohydrates, but there are numerous other foods that can also contribute to your daily carbohydrate needs. Fruits and honey provide fructose. Dairy foods contain lactose. Sucrose is found in table sugar, including some of the packets you may use to sweeten your coffee or tea. Starch is plentiful in potatoes, corn, bread, and rice, and fiber is found in all plant-derived foods.

Fats and Lipids Fats (technically known as **triglycerides**) are actually one type in a larger class of substances called **lipids.** Fats are the most common type of lipid found in foods and in your body. Once consumed, they are broken down and used to produce energy to power muscle contractions during exercise. Fat is an efficient storage form for energy, because at 9 calories per gram, it holds more than twice the energy of either carbohydrate or protein.

Excess fat in the diet is stored in fat cells located under the skin and around internal organs. In addition to fat you take in from foods, your body forms fat from excess carbohydrates and protein in the diet.

Although fat is often avoided by people who want to lose weight, you would never want to eliminate it from your diet. Dietary fat is the only source of linoleic and linolenic acids, the two fatty acids that are essential for normal growth and healthy skin. Fat also protects internal organs and assists in absorbing, transporting, and storing the fat-soluble vitamins A, D, E, and K.

Types of Fats Triglycerides are made up of three **fatty acids** (essentially, chains of carbon and hydrogen atoms) attached to a glycerol backbone. Depending on their structure, fatty acids are classified as monounsaturated, polyunsaturated, saturated, or *trans*.

Unsaturated fatty acids include monounsaturated and polyunsaturated fatty acids. They are found in plants (including nuts, seeds, grains, and vegetable oils) and are liquid at room temperature. Unsaturated fats, which contain mostly unsaturated fatty acids, are thought to be the most heart-healthy because of their effect on blood cholesterol levels. Monounsaturated fats lower LDL and polyunsaturated fats lower LDL and HDL (we'll discuss cholesterol later in the chapter).

One type of polyunsaturated fatty acid, called **omega-3 fatty acid,** is reported to lower both blood cholesterol and triglycerides. This fatty acid is found primarily in fish, especially fresh or frozen mackerel, herring, tuna, and salmon. Some researchers have argued that one or two servings per week of fish containing omega-3 fatty acids reduce the risk of heart disease (5). However, some people, in particular pregnant women and children, may need to limit their consumption of these fish because of the possibility of methlymercury contamination (see the Appreciating Diversity box on page 195).

Saturated fatty acids are solid at room temperature. They generally come from animal sources (meat and dairy products), but some (coconut oil, for example), come from plant sources. Saturated fatty acids increase LDL and levels of total blood cholesterol. High cholesterol levels, in turn, promote the buildup of fatty plaque in the coronary arteries, which can eventually lead to heart disease (Chapter 10).

Trans fatty acids, found primarily in baked and fried foods, but also naturally in some animal foods (see **Figure 8.2** on page 195), tend to raise total cholesterol and LDL levels in the blood. For this reason, they are considered to be heart-unhealthy. The U.S. Food

APPRECIATING DIVERSITY

Should Pregnant Women Eat Fish?

Seafood can be an important part of a healthy diet during pregnancy. Fish is low in fat and a great source of high-quality protein and other nutrients. However, some fish may contain a form of mercury that could harm the nervous system of a developing fetus. Pregnant women need to know the types of fish that carry the highest risk of containing methylmercury and other contaminants so that they can avoid or reduce their intake of these fish during pregnancy.

Methylmercury is a toxin produced from inorganic mercury that gets into water after the burning of wastes and fossil fuels. It enters the food chain when fish and other aquatic organisms acquire it from the water. When larger fish eat smaller fish, the methylmercury from the smaller fish will accumulate in the larger fish's body. Thus older, larger fish have higher concentrations of methylmercury in their bodies than smaller, younger fish. Some of the highest levels of methylmercury are found in large predatory fish, such as shark, swordfish, king mackerel, and tilefish, so pregnant women should avoid these species. However, eating less than 12 ounces per week of other species, such as shellfish, canned fish, small ocean fish, or farm-raised fish, can safely provide protein and other nutrients.

In addition to the wild or farmed fish found in the local grocery store, pregnant women also need to be aware of the risks for contamination of locally caught fish. The U.S. Environmental Protection Agency (EPA) provides current advice on consuming fish from your local freshwater lakes and streams. You can also contact your state or local health department for specific consumption recommendations about fish caught or sold in your area.

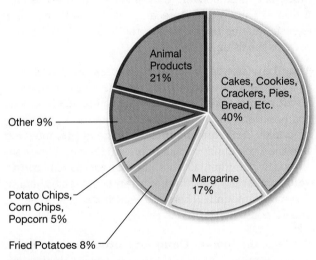

FIGURE 8.2
Major sources of *trans* fat in the diet.

Sources: National Cancer Institute. Sources of saturated fat in the diets of the U.S. population ages 2 years and older, NHANES 2005-2006; USDA and HHS. *Dietary Guidelines for Americans, 2010.* www.health.gov/dietaryguidelines.

and Drug Administration (FDA) recommends limiting the amount of *trans* fat in the diet—and even requires that food manufacturers list *trans* fat on food labels—to help consumers avoid products that contain it. Some U.S. cities, including New York and Philadelphia, have banned or greatly restricted the use of *trans* fats in restaurants. As more is learned about the effects of *trans* fats on health, food manufacturers and restaurateurs are likely to phase it out of their products.

Worried about mercury in your fish? Watch *Which Fish Is Safest to Eat?* at **www.pearsonhighered.com/powers.**

SEE IT! VIDEOS

complex carbohydrates Long chains of sugar units linked together to form starch or fiber.

starches Long chains of glucose units; commonly found in foods such as corn, grains, and potatoes.

fiber A stringy, nondigestible complex carbohydrate found in whole grains, vegetables, and fruits.

soluble fiber Viscous fiber found in oats, barley, peas, and citrus fruits.

insoluble fiber Type of fiber found in whole wheat and vegetables.

fats (triglycerides) The form of lipid that is broken down in the body and used to produce energy to power muscle contractions during exercise.

lipids A group of insoluble compounds that include fats and cholesterol.

fatty acids The basic structural unit of triglycerides; they are important nutritionally not only because of their energy content, but also because they play a role in cardiovascular disease.

unsaturated fatty acid A type of fatty acid that comes primarily from plant sources and is liquid at room temperature.

omega-3 fatty acid A type of unsaturated fatty acid that lowers both blood cholesterol and triglycerides and is found abundantly in some fish.

saturated fatty acid A type of fatty acid that comes primarily from animal sources and is solid at room temperature.

***trans* fatty acid** A type of fatty acid that increases cholesterol in the blood and is a major contributor to heart disease.

Other Types of Lipids In addition to fat, there are two other forms of lipids: **phospholipids** and **sterols.** Phospholipids are important components of cell membranes and play a key role in emulsification. The most common sterol, **cholesterol,** is an important component of cells and is used to manufacture certain types of hormones, including some male and female sex hormones.

Lipoproteins are combinations of protein, triglycerides, and cholesterol. Although lipoproteins exist in several forms, the two primary types are low-density lipoproteins (LDL cholesterol) and high-density lipoproteins (HDL cholesterol). LDL, or "bad," cholesterol consists of a limited amount of protein and triglycerides but contains large amounts of cholesterol. It is associated with promoting fatty plaque buildup in the arteries of the heart, which is the primary cause of heart disease. In contrast, HDL, or "good," cholesterol is primarily composed of protein, has limited amounts of cholesterol, and is associated with a low risk of heart disease. (We discuss HDL and LDL cholesterol again in Chapter 10.)

Fats and Lipids in Foods You can find "good" fats, including the two essential fatty acids, in fish, seeds, nuts, and vegetable oils. Unhealthy, saturated fats are found in fatty meats, butter, lard, fried foods, and many baked items. These items should be avoided or eaten only in limited amounts.

complete proteins Proteins containing all the essential amino acids; found only in soy and animal foods (meats and dairy products).

incomplete proteins Proteins that are missing one or more of the essential amino acids; found in plant sources such as nuts and legumes.

phospholipid A type of lipid that contains phosphorus and is an important component of cell membranes.

sterol A type of lipid that does not contain fatty acids; cholesterol is the most commonly known sterol.

cholesterol A type of lipid that is necessary for cell and hormone synthesis. Found naturally in animal foods, but made in adequate amounts in the body.

lipoproteins Combinations of protein, triglycerides, and cholesterol in the blood that are important because of their role in influencing the risk of heart disease.

amino acids The building blocks of protein. There are 20 different amino acids that can be linked in various combinations to create different proteins.

essential amino acids The nine amino acids that cannot be manufactured by the body and must therefore be consumed in the diet.

nonessential amino acids Eleven amino acids that the body can make and are therefore not necessary in the diet.

Dietary cholesterol is present in many foods from animal sources, including meats, shellfish, and dairy products. Although your body needs some cholesterol for normal functioning, you actually don't need to consume cholesterol from foods, because your body can make all that it needs. In fact, diets high in saturated fats cause the body to produce more than normal amounts of cholesterol.

 Should restaurants be forced to post calorie counts? Watch *You Are What You Eat* at www.pearsonhighered.com/powers.

SEE IT! VIDEOS

Proteins The primary role of protein is to serve as the structural unit to build and repair body tissues, including muscle and connective tissue. Proteins are also important for the synthesis of enzymes, hormones, and antibodies. These compounds regulate body metabolism and provide protection from disease.

As mentioned earlier, proteins are not usually a major fuel source. However, if your dietary intake of carbohydrates is too low (such as during a diet or fast), proteins can be converted to glucose and used as fuel. If you consume adequate amounts of carbohydrates, excess calories from dietary protein are stored in adipose tissue as an energy reserve.

The Structure of Proteins The basic structural units of proteins are called **amino acids.** There are 20 different amino acids, and they can be linked in various combinations to create different proteins with unique functions. Some are **essential amino acids,** meaning that the body cannot make them and they must be consumed in the diet. Others are **nonessential amino acids,** meaning that the body can synthesize them in adequate amounts. There are 9 essential amino acids, and 11 nonessential amino acids.

Protein in Foods **Complete proteins** contain all of the essential amino acids and are present only in animal foods and soy products. **Incomplete proteins** are missing one or more of the essential amino acids and are present in numerous vegetable sources. Vegetarians, who avoid animal foods, must be careful to eat a variety of foods so that they consume all of the essential amino acids.

Because of its role in building body tissue, protein is particularly important during periods of rapid growth, such as adolescence. Adolescents need to take in more than 12% of their calories from protein (the recommended amount for adults). For adolescents, the recommended dietary allowance (RDA) for proteins is 1 gram per kilogram of body weight (3). The recommendation decreases to 0.8 g/kg in women and 0.9 g/kg in men at the end of adolescence (see **Figure 8.3** on page 197).

Because the average person in industrialized countries consumes more than enough protein, the nutritional problem associated with protein intake is one of excess. Protein foods from animal sources are often high

Calculating Your Protein Needs	Example (Adult Female)
1. Determine your body weight	1. An adult female weighs 132 pounds.
2. Convert pounds (lb) to kilograms (kg) by dividing number of pounds by 2.2	2. 132 / 2.2 lb/kg = 60 kg
3. Multiply by 0.8 (adult females) or 0.9 (adult males) to get an RDA in grams/day	3. 60 kg × 0.8 g/kg = 48 g
	A 132 pound female needs to consume 48 grams of protein per day.

FIGURE 8.3
Estimated daily protein needs for adults. You can calculate the number of grams of protein you should consume daily.

in fat (and high in calories), which can lead to increased risk of heart disease, cancer, and obesity.

Micronutrients

Micronutrients include **vitamins** and **minerals.** Though needed in smaller amounts, micronutrients are as important to body function as macronutrients and are required to sustain life. Although they do not supply energy, they are essential to the breakdown and use of the macronutrients.

Vitamins Vitamins play a key role in many bodily functions, including the regulation of growth and metabolism. Some vitamins are soluble in water; others are soluble in fat. Water-soluble vitamins include the B vitamins and vitamin C. These vitamins are generally not stored in the body and can be eliminated by the kidneys. Vitamins A, D, E, and K are fat soluble. They are stored in body fat and can therefore accumulate to toxic levels. Table 8.2 on page 198 lists some functions and dietary sources of both water-soluble and fat-soluble vitamins.

In addition to their essential roles in body processes, some vitamins and minerals may also protect against tissue damage (3, 6). This has important implications for individuals engaged in an exercise program. This potential new role for micronutrients is discussed later in this chapter.

Minerals Minerals are chemical elements such as sodium and calcium that are required by the body for normal function. Like vitamins, minerals play important roles in regulating key body functions, such as the conduction of nerve impulses, muscular contraction, enzyme function, and maintenance of water balance. Minerals serve a structural function as well; calcium, phosphorus, and fluoride all are important components in bones and teeth.

Three minerals that play important roles in the body are calcium, iron, and sodium. Calcium is important in bone formation. A deficiency of calcium contributes to the development of the bone disease called **osteoporosis.** A deficiency of dietary iron may lead to iron-deficiency **anemia,** which results in chronic fatigue. High sodium intake has been associated with hypertension, a major risk factor for heart disease.

Table 8.3 on page 199 summarizes several key minerals and their functions.

Vitamin and Minerals in Foods Though a few vitamins, including A, D and K, can be made in the body, most must be consumed in foods. If you're eating a balanced diet with plenty of fresh fruits, vegetables, and whole grains, and some lean meat and poultry, you're likely getting all of the vitamins and minerals that you need. (See Tables 8.2 and 8.3 for specific food sources for these and other vitamins and minerals.) In general, the more brightly colored the fruit or vegetable, the higher its vitamin and mineral content. Note that some water-soluble vitamins can be destroyed during cooking or

vitamins Micronutrients that play a key role in many body functions, including the regulation of growth and metabolism. They are classified according to whether they are soluble in water or fat.

minerals Chemical elements (e.g., sodium and calcium) that are required by the body in small amounts for normal functioning.

osteoporosis Bone disease in which the mineral content of bone is reduced and the bone is weakened and at increased risk of fracture.

anemia Deficiency of red blood cells and/or hemoglobin that results in decreased oxygen-carrying capacity of the blood.

TABLE 8.2   Selected Vitamins: Food Sources, Functions, and Deficiency and Toxicity Symptoms

Vitamin	Selected Food Sources	Selected Functions	Deficiency Symptoms	Toxicity Symptoms
Fat-soluble				
A	Liver, spinach, carrots, sweet potatoes; other orange and green leafy vegetables	Necessary for vision, bone growth, fertility	Night blindness, impaired immunity, infertility	Birth defects, loss of appetite, blurred vision, hair loss, liver damage
D	Fortified milk; produced in the skin under sunlight	Regulates blood calcium levels; bone health; cell differentiation	Rickets in children, bone weakness and increased fractures in adults	Hypercalcemia, calcium deposits in kidney and liver
E	Vegetable oils, whole grains, nuts, seeds	Antioxidant; improves absorption of vitamin A	Anemia, impaired nerve transmission, muscle weakness	Inhibited blood clotting
K	Green leafy vegetables; cabbage, cauliflower	Helps with blood clotting	Reduced ability to form blood clots	No known symptoms
Water-soluble				
Thiamin (B$_1$)	Whole grains, organ meat, lean pork	Coenzyme in carbohydrate metabolism and some amino acid metabolism	Beriberi, weight loss, confusion, muscle weakness	No known symptoms
Riboflavin (B$_2$)	Dairy products, enriched breads and cereals, lean meats, poultry, fish	Coenzyme; helps maintain mucous membranes	Sore throat, swelling of the tongue, anemia	No known symptoms
Niacin (B$_3$)	Eggs, poultry, fish, milk, whole grains, nuts, enriched breads and cereals	Coenzyme in carbohydrate and fatty acid metabolism; plays role in DNA replication and repair and cell differentiation	Pellagra, rash, vomiting, constipation or diarrhea	Flushing, liver damage, glucose intolerance, blurred vision
Vitamin B$_6$	Eggs, poultry, fish, whole grains, liver, kidney, pork	Coenzyme involved in amino acid and carbohydrate metabolism; synthesis of blood cells	Dermatitis, anemia, convulsions	Skin lesions
Vitamin B$_{12}$	Meat, fish, poultry, fortified cereals	Coenzyme that assists with blood formation and nervous system function	Pernicious anemia, pale skin, fatigue, shortness of breath, dementia	No known symptoms
Folate	Green leafy vegetables, yeast, oranges, whole grains, legumes	Coenzyme involved in DNA synthesis and amino acid metabolism	Macrocytic anemia, weakness and fatigue, headache, neural tube defects in developing fetus	Masks symptoms of vitamin B$_{12}$ deficiency; neurological damage
Vitamin C	Citrus fruits, peppers, spinach, strawberries, tomatoes, potatoes	Antioxidant; assists with collagen synthesis; enhances immune function; enhances iron absorption	Scurvy, bleeding gums and joints, loose teeth, depression, anemia	Nausea and diarrhea, nosebleeds, abdominal cramps

Source: Thompson, Janice; Manore, Melinda, *Nutrition: An Applied Approach, 3rd Ed.,* © 2012. Reprinted and Electronically reproduced by permission of Pearson Education, Inc., Upper Saddle River, New Jersey.

TABLE 8.3 Selected Minerals: Food Sources, Functions, and Deficiency and Toxicity Symptoms				
Mineral	Selected Food Sources	Selected Functions	Deficiency Symptoms	Toxicity Symptoms
Major minerals				
Calcium	Milk and milk products; sardines; dark green leafy vegetables; fortified orange juice	Builds bones and teeth; helps maintain acid–base balance; maintains normal nerve transmission	Osteoporosis, bone fractures, convulsions and muscle spasms, heart failure	Can interfere with the absorption of iron, zinc, and magnesium; shock, fatigue, kidney failure
Phosphorus	Meat, poultry, fish, eggs, milk, soft drinks	Maintains fluid balance; plays a role in bone formation	Muscle weakness or damage, bone pain, dizziness	Muscle spasms, convulsions, low blood calcium levels
Magnesium	Grains, legumes, nuts (especially almonds and cashews), seeds, soybeans	Essential component of bone tissue; bone growth; supports muscle contraction and blood clotting	Hypomagnesemia, resulting in low blood calcium levels, muscle cramps, spasms, or seizures; chronic diseases such as heart disease, high blood pressure, and osteoporosis	Diarrhea, nausea, abdominal cramps
Potassium	Potatoes, bananas, tomato juice, orange juice	Regulates muscle contraction and transmission of nerve impulses; maintains blood pressure	Muscle weakness, paralysis, confusion	Muscle weakness, irregular heartbeat, vomiting
Sodium	Salt, soy sauce, fast foods and processed foods	Maintains acid–base balance; assists with nerve transmission and muscle contraction	Muscle cramps, dizziness, fatigue, nausea, vomiting, mental confusion	Water retention; high blood pressure; may increase loss of calcium in urine
Trace minerals				
Iron	Meat and poultry; green leafy vegetables; fortified grain products	Assists with oxygen transport in blood and muscle; conenzyme for energy metabolism	Anemia, fatigue, depressed immune function, impaired memory	Nausea, vomiting, diarrhea, dizziness, rapid heartbeat, death
Zinc	Whole grains, meat, liver, seafood	Coenzyme for hemoglobin production; plays role in cell replication, protein synthesis	Growth retardation, diarrhea, delayed sexual maturation, hair loss	Intestinal pain, nausea, vomiting, loss of appetite, diarrhea; headache, depressed immune function
Iodine	Iodized salt, seafood, processed foods	Synthesis of thyroid hormones; temperature regulation	Goiter (enlargement of the thyroid gland), hypothyroidism; deficiency during pregnancy can cause birth defects	Goiter
Fluoride	Fluoridated water, tea, fish	Maintains health of bones and teeth	Dental cavities and tooth decay; lower bone density	Teeth fluorosis (staining and pitting of the teeth); skeletal fluorosis
Selenium	Organ meats, such as liver and kidney; pork; seafood	Antioxidant; immune function; assists in production of thyroid hormone	Keshan disease, impaired immune function, infertility, muscle pain	Brittle hair, skin rashes, weakness, cirrhosis of the liver

Source: Thompson, Janice; Manore, Melinda, *Nutrition: An Applied Approach, 3rd Ed.,* © 2012. Reprinted and Electronically reproduced by permission of Pearson Education, Inc., Upper Saddle River, New Jersey.

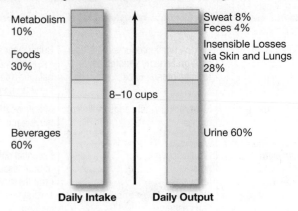

Daily Water Balance in the Body

FIGURE 8.4
The amount of water you consume in food and beverages and that you produce during metabolism is about equal to the amount you excrete in urine, sweat, and feces and through exhalation and insensible water loss.

requirements. **Figure 8.4** compares the sources of water intake and output in the average person.

MAKE SURE YOU KNOW...

- Nutrition is the study of food and its relationship to health and disease.

- Carbohydrates, fat, and protein are the three calorie-containing macronutrients. A well-balanced diet is composed of approximately 58% complex carbohydrates, 30% fat, and 12% protein.

- The kilocalorie is a unit of measure for the energy in food or the energy expended by the body. The kilocalorie is more commonly referred to as the calorie.

- Carbohydrates are the primary source of fuel for the body. Glucose is the most important of the simple carbohydrates, and all other simple and complex carbohydrates must be converted to glucose before being used by the body. Starch and fiber are complex carbohydrates.

- Fats are the most common form of lipid in foods and in the body. All excess calories consumed in the diet will eventually be converted to fat for storage. Dietary cholesterol and *trans* fat are heart-unhealthy, and you should limit or avoid your consumption of foods containing them.

- Proteins, which are made up of amino acids, are the key structural unit for building and repairing cells. All amino acids either are made by the body (nonessential amino acids) or must be consumed in the diet (essential amino acids).

- Vitamins serve many important functions in the body, including facilitating metabolism. The B vitamins and vitamin C are water soluble and are not generally stored by the body. Vitamins A, D, E, and K are fat soluble and can be stored in the body.

- Minerals are chemical elements in foods that, like vitamins, play important roles in many body functions. The mineral

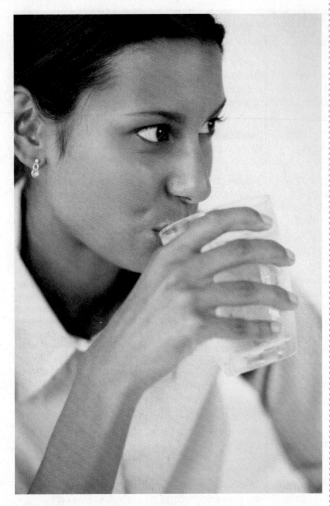

Water is a key ingredient in a healthy diet.

processing, so minimal cooking (such as by steaming, rather than boiling) and eating fresh rather than canned produce will provide higher amounts of micronutrients.

Water

Water makes up approximately 60%–70% of your body, and it is important for everything from temperature regulation, digestion, absorption, and blood formation to waste elimination. Water is especially important for physically active people. A person engaged in heavy exercise in a hot, humid environment can lose 1–3 liters of water per hour through sweating (7). Losing as little as 5% of body water causes fatigue, weakness, and the inability to concentrate; losing more than 15% can be fatal. (Chapter 12 provides guidelines for maintaining proper hydration during exercise training.)

You should consume 8–10 cups of water per day through foods and beverages. Drinking water throughout your day will help you meet this goal, as will eating food with high water content, such as fruits and vegetables. People who experience excess sweating, diarrhea, or vomiting or who donate blood may have higher water calcium is important for bone health, iron is important for healthy blood, and too much sodium can have a negative effect on heart health.

- Approximately 60%–70% of body weight is water. You should consume 8–10 cups of water from foods and beverages each day.

What Are the Guidelines for a Healthy Diet?

Nutrition may seem like a complex subject, but the basics of consuming a healthy diet are fairly simple: Balance the calories, eat a variety of foods, and consume less-healthy foods only in moderation. Additionally, everyone should strive to be physically active.

To make these points more clear, and to provide specific guidance in these areas, several national health agencies have suggested guidelines for healthy diets. For instance, the U.S. Department of Agriculture (USDA) released the *2010 Dietary Guidelines for Americans* in January 2011. These guidelines are focused around two main concepts: First, individuals should maintain calorie balance over time to achieve a healthy weight. Second, individuals should focus on consuming nutrient-dense foods and beverages. Recommendations and specific key points of advice related to these concepts include the following:

- Consume foods and drinks to meet, not exceed, calorie needs. Choose foods that limit the intake of saturated and *trans* (solid) fats, cholesterol, added sugars, salt, and alcohol.

- Maintain appropriate calorie balance during each stage of life.

- Engage in regular physical activity. Avoid physical inactivity.

- Consume sufficient amounts of fruits, vegetables, and whole grains while staying within energy needs. Make half of your plate fruits and vegetables.

- Consume less than 10% of energy intake from saturated fats and less than 300 mg per day of cholesterol; consume as little *trans* fat as possible.

- Choose fiber-rich fruits, vegetables, and whole grains often. Make at least half of your grain whole grains.

- Choose and prepare foods and beverages with little added sugars or caloric sweeteners.

- Consume less than 1 tsp of salt per day.

- If you choose to drink alcohol, do so only in moderation.

- Take proper food safety precautions.

- Account for all food and beverages consumed. Take note of how they fit into a healthy eating plan

Let's explore some of these guidelines in more depth and discuss additional tools you can use, including

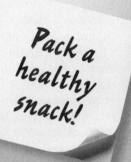

People report that they are more successful in making healthy eating choices when they plan ahead. Consider the following strategies as you plan your consumption for one day.

- Plan to eat something every 2–3 hours. Maintaining steady blood sugar is known to be helpful in reducing cravings.

- To ensure you eat at least 5 servings of fruits and/or vegetables during the day, think about fruits and vegetables you can pack to take along with you. And make sure to take your healthy snacks before you leave in the morning!

- Carefully measure your portions so that they represent actual serving sizes. Be intentional about the items and the amounts you consume.

- Stay hydrated! Hydration is an important strategy in good nutrition. Plan your water intake to match each time you eat.

Pack a healthy snack!

ChooseMyPlate.gov, to plan a healthy diet. You can also use the sample program on pages 218–219 to plan your weekly food intake.

 SEE IT! VIDEOS Learn about sugar's "triple threat." Watch *How Much Sugar?* at **www.pearsonhighered.com/powers.**

 LIVE IT! ASSESS YOURSELF Assess your eating habits with the *Your Eating Habits and Extra Calories* Take Charge of Your Health! Worksheet online at **www.pearsonhighered.com/powers.**

Eat More Fruits, Vegetables, and Whole Grains

Choosing unprocessed foods that are modest in calories and low in fat and sodium is the best way to create a healthy diet. This means doing much of your grocery shopping in the produce aisle (and perhaps stopping by the meat or seafood counter) and buying whole-grain bread and cereal products. When you eat out with friends or dine with your family, try to keep your portions of fatty meats and high-sugar desserts small, and load up on the undressed fruits and vegetables. Similarly, when you're in need of a midmorning or late-afternoon snack, reach for a banana, whole-grain crackers, or air-popped popcorn rather than a bag of chips or chocolate bar.

Once you've adopted these healthy eating strategies, you're likely to see the benefits quickly. You will have more energy and feel less lethargic in the afternoon, and you may even lose weight. Over the long term, you will have a lower risk for many chronic diseases and conditions.

 Assess your shopping habits with the *Grocery Shopping List* Take Charge of Your Health! Worksheet online at **www.pearsonhighered.com/powers.**

LIVE IT! ASSESS YOURSELF

Watch Your Intake of Calories, Sugar, Alcohol, Fat, and Sodium

With the rise in rates of overweight and obesity in the United States, it's clear that the balance of "calories in" versus "calories out" has become an issue for many individuals. Several factors are increasing calorie consumption. For example, people consume a lot of simple sugars, often in the form of sucrose (table sugar) or high fructose corn syrup (a commercial sweetener), which are used to make cakes, candies, and ice cream, as well as to sweeten beverages, cereals, and other foods. The problem with simple sugars is that they often contain many calories but few micronutrients (which is why they're called "empty calories"). An estimated half of the dietary carbohydrate intake of the average U.S. citizen is in the form of simple sugars (3).

The amount of sugar in sweets adds a tremendous amount of calories to the diet. This leads to obesity, which contributes to many health problems (e.g., diabetes). Sugar in sweets also leads to tooth decay. Although brushing your teeth after eating sweets can prevent this problem, it will not solve the other problems related to overconsumption of sugar. One way to trim your sucrose intake is to use sugar substitutes instead of sugar to sweeten some foods or beverages. Artificial sweeteners such as saccharin®, aspartame®, or sucralose® add sweetness with little or no calories.

Alcohol, if consumed in excess, is another source of empty calories that can undermine an otherwise healthy diet. Chronic alcohol consumption also tends to deplete the body's stores of some vitamins, possibly leading to severe deficiencies. Drinking too much alcohol can displace other, healthier foods in the diet by making you too full to eat or causing you to forget to eat. Finally, alcohol significantly increases your risk of accidents and injury. When it comes to drinking alcohol, the best plan is to avoid it or, if you do drink, to do so only in moderation.

consider this!

The average American consumes more than 80 pounds of table sugar and 45 pounds of high fructose corn syrup each year.

Another factor behind the rise in overweight and obesity in the United States is the high amount of fat in many people's diets. Foods high in fat not only tend to be rich in cholesterol, but also contain over twice as many calories per gram as carbohydrate or protein (9 calories/gram versus 4 calories/gram). Limiting fat in the diet helps limit calories and also reduces the risk of heart disease. Both saturated and unsaturated fats are linked to heart disease, obesity, and certain cancers.

When cutting fat from your diet it is important to look at food labels. Look for items that are low in fat or choose nonfat alternatives when available. Also, consider how you prepare food. Baking and broiling are better than frying. Processed foods are often high in fat and sodium, and many dairy products are high in fat. Heavy, cream-based sauces and dressings can add a lot of fat to an otherwise healthy meal. And you can offset one high-fat meal by making sure your other meals are low in fat. Table 8.4 provides guidelines to help you cut your dietary fat intake.

TABLE 8.4 Examples of Low or Non-Fat Alternatives	
High-Fat Choice	**Low or Nonfat Option**
Whole milk	1% or skim milk
Whole milk cheeses	Part skim or fat-free
Fried chicken with the skin	Skinless baked or broiled chicken
Creamy Italian or ranch dressing	Lite Italian or a vinaigrette dressing
Mayonnaise	Mustard
Alfredo sauce	Marinara sauce
Shortening or butter	Cooking spray or olive oil

Having less cholesterol in your diet will help lower your blood cholesterol, which in turn will lower your risk of heart disease. Research has shown that a 1% reduction in dietary cholesterol results in a 2% reduction in risk (Chapter 10). Additionally, many foods that are high in cholesterol are also high in fat (and therefore calories).

Although salt (sodium chloride) is a necessary micronutrient, the body's daily requirement is small (less than ¼ teaspoon, although very active people who perspire a great deal may need over 1½ teaspoons per day). Most people consume much more sodium than they need, however, and this increased intake is putting them at increased risk for high blood pressure (hypertension). You might be surprised just how much salt is in many of your foods. For example, **Figure 8.5** illustrates the "hidden" salt in an average pizza.

As mentioned, consuming too much sodium can be a complicating factor for people with high blood

pressure. In countries where salt is not added to foods, either during cooking or at the table, high blood pressure is virtually unknown (8). Even if you don't already have high blood pressure, you should limit salt in your diet to only the minimal daily requirements.

 Assess your fat intake with the *Cutting out the Fat* Take Charge of Your Health! Worksheet online at **www.pearsonhighered.com/powers.**

LIVE IT! ASSESS YOURSELF

Use the Recommended Dietary Allowances, MyPlate, and Food Labels to Plan Healthy Meals

The National Academy of Sciences has established guidelines concerning the quantities of each micronutrient required to meet the minimum needs of most individuals (9). Recommended Dietary Allowances (also known as RDAs) are the daily amounts of the different food nutrients the Academy deems adequate for healthy individuals (see Table 8.5 on pages 204–205).

However, even today, RDAs for some nutrients are not known. Thus, the Academy has issued additional indices to guide people in monitoring their diets. They refer to these indices as Dietary Reference Intakes (DRIs). DRIs are divided into four categories, each of which addresses a different nutritional issue:

1. *Recommended Dietary Allowance (RDA)*. The RDAs are the amount of nutrient that will meet the needs of almost every healthy person in a specific age and gender group. Also, the latest RDAs are meant to reduce disease risk, not just prevent deficiency.

Ingredients	Mg sodium
Crust	
Pre-made from Pillsbury Hot Roll Mix (whole box)	1536
Sauce	
8 oz. Contadina Pizza Sauce	1350
Toppings	
Mozzarella (8–10 oz at 150 mg/oz)	1200–1500
Pork sausage (170 mg/oz) 6 oz	1020
Canadian bacon 2 oz	1450
Pepperoni 2 oz	1100
Black olives, 5 (sliced)	200
Mushrooms (raw sliced 1/2 cup)	5
Onion (1/2 cup raw)	6
Green pepper (1/2 cup raw)	10
Seasonings/herbs/spices (1 tsp)	500
Total = 8,677 mg sodium	

FIGURE 8.5
The amount of sodium in a typical medium pizza with "the works" will probably surprise you. Even if you eat only two slices, you are still likely consuming more than 1000 mg of sodium! Note, though, that cutting back on the meat toppings and loading up on the veggies will significantly lower the sodium.

consider this!

The average American consumes between 3 and 10 teaspoons of salt per day.

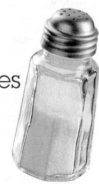

2. *Adequate Intake (AI)*. This value is used when the RDA is not known because the scientific data aren't strong enough to produce a specific recommendation, yet there is enough evidence to give a general guideline. Thus, the AI is an "educated guess" at what the RDA would be if it were known.

TABLE 8.5	Recommended Dietary Allowances of Micronutrients											
	Elements											
Life Stage Group	Calcium (mg/d)	Phosphorus (mg/d)	Magnesium (mg/d)	Iron (mg/d)	Zinc (mg/d)	Selenium (μg/d)	Iodine (μg/d)	Copper (μg/d)	Manganese (mg/d)	Fluoride (mg/d)	Chromium (μg/d)	Molybdenum (μg/d)
Infants												
0 to 6 mo	200*	100*	30*	0.27*	2*	15*	110*	200*	0.003*	0.01*	0.2*	2*
6 to 12 mo	260*	275*	75*	11	3	20*	130*	220*	0.6*	0.5*	5.5*	3*
Children												
1–3 y	700	460	80	7	3	20	90	340	1.2*	0.7*	11*	17
4–8 y	1000	500	130	10	5	30	90	440	1.5*	1*	15*	22
Males												
9–13 y	1300	1250	240	8	8	40	120	700	1.9*	2*	25*	34
14–18 y	1300	1250	410	11	11	55	150	890	2.2*	3*	35*	43
19–30 y	1000	700	400	8	11	55	150	900	2.3*	4*	35*	45
31–50 y	1000	700	420	8	11	55	150	900	2.3*	4*	35*	45
51–70 y	1000	700	420	8	11	55	150	900	2.3*	4*	30*	45
>70 y	1200	700	420	8	11	55	150	900	2.3*	4*	30*	45
Females												
9–13 y	1300	1250	240	8	8	40	120	700	1.6*	2*	21*	34
14–18 y	1300	1250	360	15	9	55	150	890	1.6*	3*	24*	43
19–30 y	1000	700	310	18	8	55	150	900	1.8*	3*	25*	45
31–50 y	1000	700	320	18	8	55	150	900	1.8*	3*	25*	45
51–70 y	1200	700	320	8	8	55	150	900	1.8*	3*	20*	45
>70 y	1200	700	320	8	8	55	150	900	1.8*	3*	20*	45
Pregnancy												
14–18 y	1300	1250	400	27	12	60	220	1000	2.0*	3*	29*	50
19–30 y	1000	700	350	27	11	60	220	1000	2.0*	3*	30*	50
31–50 y	1000	700	360	27	11	60	220	1000	2.0*	3*	30*	50
Lactation												
14–18 y	1300	1250	360	10	13	70	290	1300	2.6*	3*	44*	50
19–30 y	1000	700	310	9	12	70	290	1300	2.6*	3*	45*	50
31–50 y	1000	700	320	9	12	70	290	1300	2.6*	3*	45*	50

3. *Estimated Average Requirement (EAR).* This is a value that is estimated to satisfy the needs of 50% of people in a given age group. It is primarily used to establish the RDA. In addition, it is used for evaluating and planning the diets of large groups of people (such as the army), not individuals.

4. *Tolerable Upper Intake Level (UL).* This is the maximal amount that a person can take without risking "adverse health effects." Anything above this amount might result in toxicity. In most cases,

this number refers to the total intake of the nutrient—from foods, fortified foods, and nutritional supplements.

Once you know the recommended daily allowances for nutrients, the key question is how to choose foods to meet these goals.

MyPlate MyPlate, developed by the USDA, is the latest visual guide to eating healthy. It is a placemat that represents the proportion each food group should have

TABLE 8.5 Recommended Dietary Allowances of Micronutrients (Continued)

							Vitamins							
Life Stage Group	Vitamin A (μg/d)[a]	Vitamin D (μg/d)[b]	Vitamin E (mg/d)[c]	Vitamin K (μg/d)	Thiamin (mg/d)	Riboflavin (mg/d)	Niacin (mg/d)[d]	Pantothenic Acid (mg/d)	Biotin (μg/d)	Vitamin B$_6$ (mg/d)	Folate (μg/d)[e]	Vitamin B$_{12}$ (μg/d)	Vitamin C (mg/d)	Choline (mg/d)
Infants														
0 to 6 mo	400*	400*	4*	2.0*	0.2*	0.3*	2*	1.7*	5*	0.1*	65*	0.4*	40*	125*
6 to 12 mo	500*	400*	5*	2.5*	0.3*	0.4*	4*	1.8*	6*	0.3*	80*	0.5*	50*	150*
Children														
1–3 y	300	600	6	30*	0.5	0.5	6	2*	8*	0.5	150	0.9	15	200*
4–8 y	400	600	7	55*	0.6	0.6	8	3*	12*	0.6	200	1.2	25	250*
Males														
9–13 y	600	600	11	60*	0.9	0.9	12	4*	20*	1	300	1.8	45	375*
14–18 y	900	600	15	75*	1.2	1.3	16	5*	25*	1.3	400	2.4	75	550*
19–30 y	900	600	15	120*	1.2	1.3	16	5*	30*	1.3	400	2.4	90	550*
31–50 y	900	600	15	120*	1.2	1.3	16	5*	30*	1.3	400	2.4	90	550*
51–70 y	900	600	15	120*	1.2	1.3	16	5*	30*	1.7	400	2.4	90	550*
>70 y	900	700	15	120*	1.2	1.3	16	5*	30*	1.7	400	2.4	90	550*
Females														
9–13 y	600	600	11	60*	0.9	0.9	12	4*	20*	1	300	1.8	45	375*
14–18 y	700	600	15	75*	1	1	14	5*	25*	1.2	400	2.4	65	400*
19–30 y	700	600	15	90*	1.1	1.1	14	5*	30*	1.3	400	2.4	75	425*
31–50 y	700	600	15	90*	1.1	1.1	14	5*	30*	1.3	400	2.4	75	425*
51–70 y	700	600	15	90*	1.1	1.1	14	5*	30*	1.5	400	2.4	75	425*
>70 y	700	800	15	90*	1.1	1.1	14	5*	30*	1.5	400	2.4	75	425*
Pregnancy														
14–18 y	750	600	15	75*	1.4	1.4	18	6*	30*	1.9	600	2.6	80	450*
19–30 y	770	600	15	90*	1.4	1.4	18	6*	30*	1.9	600	2.6	85	450*
31–50 y	770	600	15	90*	1.4	1.4	18	6*	30*	1.9	600	2.6	85	450*
Lactation														
14–18 y	1200	600	19	75*	1.4	1.6	17	7*	35*	2	500	2.8	115	550*
19–30 y	1300	600	19	90*	1.4	1.6	17	7*	35*	2	500	2.8	120	550*
31–50 y	1300	600	19	90*	1.4	1.6	17	7*	35*	2	500	2.8	120	550*

Source: Adapted from Thompson, Janice; Manore, Melinda, *Nutrition: An Applied Approach, 3rd Ed.*, © 2012. Reprinted and Electronically reproduced by permission of Pearson Education, Inc., Upper Saddle River, New Jersey.

Note: This table is adapted from the DRI reports; see www.nap.edu. It lists Recommended Dietary Allowances (RDAs), with Adequate Intakes (AIs) indicated by asterisks (*). RDAs and AIs may both be used as goals for individual intake. RDAs are set to meet the needs of almost all (97% to 98%) individuals in a group. For healthy breastfed infants, the AI is the mean intake. The AI for other life stage and gender groups is believed to cover the needs of all individuals in the group, but lack of data prevent being able to specify with confidence the percentage of individuals covered by this intake.

[a]Given as retinal activity equivalents (RAE).

[b]Also known as calciferol. The DRI values are based on the absence of adequate exposure to sunlight.

[c]Also known as α-tocopherol.

[d]Given as niacin equivalents (NE), except for infants 0–6 months, which are expressed as performed niacin.

[e]Given as dietary folate equivalents (DFE).

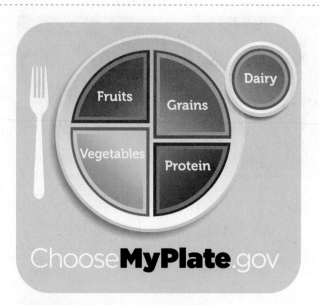

FIGURE 8.6
The USDA's MyPlate food guidance system reminds you to eat a varied diet with lots of nutrient-dense foods and to incorporate physical activity into your daily routine.

Source: www.choosemyplate.gov

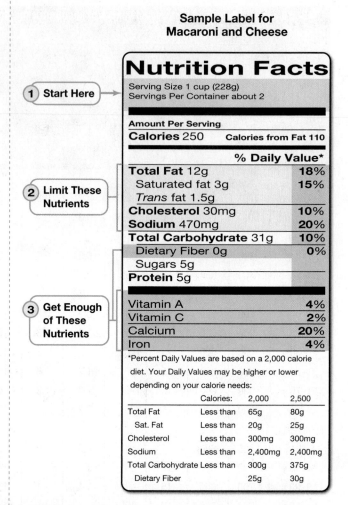

FIGURE 8.7
The Nutrition Facts label can help you select foods that are low in fat, cholesterol, sodium, and calories and that are adequate in protein, vitamins A and C, iron, and calcium. The % Daily Value (DV) helps you determine how good a source a food is for a given nutrient. In general, foods with less than 5% of the DV are considered low in a nutrient, whereas those with more than 20% of the DV are considered high in that nutrient.

Source: U.S. Department of Agriculture. *Dietary Guidelines for Americans 2000.* Washington, DC: U.S. Government Printing Office.

on a healthy plate, thus serving as a reminder about making healthy choices when eating (**Figure 8.6**). For instance, you can see that half of the plate is comprised of fruits and vegetable, fitting with 2010 Dietary Guidelines.

Another tool that the consumer can use when making food choices is the food label that's required on almost all packaged foods (**Figure 8.7**). Among the important information contained on the label is the number of calories per serving, a list of ingredients found in the food (listed in order of the amount contained), the amount of sodium and fat per serving, and the percent **Daily Values** of total fat, carbohydrate, and protein.

Now that we have presented the guidelines for a healthy diet, let's put these principles into practice and construct a day's healthy diet. As we discuss the steps for choosing the right foods, refer to Table 8.6 on page 207, which presents a sample of a healthful 1-day diet for a college-aged woman weighing 132 pounds and with light to moderate daily activities. Her projected daily caloric need is approximately 1980 calories (see Figure 9.1 in Chapter 9 to estimate daily calorie needs based on activity level). To use of this diet plan for yourself, adjust the quantities accordingly.

Breakfast A healthy breakfast might include a grapefruit, whole-grain cereal, skim milk, and a banana. This meal would provide two fruits, one bread/cereal, and one dairy product to start the day. The breakfast is low in fat, cholesterol, and sodium. A quarter of her protein need is met, as well as over 40% of her calcium and iron needs. The fruits alone provide almost all of the recommended vitamin A and C intake for the day.

Snack A morning snack adds some energy and helps to suppress the appetite before lunch. You might choose a second dairy product for the day (in this example, low-fat yogurt) that provides 115 calories of energy and lots of calcium. A handful of almonds adds some protein, and is good source of fiber.

Lunch For lunch, a turkey sandwich (made with low-sodium turkey) on whole-wheat bread and a handful of baby carrots will provide one serving of meat, two more servings of breads/cereals, and one vegetable. Adding lettuce and tomato to the sandwich will provide additional vegetables with few calories and extra vitamins and minerals. This lunch provides a low-calorie meal with lots of protein, vitamin A, and iron.

TABLE 8.6	Sample Diet for a College-Aged Female Weighing 132 Pounds, Assuming Light to Moderate Daily Activities								
	kcal	Fat (g)	Cholesterol (mg)	Sodium (mg)	Carbohydrate (g)	Protein (g)	Vitamin A (RE)*	Vitamin C (mg)	Calcium (mg)
Breakfast									
½ grapefruit	41	0	0	0	10	1	59	44	15
Whole-grain cereal (1 cup)	114	0.5	0	207	29	2	155	16	104
Skim milk (1 cup)	83	0	5	103	12	8	149	0	299
1 banana	105	0	0	1	27	1	4	10	6
Snack									
Low-fat yogurt (4 oz.)	115	1	5	66	22	5	11	0	172
Almonds, dry roasted w/o salt added (1 oz.)	169	14	0	0	5	6	0	0	75
Lunch									
Turkey sandwich: whole-wheat bread with lettuce, tomato and mustard	199	1.6	19	446	27	15	67	7	81
Baby carrots (8)	33	0	0	55	8	1	668	5	26
Snack									
Trail mix with nuts, seeds, and dried fruit (½ cup)	176	7	0	2	13	6	0	0	30
Mozzarella string cheese stick, low sodium (1)	78	4.5	15	4	1	8	38	0	205
Dinner									
Whole-wheat pasta with meatless tomato sauce 1½ cups)	363	8	3	818	62	11	99	3	56
Mushrooms (½ cup)	22	0	0	2	4	2	0	3	5
Whole-wheat dinner rolls (2)	149	2.7	0	268	29	5	0	0	59
Broccoli (2 spears)	26	0	0	30	5	2	57	48	30
Fruit salad (1 cup)	93	0	0	2	24	1	28	26	14
Evening Snack									
Skim milk (1 cup)	83	0	0	103	12	8	149	0	299
Multigrain pretzels (½ cup)	76	0	0	2	16	2	0	0	6
Totals	1925	51	52	2110	302	85	1486	163	1481
RDA	1980	<30%	<300	<2300	<58%	48	700	75	1000
% of RDA	97	9	17	92	105	177	212	217	148

*RE = retinol equivalents

Snack A light snack of trail mix made with nuts, seeds, and dried fruit will provide fiber and protein. Choose trail mix carefully, as some can have a lot of fat. A low-sodium, part-skim mozzarella cheese stick is another source of dairy that is loaded with calcium.

Dinner The final meal of the day, whole-wheat pasta with meatless tomato sauce and mushrooms, adds more vegetables and whole grains. Broccoli and the fruit salad add vitamins A and C and calcium.

Evening Snack A handful of multigrain pretzels and a glass of skim milk is a low-calorie, low-fat option when you need a boost during your evening study time.

Watch for Special Dietary Considerations

Some people have special dietary considerations that affect their needs for certain nutrients. Strict vegetarians, for example, need to monitor their intake of protein,

Daily Values Standard values for nutrient needs, used as a reference on food labels. The Daily Values may not exactly reflect the true nutrient needs for all people.

calcium, and some vitamins, and children and pregnant women need to be sure to consume enough iron to help with growth. Let's take a look at some of these nutrient considerations.

Vitamins: B$_{12}$, D, and Folate Though most people will not need vitamin supplements if they are eating a healthy diet, people who have increased nutrient needs or special circumstances may benefit from enriched or fortified foods, a multivitamin, or other vitamin supplement. For example, strict vegetarians (vegans), who eat no animal foods, need to be sure to get enough vitamin B$_{12}$ (which is found primarily in animal products) through fortified foods, such as breakfast cereals, or by taking a supplement. Vegetarians who do not get 15 to 30 minutes of exposure to sunlight every few days may also need to take a vitamin D supplement.

Pregnant women need to be sure to consume enough folic acid, usually through a supplement, to reduce the risk of birth defects in their growing babies. And some older individuals, who may have depressed appetites or may not be able to cook or consume meals easily, may be advised to take a multivitamin to ensure that they meet their needs.

Other individuals also might benefit from vitamin supplementation:

- People with chronic illnesses that depress the appetite or the absorption of nutrients
- People on medications that affect appetite or digestion
- Athletes engaged in a rigorous training program
- Lactating women
- Individuals on prolonged low-calorie diets

Minerals: Iron and Calcium Iron is an essential component of red blood cells, which carry oxygen to all our tissues for energy production. An iron deficiency can result in decreased oxygen transport to tissues and thus an energy crisis. Getting enough iron can be a problem for women who are menstruating, pregnant, or nursing. Indeed, only half of all women of child-bearing age get the necessary 15 mg of iron per day (3). Five percent suffer from iron-deficiency anemia. Although these individuals should not take iron supplements unless their physician prescribes them (because the body excretes very little iron, there is a potential for toxicity if too much is consumed), they can modify their diets to ensure getting the RDA of iron. The following dietary modifications can help meet this requirement:

- Eat legumes, fresh fruits, whole-grain cereals, and broccoli, all of which are high in iron.
- Also eat foods high in vitamin C, which helps iron absorption.

- Eat lean red meats high in iron at least two or three times per week.
- Eat iron-rich organ meats, such as liver, once or twice per month.
- Don't drink tea with your meals; it interferes with iron absorption.

Another mineral, calcium, is the most abundant mineral in the body and is essential for building bones and teeth, as well as for normal nerve and muscle function. Adequate calcium is especially important for pregnant or nursing women. There is some evidence that calcium may help prevent colon cancer (3).

The most recent RDAs call for a significant increase in calcium intake for both sexes beginning at age 9. Children between 9 and 18 years of age should consume a 1300 mg of calcium each day. Adequate calcium intake during those years may be a crucial factor in preventing osteoporosis in later years, which strikes one in two women and one in five men over the age of 50 (10). Adults over age 18 should consume 1000 mg of calcium per day.

The following recommendations can help you get the calcium you need:

- Add low-fat or nonfat dairy products to your diet.
- Choose other calcium-rich alternatives, such as canned fish (with the bones, packed in water), turnip and mustard greens, and broccoli.
- Eat foods rich in vitamin C to boost absorption of calcium.
- Use an acidic dressing, made with citrus juices or vinegar, to enhance calcium absorption from salad greens.
- Add a supplement if you can't get enough calcium in the foods you like. However, beware of supplements made with dolomite or bone meal, because they may be contaminated with lead.

Vegetarian Diet

People choose a vegetarian diet for a variety of reasons including health, religion, or animal rights. Vegetarian diets are healthy diets, but it is important to know how to plan for meals that will meet the body's need for protein, iron, calcium, vitamin B$_{12}$, and other nutrients that are found in high quantities in animal sources. Because B$_{12}$ is primarily found in animal sources, there might be a need for vegetarians to supplement this vitamin, especially vegans, who do not include any food or beverages from animal sources in their diets. Pesco-vegetarian diets include fish, but not other types of meat. Those who consume a lacto-vegetarian diet include dairy products, and ovo-lacto-vegetarians include eggs and dairy products in their diets. Depending on the type of vegetarian, more effort and a greater variety of options

What Is the Glycemic Index and When Is it Helpful?

Low-carbohydrate diets are based on the notion that some carbohydrate-rich foods cause a dramatic increase in blood insulin level, which results in increased storage of fat, and a decrease in blood glucose that increases appetite. The diets are based on the **glycemic index** (GI) of foods, a measure of the effect a given food will have on the amount of glucose in the blood after the food is eaten. The concept is that eating foods with a low glycemic index results in less glucose fluctuation in the blood after a meal, which in turn stabilizes insulin levels and appetite. The typical reference for the GI is pure glucose, which has a GI of 100.

The GI of a food is not always easy to predict. Although some foods that contain simple sugars, such as candy, will logically have a higher GI, some foods with natural sugar, such as an apple (which is high in fructose) will have a lower GI. Additionally, the way the food is prepared and its fat and fiber content can affect its GI ranking. Instant mashed potatoes, white bread, and white rice have higher GIs than oat bran or kidney beans.

The glycemic index can be useful for some individuals, such as people with diabetes, to help them avoid fluctuations in blood glucose levels. In general, if you want to eat foods with lower, rather than higher, GIs, follow these guidelines:

- Eat breakfast cereals made of oats, barley, and bran.
- Eat dense, chewy breads made with whole seeds, not white bread.
- Eat fewer potatoes, but more al dente pasta.
- Choose basmati rather than white rice.
- Enjoy all types of vegetables.
- Eat plenty of salad vegetables with vinaigrette dressing.
- Balance a meal containing high-GI foods with extra low-GI foods.
- Add food acids (such as citrus fruits) to help slow stomach emptying and reduce the glycemic response.
- Eat fewer sugary foods, such as cookies, cakes, candy, and soft drinks.

Glycemic Index Range		
	Range	Example Foods
Low GI	0–55	Apples, oranges, bananas
Medium GI	56–69	White rice, ice cream
High GI	70–100	White bread, crispy rice cereal

may be required to meet nutritional needs. Using the SuperTracker tools on ChooseMyPlate.gov can assist in planning meals that will provide the recommended amounts of nutrients.

MAKE SURE YOU KNOW...

- The basic guidelines for a healthy diet are to eat adequate amounts of fruits, vegetables, and whole grains and to watch your intake of calories, sugar, alcohol, fat, and sodium. If you choose to drink alcohol, do so only in moderation.
- Recommended Dietary Allowances (RDAs), Dietary Reference Intakes (DRIs), and the USDA's MyPlate are tools you can use to plan a healthy diet. You can use food labels to choose foods that are low in calories, fat, sodium, and sugar.
- Some people, including children, pregnant and lactating women, and strict vegetarians, may have special nutrient needs and may therefore benefit from choosing enriched or fortified foods and/or taking a vitamin or mineral supplement.
- There are multiple types of vegetarian diets, and these can be very healthy options. However, it is important for those who choose a vegetarian diet to make sure their diet provides the recommended amounts of nutrients that are commonly found in large quantities in animal sources of food.

How Does Nutrition Affect Physical Fitness?

Think about the last magazine, TV, or online ad you saw for a nutrition-related product. Do you remember what was said about the product, and did you question whether it was true? The reality is that much of what you see and hear in such advertisements is not based on sound research and, in some cases, is entirely made up. Often, successful athletes endorse various nutritional products and convince the public that a particular food or beverage is responsible for their success. Even though most of the claims made in commercial endorsements are not supported by research, the claims often become accepted as fact.

The truth is, there are no miracle foods to improve physical fitness or exercise performance. Although your energy needs change when you become more physically

glycemic index A ranking system for carbohydrates based on a food's effect on blood glucose levels.

STEPS FOR ▸ BEHAVIOR CHANGE

Are you a fast food junkie?

Although eating at fast-food restaurants is generally not a healthy habit, there are choices you can make to improve your diet. Take the following quiz to assess your current behavior.

Y N

☐ ☐ Do you typically order the largest size on the menu?

☐ ☐ Do you always order a burger or fried fish or fried chicken sandwich?

☐ ☐ Do you always get french fries as a side?

☐ ☐ Is soda your "default" beverage for washing down your meal?

☐ ☐ Are your fast-food sandwiches and salads typically loaded up with mayonnaise, creamy dressings, or other high-fat sauces?

If you answered yes to more than two of these questions, you're probably consuming major amounts of fat and calories with every fast food meal. Fortunately, there's a lot you can do to improve the nutritional quality of your next fast food meal, without forgoing the drive-through altogether.

TIPS FOR THE NEXT TIME YOU'RE AT THE FAST FOOD COUNTER

Tomorrow, you will:

☑ Review menus of your favorite fast food restaurants to check the calorie and nutrient content of your typical order.

☑ Select alternate items to replace any items that do not fit with your new healthier dietary plan.

Within the next 2 weeks, you will:

☑ Make healthier choices when you go to a fast food restaurant. For example, you can order the small-sized items, and pass on the offer to "supersize" your meal. Consider these numbers: Depending on the restaurant, a double cheeseburger may contain 600–700 calories, 30–40 grams of fat, 120–140 mg of cholesterol, and 1000–1200 mg of sodium! You'll be surprised how satisfied you'll be with just a single burger and a small order of fries, and you'll save yourself a ton of calories.

☑ Forgo the sauces and creamy salad dressing. A typical tablespoon of tartar sauce contains about 20 grams of fat and 220 mg of sodium, and a tablespoon of mayonnaise will add 100 calories and 11 grams of fat to your sandwich.

☑ Order grilled meat instead of fried. Breaded chicken typically contains double the amount of fat in a broiled piece.

☑ Choose healthier sides: Try ordering a small salad instead of french fries, or a fruit cup rather than apple pie for dessert.

☑ Skip the soda or milkshake. Drink water, nonfat milk, or 100% juice with your meal.

By the end of the semester, you will:

☑ Decrease the number of times per week you eat at fast food restaurants.

---

active, you should be careful of compensatory eating. This habit occurs when people assume they can eat anything they want because they are exercising, a common pattern among new exercisers. Often they eat in excess of their energy needs and fail to lose weight when that is a goal, and in some cases even gain weight. In the sections that follow we discuss the specific nutritional needs of individuals in a regular exercise program.

Carbohydrates Are Used for Energy during Exercise

You need more fuel during exercise than when you're sedentary. Recall that carbohydrates and fats are the primary fuels used to provide energy for exercise. Because even very lean people have a large amount of energy stored as fat, lack of fat for fuel is not a problem during exercise. In contrast, the carbohydrate stores in the liver and muscles can reach critically low levels during intense or prolonged exercise (7).

Because carbohydrates play a critical role in providing energy during exercise, some exercise scientists have suggested that people participating in daily exercise programs should increase the complex carbohydrates in their diet from 58% to 70% of the total calories consumed (fat intake is then reduced to 18% of total caloric intake) (7). If exercise is intense, carbohydrates can be depleted from the liver and muscles, resulting in fatigue. The intensity of the exercise determines

Percent V̇O₂max	<30%	40-60%	75%	>80%
Fuel Used During Aerobic Exercise	Mostly fat stores	Fat and carbohydrate equally	Mainly carbohydrate	Nearly 100% carbohydrate

FIGURE 8.8 The influence of exercise intensity on fuel use.

whether carbohydrates or fat is the predominant source of energy production (7, 11) **(Figure 8.8)**.

In most cases, the energy you use during your workout comes from energy stored from meals eaten the previous day. Hence, products such as sports drinks and gels may not be as useful for energy during exercise as they are marketed to be. In fact, sugared sports drinks can cause a rapid rise in blood glucose, which promotes hormonal changes that reduce blood glucose to levels below normal and results in feelings of fatigue (7).

Increasing the percentage of complex carbohydrates in the diet and maintaining sufficient caloric intake can ensure that an adequate supply of energy from carbohydrates is stored in the muscles and the liver to meet the needs of a rigorous exercise training program.

Protein Needs Can Be Met with a Healthy Diet

Many bodybuilders consume large quantities of protein in supplements, in addition to the protein they take in through their normal diet, because they think this will promote muscular growth. Unfortunately, they're drinking those shakes and eating those bars largely in vain, because research has shown that a normal, well-balanced diet meets the protein requirements of most bodybuilders (12, 13). The increased caloric needs of someone in a strength-training program should come from additional amounts of nutrient-dense foods and not simply from additional protein. This strategy supplies not only the extra macronutrients, but also the micronutrients necessary for energy production.

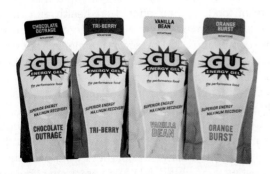

Products such as sports gels and drinks are sometimes used by athletes during competition. Usually, these are unnecessary. Use caution when using them, and make sure they are appropriate for your situation.

High Vitamin Intake Does Not Improve Performance

Some vitamin manufacturers have argued that megadoses of vitamins can improve exercise performance. This belief is based on the notion that exercise increases the need for energy and, because vitamins are necessary for the breakdown of foods for energy, an extra load of vitamins should be helpful. There is no evidence to support this claim (14). The energy supplied for muscle contraction is not enhanced by vitamin supplements. In fact, megadoses of vitamins may interfere with the delicate balance of other micronutrients and can be toxic as well (3). For example, excess vitamin A can cause problems in unborn babies, including damage to the nervous system and eyes, as well as cleft palate.

Antioxidants Help Prevent Oxidative Damage

Antioxidants are vitamins and micronutrients that protect cells by preventing a process called *oxidation*. (Oxidation is the same process that causes iron to rust over time. In fact, you can think of oxidation in the body as something like rusting from the inside.) Antioxidants work by combining with, and neutralizing, **free radicals** before they can damage cells. Excess production of free radicals has been implicated in cancer, lung disease, heart disease, and even the aging process (15). Therefore, increasing the level of antioxidants may be beneficial to health. Several micronutrients, including vitamins A, E, and C, beta-carotene, zinc, and selenium, have been identified as potent antioxidants.

Recent research suggests that the increased muscle metabolism associated with exercise may increase free radical production (16). Several studies have shown that this increase in free radicals may contribute to fatigue and perhaps even muscle damage.

Preliminary studies have indicated that antioxidants, primarily vitamin E, play a positive role in neutralizing exercise-produced free radicals. In fact, recent reports have demonstrated a reduction in muscle damage following administration of antioxidants (16). Several researchers have suggested that an additional 400 IU of vitamin E be consumed daily to protect against free radical

antioxidants Molecules that neutralize free radicals, thereby preventing them from causing damage to cells.

free radicals Oxygen molecules that can potentially damage cells.

COACHING Corner

Are you really hungry? Use the following tips to understand when it's time to eat.

- Are you hungry enough to eat an apple, carrot, peach, or any other fruit/vegetable? If so, then your body is likely signaling that you need to eat. If not, then you may just be bored.

- At the moment you are about to consume something you had not planned to, reflect for a moment to determine if something has triggered your perceived need to eat. Are you eating because food is available or are you actually hungry?

- While eating, take a few moments to sit and analyze whether you are still hungry or if you are eating simply because there is more on the plate. Try to recognize the point where you feel satisfied, and be content saving the rest of the meal for later.

- Improving the quality of your food will often result in an easy reduction in the quantity. Eat foods that are flavorful, rich in nutrients, and unrefined, and you'll need less to feel full.

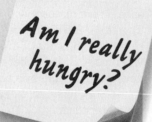

damage. However, you should consult a nutritionist before consuming more than the RDA of fat-soluble vitamins. Remember: Fat-soluble vitamins are stored in the body, and their accumulation may lead to toxicity.

MAKE SURE YOU KNOW...

- The amount of carbohydrate and fat used as fuel during exercise will vary according to the intensity of the exercise.
- The extra energy needed for strength training should not come solely from increased protein intake.
- Excess vitamin intake does not improve exercise performance.

- Antioxidants help prevent free radicals from damaging cells. To date, vitamins A, E, and C, beta-carotene, zinc, and selenium have been identified as potent antioxidants.

Do Supplements Provide an Edge for Health and Performance?

As previously mentioned, athletes aren't the only ones who might consider taking supplements. Many less-active individuals also use (or consider using) vitamins, minerals, herbs, enzymes, amino acids, or other compounds in pill, powder, or tablet form to improve health and wellness. Over the past decade, the use of nutritional and pharmaceutical supplements has become common in the United States. The search for a speedy path to health, wellness, and fitness led Americans to spend approximately $28.1 billion on nutritional supplements in 2010 (1). As a result, the U.S. government has been closely examining how this industry is regulated. In the following sections we examine how supplements are regulated and which ones might have the potential to be beneficial.

The Role of Supplements in a Healthy Diet

The FDA estimates that more than 25,000 products are available as dietary supplements. There is no scientific evidence to validate most of the claims that supplements improve health or exercise performance. Some of the more popular supplements currently marketed for improving health and enhancing exercise performance are listed in Table 8.7 on page 213.

The relationship between diet and disease highlights the importance of consuming adequate amounts of nutrients while avoiding dietary excesses. However, not much is known about newly discovered, unclassified, and naturally occurring micronutrient components of food or their effects on health and disease. For example, several studies have identified numerous plant compounds, called phytochemicals, that—when ingested by humans in small amounts—may protect against a variety of diseases. We still don't know whether the large amounts of phytochemicals typically present in supplements are safe or effective. (See the Closer Look box on page 214.) Given our current incomplete knowledge, eating a wide variety of foods and avoiding excessive use of dietary supplements are the best ways to obtain adequate amounts of beneficial food components.

TABLE 8.7 Comparison of Dietary Supplements

Supplement	Origin	Benefits Claimed	Evidence of Effectiveness
Caffeine	Compound found in coffee, cola, chocolate, candy, stimulants, weight-loss products.	Used to increase muscle fiber activation to increase strength, or to increase fat metabolism and endurance.	Increases endurance in events lasting more than 20 minutes. No consistent effects on strength.
Carbohydrates	Component of most food. Usually found as a dietary supplement in the form of beverages or bars.	Increase in stored glucose in muscle and liver and increase in endurance.	Improves endurance in events longer than 90–120 minutes. Also helps restore glucose after exercise.
l-carnitine	Made by the body and ingested in meat products.	Increases transport of fat in cells, reduces lactate accumulation.	Carnitine is in adequate supply in the cells, and additional amounts provide no benefit before, during, or after exercise.
Chromium picolinate	Trace element found in several foods; picolinate is added to supplements to aid absorption.	Helps insulin action and is thought to aid glucose metabolism, blood fats, and have anabolic effects.	No good evidence for any benefits. *Side effects: Stomach upset, anemia, genetic damage, kidney damage.*
Coenzyme Q-10	Made by the body as a component of the biochemical pathway that makes adenosine triphosphate (ATP).	Enhances ATP production.	No evidence suggests a benefit during or after exercise.
Creatine	Made by the body and also found in meat products.	Decreases fatigue in short, intense exercise. Increases muscle size and strength.	Increases endurance in short, intense exercise. Causes water gain in muscle but not increases in strength.
Echinacea	Herbal supplement.	Reduces duration of colds, boosts immune system, heals wounds.	Some evidence suggests it may be beneficial for these conditions. *Side effects: Uncommon, but possible GI upset, chills, nausea.*
Ginkgo biloba	Extracts of dried leaves of *Ginkgo* plant.	Used for antioxidant properties and to improve blood flow and memory.	Does have antioxidant properties that may be beneficial in improving blood flow, improving neural function, and reducing production of stress hormones. *Side effects: Nausea, headache, dizziness, skin rash, hemorrhage if used with blood thinners.*
St. John's wort	Plant extract.	Used to treat depression and external wounds, burns, and muscle aches.	Some evidence suggests that it is beneficial for treating these conditions.

Regulation of Supplements

Dietary supplements are not regulated in the same way that foods and prescription and over-the-counter drugs are regulated. The difference is that foods and drugs are tested and approved by governmental agencies (such as the FDA), whereas supplements are not. Manufacturers, not the government, are responsible for the safety of supplements. Supplement manufacturers are not required to get FDA approval before they market their products, and the FDA does not test supplements. Rather, the manufacturers are expected to ensure that the products are safe and effective.

However, the claims made on supplement labels are regulated. Supplement manufacturers are allowed to claim effects on the "structure or function" of the body, but they are not allowed to make claims concerning the treatment, prevention, cure, or diagnosis of disease. The FDA instituted the "structure/function rule"

in 2000 to distinguish disease claims from structure/function claims. Disease claims require evidence of safety and benefits to be demonstrated to the FDA prior to marketing; structure/function claims do not. The rule prohibits both express disease claims (e.g., "prevents heart disease") and implied claims (e.g., "prevents bone fragility in postmenopausal women") without prior FDA review. However, the rule permits health-maintenance claims (e.g., "maintains healthy bones"), other claims not related to disease (e.g., "for muscle enhancement"), and claims for the relief of common minor symptoms associated with life stages (e.g., "for common symptoms of PMS").

Since its release, the rule has been modified both to expand the number of acceptable structure/function claims and to narrow the definition of *disease* to disallow structure/function claims pertaining to aging, pregnancy, menopause, and adolescence. Supplement

Do Phytochemicals Protect Against Disease?

Besides nutrients, plant foods—legumes, vegetables, fruits, and whole grains—contain a whole other "crop" of chemicals called phytochemicals (*phyto* means "plant"). These substances, which plants produce naturally to protect themselves against viruses, bacteria, and fungi, may help protect us from diseases as well.

Phytochemicals include hundreds of naturally occurring substances, including carotenoids, flavonoids, indoles, isoflavones, capsaicin, and protease inhibitors. And just as with vitamins and minerals, different plant foods contain different kinds and amounts of phytochemicals.

Certain phytochemicals appear to protect against some cancers, heart disease, and other chronic health conditions. Until more is known, the nutrition bottom line still applies: Eat a wide variety of fruits, vegetables, legumes, and whole grains, and count on food, not diet supplements, to get the nutrients your body needs. That way, you'll reap the potential benefits of the many phytochemicals found in all kinds of plant foods.

Source: Heber, D. Vegetables, fruits and phytoestrogens in the prevention of diseases. *Journal of Postgraduate Medicine* 50(2):145–149, 2004.

manufacturers are required to document evidence for any structure/function claims they make. However, the FDA neither examines nor substantiates the legitimacy of this documentation. Manufacturers must also include on their labels a disclaimer stating that their dietary supplements are not drugs and received no FDA approval before marketing. In addition, manufacturers must notify the FDA of a product claim within 30 days of marketing it. All this means that the consumer is ultimately responsible for determining whether a given supplement is needed or safe (see the Consumer Corner box on page 215).

MAKE SURE YOU KNOW...

- Supplements should never replace foods as major sources of dietary nutrients.
- Supplements are not tested or approved by the FDA or other governmental body. However, the FDA does mandate that the only claims that can be made about supplements must relate to effects on "structure or function" of the body. Manufacturers are allowed to make no label claims about the effects of a supplement on disease.
- Because dietary supplements are poorly regulated, consumers should be cautious when choosing and using such supplements.

Topics in Food Safety and Technology

The quality of your food choices and an adequate (but not too high) calorie intake are two aspects of a healthy diet. Ensuring the foods you eat are safe and free from contamination is another component of eating well. Let's discuss the specifics of food safety and technology next.

Foodborne Illness

If a food carries a disease-causing microorganism, such as a bacterium, consuming the food can potentially make you sick. According to the Institute of Food Technologists, approximately 80 million cases of foodborne bacterial disease occur each year. These illnesses produce nausea, vomiting, and diarrhea from 12 hours to 5 days after infection (17). The severity of the illness depends on the microorganism ingested and the victim's overall health. Foodborne infections can be fatal in children, people with compromised immune systems, or other people in ill health.

Two types of foodborne illness that you may have heard about are *Salmonella* contamination and botulism. The *Salmonella* bacterium is usually found in raw or undercooked chicken and eggs and in processed meats. The relatively uncommon but sometimes fatal botulism usually results from improper home-canning procedures. A particular strain of the *Escherichia coli* bacterium, O157:H7, is sometimes found in contaminated raw or undercooked ground beef and can lead to bloody diarrhea, among other symptoms.

To reduce your risk of contracting foodborne illness, follow these guidelines:

- Select foods that appear clean and fresh.
- Wash produce thoroughly with running water; use a vegetable brush on firm fruits and vegetables.
- Drink only pasteurized milk and juices.
- Don't eat raw eggs.
- When storing perishable foods for future consumption, keep them cold or frozen to prevent bacterial growth.
- Cook all meat products, such as chicken, pork, and ground beef, thoroughly. When dining out, order meats well done.

Detecting Supplement Fraud

Most of the dietary supplements on the market today are useless. These products often do nothing more than cheat consumers out of their money or steer them away from products that have been proven useful. Some supplement products may do more harm than good.

How can you avoid being scammed by the maker of a worthless supplement? Marketers have sophisticated ways of making their products attractive to potential buyers, but you can protect yourself by learning about marketing ploys. Beware of the following techniques, claims, or catch-phrases:

- **The product "does it all."** Be suspicious of any supplement that claims to have multiple benefits. No one product is likely to be capable of so great a range of effectiveness.

- **The product is supported by personal testimonials.** Testimonials are often simply stories that have been passed from person to person, and sometimes they are completely made up. Because testimonials are difficult to prove, they may be a "tip" to the possibility of fraud.

- **The product provides a "quick fix."** Be skeptical of products that claim to produce immediate results. Tip-offs include ambiguous language such as, "Provides relief in days," or "You'll feel energized immediately." Unscrupulous marketers use such phrases to protect themselves against any subsequent legal action.

- **The product is "natural."** The term *natural* suggests that the product is safer than conventional treatments. Any product—synthetic or natural—that is potent enough to produce a significant physiological effect is potent enough to cause side effects.

- **The product is "a new, time-tested treatment."** A product is usually one or the other, but be suspicious of any product that claims to be both a breakthrough and a decades-old treatment. If a product that claims to be an "innovation" or a "new discovery" were really so revolutionary, it would be widely reported in the media and prescribed by health professionals, not featured in obscure ads.

- **Your "satisfaction is guaranteed."** Money-back guarantees are often empty promises. The makers of this claim know most people won't go to all the trouble involved in trying to get a refund of only $9.95 or so.

- **The product's ads contain meaningless medical jargon.** The use of scientific-sounding terms such as "aerobic enzyme booster" may seem impressive and may even contain an element of truth, but these terms likely cover up a lack of scientific data concerning the product.

Always ask yourself, "Does this claim seem too good to be true?" If it does, then the product is probably a fraud. If you're still not sure, talk to your doctor or other health professional. The Better Business Bureau or your state attorney general's office can tell you whether other consumers have lodged complaints about a product or its marketers. If a product is promoted as being helpful for a specific condition, check with the appropriate professional group—for example, consult the American Heart Association about products that claim some effectiveness concerning heart disease.

- Cook all shellfish thoroughly; steaming them open may not be sufficient.

- Avoid raw fish; it may contain parasitic roundworms. Keep fish frozen, and cook until well done.

- Use separate sets of cutting boards and utensils (e.g., knives) for meat and produce; chopping raw meat and vegetables with the same knife, without washing it thoroughly first, can lead to cross-contamination.

- Wash utensils, plates, cutting boards, knives, blenders, and other cooking equipment with soap and very hot water after each use.

See the Closer Look box on page 216 for more about minimizing your risk for foodborne illness.

Food Additives

Food additives are used by manufacturers for a variety of reasons: to improve nutritional quality, as a preservative to maintain freshness and/or increase shelf life, to improve taste or color, or to make it more appealing in some other way. Among the most commonly used additives are sugar, salt, and corn syrup. Other additives, such as monosodium glutamate (MSG) and sulfites, may cause a reaction in people who are particularly sensitive to them. Nitrites, which are found in bacon, sausages, lunch meats, and other processed foods, may also form cancer-causing agents (nitrosamines) in the body. If you think you are sensitive to a particular food additive, read

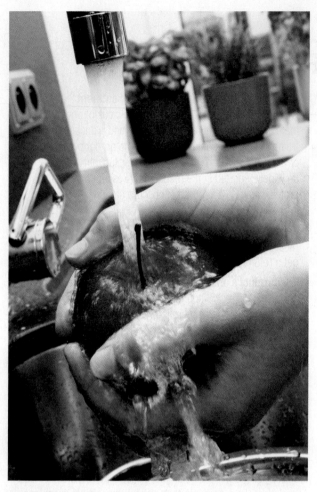

Washing fresh produce under running tap water will help you avoid foodborne illness.

labels carefully and avoid foods that contain additives to which you are likely to have a reaction.

Antibiotics, Hormones, and Organically Grown Foods

As consumers become more aware of the quality of the foods they eat, they are buying increasing quantities of **organic** foods. *Organic,* in this context, refers to foods that are grown without the use of pesticides, hormones, antibiotics, or chemical fertilizers. Currently, the United States, the European Union, Japan, and many other countries require producers to obtain certification to market food as organic (see **Figure 8.9** on page 217).

Livestock animals raised on factory farms are often treated with high doses of antibiotics to ward off potential infections. Though there is little evidence to support the view, some people are concerned that eating meat or drinking milk from these animals could lead to the development of antibiotic-resistant bacteria in humans.

Farmers also often use hormones in animals to increase production of meat and milk. Most notably, a form of growth hormone, bovine somatotropin, has been used to increase milk production in dairy cows. Some people fear that hormones in food may cause health problems, including cancer, in humans. Many supermarkets are restricting the sale of milk produced with the aid of hormone supplements.

Should you buy organic foods? This is a decision you have to make for yourself. However, be aware that there is no research to support the idea that organic foods are nutritionally superior to nonorganic foods, and

---

A CLOSER LOOK

Keep Hot Foods Hot and Cold Foods Cold to Avoid Foodborne Illness

Whether from restaurants, supermarkets, or quick-service establishments, take-out foods have become a part of our way of life. But to avoid foodborne illnesses, you must keep these foods at the appropriate temperature. The next time you order take-out or bring a hot or cold food to a party or family function, keep the following recommendations in mind.

For Hot Foods

- Keep hot foods above 140°F. You can cover food with foil (to keep it moist) and keep it warm—140°F or above—in the oven (check the food's temperature with a meat thermometer). Using a slow cooker is another option for some foods. It's best to eat food within 2 hours of preparation.
- If the food won't be eaten for more than 2 hours, refrigerate it in shallow, covered containers. Before serving, reheat it in an oven to 165°F or until it's hot and steaming. If you

prefer, reheat food in a microwave oven—cover and rotate—and then let it stand for 2 minutes to ensure thorough, even heating.

For Cold Foods

- Keep cold foods at 40°F or below.
- If cold foods are not eaten right away, refrigerate them as soon as possible.
- Discard any foods kept at room temperature for more than 2 hours. If conditions are warmer than 90°F, toss the food after only 1 hour.
- Transport and store cold foods in chilled, insulated coolers.
- If you're going to put out a deli platter, keep it on a bowl of ice.

Source: USDA Food Safety and Inspection Service. *Cooking for Groups: A Volunteer's Guide to Food Safety.* Item #604H, Pueblo, CO 81009.

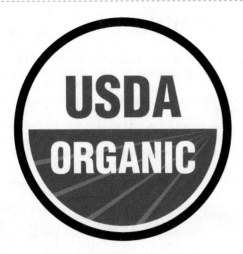

FIGURE 8.9   Organic food symbol

organic foods tend to be more expensive than their non-organic counterparts.

 How did the farmers' market revival happen? Watch *Going Green* at **www.pearsonhighered.com/powers.**

SEE IT!
VIDEOS

Irradiated and Bioengineered Foods

Irradiation is sometimes used to kill microorganisms in foods and to prolong the shelf life of the food (17). In fact, irradiated food can be stored for years in sealed containers at room temperature without spoiling. In addition, irradiation can delay the sprouting of vegetables such as potatoes and onions and delay the ripening of fruits such as bananas, tomatoes, and avocados. This can result in significant cost savings.

Are these irradiated foods safe to eat? Currently, all research indicates that the foods are safe and that nutritional content is maintained, but only limited data exist (17). Irradiated foods must carry a seal of approval to inform consumers that they have been treated **(Figure 8.10)**.

Another practice that has become controversial is the use of bioengineered foods. Bioengineering involves inserting the genes from one plant or animal species into another plant or animal's DNA to achieve a desired trait. Food crops such as corn and tomatoes have been bioengineered to improve yields, pest resistance, and

FIGURE 8.10   Irradiated food symbol

longevity (which improves the crops' ability to be shipped long distances). Although the benefits of bioengineering can be great, the practice is considered unproven, and possibly unsafe, in some countries.

MAKE SURE YOU **KNOW...**

- Proper food storage and preparation are the keys to preventing foodborne illness. Select foods that appear clean and fresh; keep foods cold or frozen to prevent bacteria from growing; clean fresh fruits, vegetables, and meats thoroughly; cook all meats thoroughly; order meats well done when dining out.

- The use of the word *organic* on food labels is strictly regulated; organic foods are grown without the use of pesticides and other chemicals.

- Irradiation and bioengineering are two forms of food technology that are used to enhance food safety and to increase yields and pest resistance. Despite all indications that they are safe, both techniques remain somewhat controversial.

> **organic** Plant or animal foods that are grown without the use of pesticides, chemical fertilizers, antibiotics, or hormones.
>
> **irradiation** The use of radiation (high-energy waves or particles, including radioactivity and X-rays) to kill microorganisms that grow on or in food.

Sample Program for Changing Daily Caloric Intake

Scan to plan your individualized program for nutrition. ▶

The plan below is for an individual who needs to change the composition of daily caloric intake and reduce the overall caloric intake. (Also consider the recommendations from the MyPlate. gov dietary analysis in Laboratory 8.1.) Specific recommendations for weight loss, weight gain, or change due to an increase in physical activity will vary. Note that the plan presented does not eliminate all "bad foods," but makes recommendations for allowing sweets or foods higher in fat in moderation. Maintain the changes each week and incorporate the new changes until the recommendations from Myplate. gov are met.

You can eliminate empty calories by cutting down on soda and candy. Replace beverages with water or lower-fat options; for example, try skim milk versus 2% milk, regular coffee with skim milk versus a latte.

	Food Category	Monday	Tuesday	Wednesday	Thursday	Friday	Saturday	Sunday
Week 1	Caloric Intake	Eliminate at least 150 "empty calories"	Eliminate at least 150 "empty calories"			Eliminate at least 150 "empty calories"	Eliminate at least 150 "empty calories"	
	Beverages and Alcohol	Replace beverages with water or lower-fat options	Replace beverages with water or lower-fat options	Replace beverages with water or lower-fat options	Replace beverages with water or lower-fat options	(1) Replace beverages with water or lower-fat options (2) If you drink alcohol, limit to 1–2 drinks	Replace beverages with water or lower-fat options	Replace beverages with water or lower-fat options
	Fruits and Vegetables							
	Carbohydrates							
	Protein							
	Fats			Substitute a low-fat option for a high-fat food	Substitute a low-fat option for a high-fat food			Substitute a low-fat option for a high-fat food
	Reward							Allow a splurge of one serving of a food you enjoy

	Food Category	Monday	Tuesday	Wednesday	Thursday	Friday	Saturday	Sunday
Week 2	**Caloric Intake**							
	Beverages and Alcohol							
	Fruits and Vegetables	Increase fruit and vegetable intake, and eat a variety of fruits and vegetables		Increase fruit and vegetable intake, and eat a variety of fruits and vegetables		Increase fruit and vegetable intake, and eat a variety of fruits and vegetables	Increase fruit and vegetable intake, and eat a variety of fruits and vegetables	
	Carbohydrates		Replace refined carbohydrate choices with whole grains		Replace refined carbohydrate choices with whole grains			
	Protein	Reduce protein intake		Reduce protein intake		Reduce protein intake	Reduce protein intake	
	Fats							
	Reward							Allow a splurge of one serving of a food you enjoy
Week 3	**Caloric Intake**							
	Beverages and Alcohol	Consume water or low-fat/low-sugar beverages	Consume water or low-fat/low-sugar beverages	Consume water or low-fat/low-sugar beverages	Consume water or low-fat/low-sugar beverages	(1) Consume water or low-fat/low-sugar beverages (2) If you drink alcohol, limit to 1–2 drinks	(1) Consume water or low-fat/low-sugar beverages (2) If you drink alcohol, limit to 1–2 drinks	Consume water or low-fat/low-sugar beverages
	Fruits and Vegetables	Increase fruit and vegetable intake, and eat a variety of fruits and vegetables	Increase fruit and vegetable intake, and eat a variety of fruits and vegetables	Increase fruit and vegetable intake, and eat a variety of fruits and vegetables	Increase fruit and vegetable intake, and eat a variety of fruits and vegetables	Increase fruit and vegetable intake, and eat a variety of fruits and vegetables	Increase fruit and vegetable intake, and eat a variety of fruits and vegetables	Increase fruit and vegetable intake, and eat a variety of fruits and vegetables
	Carbohydrates	Replace refined carbohydrate choices with whole grains	Replace refined carbohydrate choices with whole grains	Replace refined carbohydrate choices with whole grains	Replace refined carbohydrate choices with whole grains	Replace refined carbohydrate choices with whole grains	Replace refined carbohydrate choices with whole grains	Replace refined carbohydrate choices with whole grains
	Protein	Replace high-fat protein sources with a lower-fat protein source	Replace high-fat protein sources with a lower-fat protein source	Replace high-fat protein sources with a lower-fat protein source	Replace high-fat protein sources with a lower-fat protein source	Replace high-fat protein sources with a lower-fat protein source	Replace high-fat protein sources with a lower-fat protein source	Replace high-fat protein sources with a lower-fat protein source
	Fats							
	Reward							Allow a splurge of one serving of a food you enjoy

SUMMARY

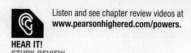

Listen and see chapter review videos at www.pearsonhighered.com/powers.

HEAR IT!
STUDY REVIEW

1. Nutrition is the study of food and its relationship to health and disease. In industrialized countries, the current primary problem in nutrition is overeating.

2. A well-balanced diet is composed of approximately 58% complex carbohydrates, 30% fat, and 12% protein. Macronutrients provide the energy (kilocalories, or calories) necessary for bodily functions. The calorie is a unit of measure of the energy value of food or the energy required for physical activity.

3. Carbohydrate is a primary fuel used by the body to provide energy. Simple carbohydrates, or sugars, include glucose, fructose, sucrose, galactose, lactose, and maltose. The complex carbohydrates consist of starches and fiber. Starches are composed of chains of glucose. Fiber is a nondigestible but essential form of complex carbohydrates contained in whole grains, vegetables, and fruits. Fiber is important in regulating digestion and forming waste products.

4. Fat is an efficient storage form for energy, because each gram contains over twice the energy of carbohydrates or protein. Fat can be derived from dietary sources or formed from excess carbohydrates and protein consumed in the diet.

5. Fats are a type of lipid. Most of the fat found in foods and in your body is in the form of triglycerides. Triglycerides consist of three fatty acids attached to a glycerol backbone. Fatty acids are classified as either saturated or unsaturated, depending on their chemical structures. Cholesterol is another form of lipid. Blood cholesterol levels can affect your risk of heart disease.

6. The primary role of protein is to serve as the structural unit for building and repairing cells in all tissues of the body. Protein consists of amino acids made by the body (11 nonessential amino acids) and those available only through dietary sources (9 essential amino acids). If you consume inadequate amounts of carbohydrates or fat, protein can be broken down and used for energy.

7. Vitamins serve many important functions in the body, including regulation of growth and metabo-

lism. The B-complex vitamins and vitamin C are water soluble and, for the most part, cannot be stored in the body. The fat-soluble vitamins A, D, E, and K can be stored in the body.

8. Minerals are inorganic chemical elements that serve many important roles in regulating body functions.

9. Approximately 60%–70% of the body is water. Water is involved in all vital processes in the body and is particularly important for physically active individuals. You need to consume 8–10 cups of water in food and beverages daily.

10. A healthy diet consists of adequate amounts of fruits, vegetables, whole grains, and lean meats and dairy products, with limited amounts of sugar, fat, and sodium. You should balance the calories you consume with the calories you expend, and if you drink alcohol, do so only in moderation. You can use the RDAs, DRIs, MyPlate, and food labels to help you choose healthy foods.

11. The intensity of exercise dictates the relative proportions of fat and carbohydrates that are used as fuel during exercise. In general, the lower the intensity of exercise, the more fat is used as fuel. Conversely, the greater the intensity of exercise, the more carbohydrates are used as fuel.

12. Antioxidants are nutrients that prevent free radicals from damaging cells. Vitamins E and C, betacarotene, zinc, and selenium have been identified as antioxidants.

13. Most people can consume adequate nutrients through a healthy diet and do not need to take supplements. However, pregnant women, strict vegetarians, older adults, and some others may benefit from a dietary supplement.

14. The key to preventing foodborne illness is to prepare, store, and cook foods properly. Select foods that appear clean and fresh; keep foods cold or frozen to prevent bacteria from growing; thoroughly clean fresh fruits, vegetables, and meats; cook all meats thoroughly, and order well-done meats when dining out.

STUDY QUESTIONS

Find more review questions online at www.pearsonhighered.com/powers.

REVIEW IT!
QUIZZES

1. What is the primary role of carbohydrates in the diet?
   a. building tissue
   b. providing energy
   c. forming hormones
   d. forming enzymes

2. The primary role of protein in the diet is to
   a. provide energy.
   b. provide hydration.
   c. build tissues.
   d. regulate hormones.

3. Water is important for
   a. providing energy.
   b. building bones.
   c. forming blood.
   d. building protein.

4. What approximate percentages of carbohydrate, fat, and protein in the diet are recommended daily?
   a. 60, 20, 20
   b. 58, 22, 20
   c. 40, 20, 40
   d. 58, 30, 12

5. Which of the following may protect the body's cells against damage during normal and elevated metabolism?
   a. proteins
   b. hormones
   c. antioxidants
   d. antibiotics

6. List the major food sources of dietary carbohydrates.

7. List the various subcategories of carbohydrates.

8. Define *triglyceride,* and discuss its use in the body.

9. Distinguish between saturated and unsaturated fatty acids.

10. What are omega-3 fatty acids?

11. What is the difference between essential and non-essential amino acids?

12. What are the classes of vitamins, and what role do vitamins play in body function?

13. Outline the role that minerals play in body function.

14. How many calories are contained in 1 gram of carbohydrate, fat, and protein, respectively?

15. Discuss the special need for carbohydrates in an individual who is engaging in an exercise training program.

16. Discuss the special need for protein in an individual who is engaging in an exercise training program.

17. Discuss the impact of the following on heart disease: high-density lipoproteins (HDL cholesterol) low-density lipoproteins (LDL cholesterol)

18. Discuss the structure/function rule pertaining to dietary supplements.

HELPFUL WEBLINKS

DO IT!
WEBLINKS

For links to the organizations and websites listed, visit
www.pearsonhighered.com/powers.

Academy of Nutrition and Dietetics
Presents nutritional resources, FAQs, links, and more. www.eatright.org

Ask the Dietician
Presents sound nutritional advice on many diet-related questions. Includes an excellent "Healthy Body Calculator" for formulating diet and exercise programs. www.dietitian.com

Fast Food Nutrition Facts
Enables you to search for fast food restaurants and find nutritional information. www.fastfoodnutrition.org

Food and Drug Administration
Home page for the FDA office dealing with food and supplement regulations. Great information on food safety and supplements. The FDA provides key information and updates about regulatory actions related to food labeling, nutrition, and dietary supplements, as well as educational materials and important announcements. www.fda.gov

FoodSafety
Gateway to government food safety information. Includes news and safety alerts, consumer advice, national food safety programs, and foodborne pathogens. www.foodsafety.gov

MedlinePlus Health Information: Vitamin and Mineral Supplements
A service of the National Library of Medicine, National Institutes of Health, that provides information on health topics, including vitamin and mineral supplements. www.nlm.nih.gov/medlineplus/vitamins.html and www.nlm.nih.gov/medlineplus/dietarysupplements.html

MyPlate
Home page for the USDA's food guidance system, which includes SuperTracker to help you track your diet and physical activity. www.choosemyplate.gov

Nutrition.gov
A federal resource that provides easy access to all online federal government information on nutrition. www.nutrition.gov

USDA Center for Nutrition Policy and Promotion
Provides guidelines for diets. www.cnpp.usda.gov

USDA Food Safety Publications
Contains articles about all aspects of safety in food preparation, storage, and handling. www.fsis.usda.gov/Factsheets/index.asp

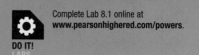
Name _____   Date _____

Analyzing Your Diet

The purpose of this exercise is to analyze your eating habits. For a 3-day period (two weekdays and one weekend day), eat the foods that typically constitute your normal diet. Use the SuperTracker feature on ChooseMyPlate.gov to chart the foods you ate that day and the amounts of each food. Select Food Tracker under Track Food & Activity. You can enter your food or search or the items you ate during the day. After you record your food intake, you can use the dietary analysis features to determine the nutrients in each food, the daily totals, and the average for the 3 days. The nutrient recommendations are based on the information you entered for your age, weight, sex, and activity level.

Select the Food Details report and click the Select All box under nutrients to see the nutrient totals for each day. This report will provide nutrient values for each item that you consumed per day. Next, select the Nutrients report for the average of your calorie and nutrient values over the 3-day period. When you create your profile, your data will be saved in SuperTracker. You can use the site to monitor your diet as you make healthy modifications. You can also print your report or save it to your computer for reference.

Compare your average intake for each of the nutrients with the recommended values based on your age, sex, and activity level. (Remember that this analysis is only as representative of your normal diet as the foods you eat over the 3-day period.) Then answer the following questions:

1. How did you do on calories? Are you taking in more or fewer calories than you should be for your sex, age, and activity level?

    _____

2. Was your fat, sodium, cholesterol, and empty calorie intake higher than it should be?

    _____

3. What nutrients did you eat in inadequate amounts?

    _____

4. What are three substitutions you could have made that would improve the quality of your diet?

    _____

RECOMMENDED DIETARY ALLOWANCES*

*   Kcal total (total daily energy expenditure) equals body weight multiplied by kcal per pound per day:

    _____ × _____ = _____

       Body weight in lb   kcal per lb per day   **kcal total (total daily**
                     (from Table 9.1 on page 232) **energy expenditure)**

*   Kcal from fat should be no more than 30% of total calories per day:

    _____ × _____ = _____

       30% (0.3)   kcal per day   **recommended MAXIMUM kcal from fat**

*   Protein intake should be 12% of total calories per day, or 0.8 to 0.9 gram per kilogram (0.36 g per pound) of body weight. (Pregnant women should add 15 g, and lactating women should add 20 g.):

    _____ × _____ = _____

       0.36 g   body weight in lb   **recommended protein intake**

*   Carbohydrate intake should be approximately 58% of total calories per day:

    _____ × _____ = _____

       58% (0.58)   kcal per day   **recommended carbohydrate intake**

    Fat <30% of diet; fiber ~30% of diet; saturated fat <10% of diet; cholesterol <300 mg; sodium <3000 mg.

*See Table 8.5 on pages 204 and 205 for vitamin and mineral RDA values.

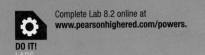
Name _____   **Date** _____

Setting Goals for a Healthy Diet

What are your three worst dietary habits? (Use your Nutrient reports from Laboratory 8.1 to help identify problems areas with your dietary habits.)

1. _____

2. _____

3. _____

Check the appropriate boxes in the table below to indicate the changes that you think you need to make to improve your diet.

	Increase	Decrease	Keep the Same
Calories			
Carbohydrates			
Fat			
Protein			
Vitamins			
Minerals			

Based on your selections above, list two short-term and two long-term SMART goals for improving your diet:

Short-term goal 1

_____

_____

Short-term goal 2

_____

_____

Long-term goal 1

_____

_____

Long-term goal 2

_____

_____

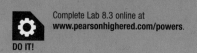
Name _____   Date _____

Planning a New Diet

The purpose of this exercise is to plan a new diet using the principles outlined in this chapter. You can also use the My Plan tool of SuperTracker. This feature will provide general recommendations, and then you can select specific foods to meet those recommendations. After completing Laboratory 8.1, you should have a general idea of how your diet may need modification. Follow the example given in Table 8.6 on page 207 and the discussion in the text to choose foods to build a new diet that meets the recommended dietary goals presented in this chapter. Fill in the chart below with the requested information obtained from Food-A-Pedia on SuperTracker or from package labels. Use the totals for each column and the RDA for each nutrient in Laboratory 8.1 or Table 8.5 on pages 204 and 205 to determine your percentage of RDA for each nutrient.

	kcal (g)	Protein (g)	Sat. Fat (g)	Chol. (mg)	Sod. (mg)	Carb. (g)	Vit. A (IU)	Vit. C (mg)	Ca (mg)	Iron (mg)	GI
Breakfast											
Lunch											
Dinner											
Totals											
RDA	*	<30%†	<10%	<300	3000	>58%	1000	60	1200	12	‡
% of RDA											

*See Table 9.1 in Chapter 9 (page 232) for determination of kcal requirements.

†Protein intake should be 0.8 g/kg of body weight (0.36 g/lb). Pregnant women should add 15 g, and lactating women should add 20 g.

‡For a complete list of the glycemic index of various foods, visit www.glycemicindex.com

Name _____ **Date** _____

Assessing Nutritional Habits

Read the following scenarios and select which option applies to you. Score your answers according to the instructions at the end.

1. You don't have time to make dinner, so you run out to get "fast food." What do you get?
   a. grilled chicken breast sandwich
   b. supersized burger

2. You go to a movie, find yourself hungry, and cannot resist a snack. Which do you buy?
   a. unbuttered popcorn
   b. candy

3. You're late for work and realize you forgot breakfast. You decide to stop and grab something to eat. What do you pick up?
   a. a banana
   b. a sausage biscuit

4. You decide to go out for a nice dinner at an Italian restaurant. What do you order?
   a. spaghetti with red sauce
   b. five-cheese lasagna

5. It's 3:00 P.M., and you didn't have much lunch and need an afternoon snack. What do you reach for?
   a. an apple
   b. M&Ms

6. You stop for ice cream. Which do you pick?
   a. a fruit sorbet
   b. regular ice cream

7. What kind of dessert would you normally choose to eat?
   a. a bowl of mixed berries with a sprinkling of sugar
   b. chocolate cake with frosting

8. What do you use to stir fry vegetables?
   a. olive oil
   b. margarine

9. Which of the following salty snacks would you prefer?
   a. pretzels
   b. potato chips

10. You want cereal for breakfast. Which would you choose?
    a. whole-grain flakes
    b. peanut butter puffs

INTERPRETATION

If you answered "b" to any of the above questions, you chose foods that are high in calories, fat, or sugar. Follow the advice in this chapter and MyPlate food guidance system to improve your food choices.

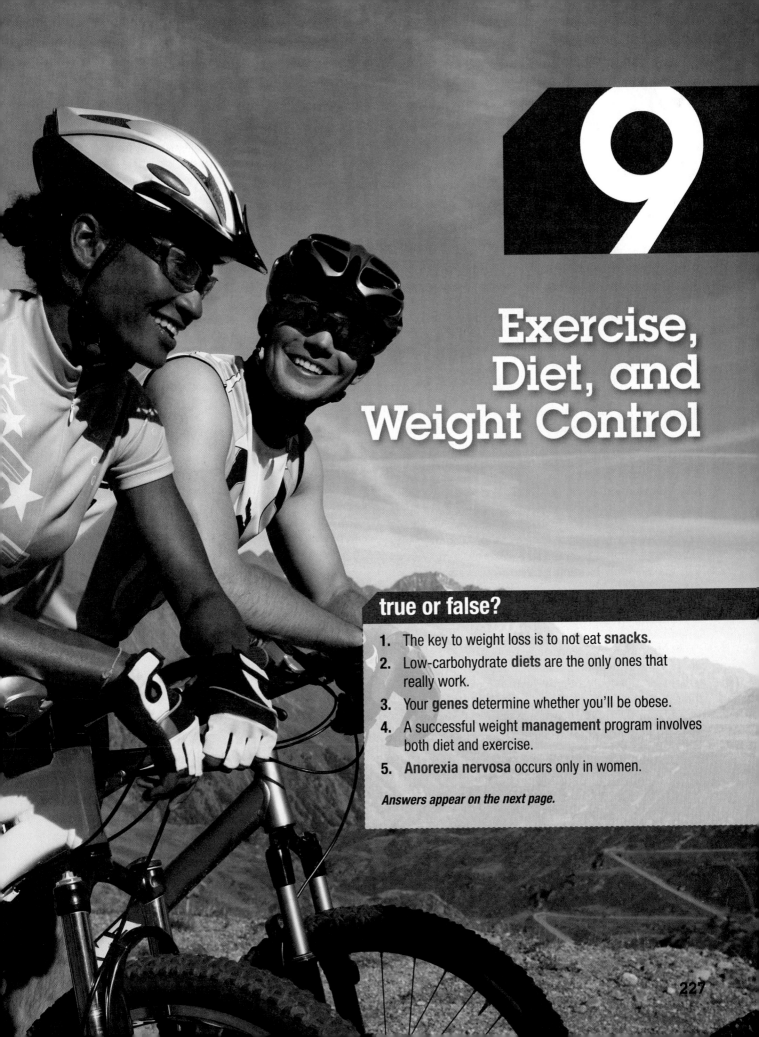

9

Exercise, Diet, and Weight Control

true or false?

1. The key to weight loss is to not eat **snacks.**
2. Low-carbohydrate **diets** are the only ones that really work.
3. Your **genes** determine whether you'll be obese.
4. A successful weight **management** program involves both diet and exercise.
5. **Anorexia nervosa** occurs only in women.

Answers appear on the next page.

227

illions of people in the United States are over-weight. In fact, over 60% of adults and 20% of children are overweight or obese (1). While the United States has the highest incidence of over-weight people in the world, obesity has become a global epidemic and is now one of the leading causes of illness worldwide (1, 2). Being overweight has been shown to be a risk factor for health problems such as diabetes, gallbladder disease, high blood pressure, high choles-terol, heart disease, and even some cancers (1). As a result of this connection between health and increased body weight, more people are trying to lose weight.

This epidemic in overweight and obesity has given birth to a multi-billion-dollar weight-loss industry in the United States. In fact, it is estimated that 50–70 million Americans go on a diet each year. As a result, consum-ers spend billions of dollars every year on diet sodas, appetite suppressants, diet books, commercial diets, and medically supervised diets in an attempt to lose weight. In addition, the number of individuals seeking gastric bypass surgery has increased markedly in the last 15 years (3). Many commercial weight-loss programs advertise that they are highly successful. Unfortunately, research has found that with no other treatment, only 5% of individuals maintain their weight loss for 5 years after completing the program (3). The good news is that long-term weight loss is achievable, and many people do successfully alter their diet and lifestyle habits to achieve a healthy weight. The key is to recognize that short-term diets and gimmicks work only temporarily and that the only solution for long-term weight loss is to change one's eating and physical activity patterns.

In this chapter, we will discuss the principles of determining an ideal body weight for health and fitness; how to use a combination of diet, exercise, and behav-ior modification to successfully reduce body fat; and the principles involved in maintaining a desirable body weight throughout life. Finally, we will look at the symp-toms and health effects of several eating disorders. We begin by revisiting the concept of optimal body weight (which you read about in Chapter 6).

What Is Your Optimal Body Weight?

Before you can decide whether you should implement a weight-loss program, you need to determine if you're currently at an optimal body weight. In general, opti-mal body fat for health and fitness in men ranges from 8% to 19%, whereas the optimal range of body fat for women ranges from 21% to 32% (4) (Chapter 6). These ranges allow for individual differences in physical activ-ity and appearance and are associated with limited risk for diseases linked to body fatness. How can you

answers

1. **FALSE** Snacking between meals can help suppress the appetite and can be a healthy strategy for weight management, as long as the snack foods are healthy. Fruits and raw vegetables make ideal snacks.
2. **FALSE** Low-carbohydrate diets may help you initially lose weight, but you'll likely regain the weight once you resume your normal carbohydrate intake.
3. **FALSE** Genetics do play a role in overweight and obesity; however, only 1%–5% of the population have genetic conditions that are the main cause of obesity. For most obese people, the condition is a result of diet and lifestyle factors.
4. **TRUE** The combination of diet and exercise is the only effective means for losing weight and maintaining the weight loss over the long term.
5. **FALSE** Anorexia nervosa can affect both men and women.

compute your desired range of body weight? The calcu-lation can be done in two simple steps; the first step is to calculate your fat-free weight. Consider the following example of a male college student who has 25% body fat and weighs 185 pounds.

Step 1. Compute fat-free weight—that is, the amount of total body weight contained in bones, organs, and muscles:

% total body weight − % fat weight = % fat-free weight

100% − 25% = 75%

This means that 75% (or 0.75, expressed as a deci-mal) of total body weight is fat-free weight. There-fore, the fat-free weight for this student is

0.75 × 185 pounds = 138.8 pounds

Step 2. Calculate the optimal weight (which for men is 8%–19% of total body weight). The formula to compute optimum body weight is

Optimum weight = fat-free weight ÷ (1 − optimal % fat)

Note that % fat should again be expressed as a deci-mal. Thus, for 8% body fat,

Optimum weight = 138.8 ÷ (1 − 0.08) = 150.9 pounds

For 19% body fat,

Optimum weight = 138.8 ÷ (1 − 0.19) = 171.3 pounds

Hence, the optimal body weight for this individual is between 150.9 and 171.3 pounds. See Labora-tory 9.1 to compute your optimal body weight, using both percentage of body fat and body mass index (from Chapter 6).

MAKE SURE YOU KNOW...

- The ranges of optimal body fat for health and fitness are 8%–19% for men and 21%–32% for women.
- You can calculate your optimal body weight using your percent body fat and current body weight.

What Factors Can Affect Weight Management?

In most obese people, being over-fat is a result of a complex interaction between internal and external (environmental) factors. Internal factors include genetics and hormonal secretions. External factors such as diet, exercise, and social settings also directly affect weight management. Let's examine these two sets of influences more closely.

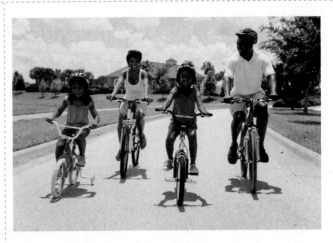

Exercise is a key component to any weight-loss program. Family and friends can help support exercise and healthy behaviors.

Genetic Factors and Hormones

There are a few rare conditions, including Prader-Willi syndrome and Bardet-Biedl syndrome, that account for extreme obesity in about 1% of the population. These two conditions are genetic disorders and are present at birth (5). Other physiological causes of obesity may be related to the release of hormones that regulate appetite, especially leptin and ghrelin, and much current research focuses on this area.

Appetite control is a function of the brain (6). More specifically, the hypothalamus is the region of the brain that houses the appetite center. This appetite control region contains sensors that monitor fat and sugar levels in the blood, including receptors that respond to specific hormones.

The hormone **leptin** is produced in fat cells and released into the blood (7). Circulating leptin depresses appetite by acting on receptors in the hypothalamus (8). Researchers working on the connection between hormones and obesity found that obese mice had very low levels of leptin; when injected with leptin, the mice became lean. Leptin was believed to be the cure-all for the obesity epidemic until it was later discovered that many obese people produce abnormally high levels of leptin. For these obese individuals, leptin is unable to depress appetite because leptin receptors in the brain have lost their ability to respond to the hormone (6). Further research has revealed that leptin also works with other hormones such as insulin (a hormone manufactured by the pancreas) to suppress appetite (6, 7).

Another hormone, called **ghrelin**, promotes feelings of hunger (8). High levels of ghrelin trigger nerve signals in the brain to promote hunger (9). Because ghrelin increases hunger, much research has been aimed toward developing ways to inhibit ghrelin production. Although controversial, there is evidence that moderate-intensity resistance and cardiorespiratory

exercise can suppress ghrelin production, thus reducing appetite (10, 11). Gastric bypass surgery has also been shown to suppress ghrelin levels (12).

In general, food in the stomach suppresses ghrelin production and release. However, foods differ in their ability to suppress ghrelin. For example, foods rich in fat are less effective in suppressing the production of ghrelin than foods containing proteins or carbohydrates (i.e., sugars) (8). Proteins are the best foods at suppressing ghrelin. Consumption of a high-carbohydrate meal suppresses ghrelin production initially, but this effect is short-lived and ghrelin manufacture rapidly rises after such a meal (8).

 LIVE IT! ASSESS YOURSELF Assess your diet with the *All-or-Nothing Thinking and "Safe Foods" versus "Forbidden Foods"* Take Charge of Your Health! Worksheet online at **www.pearsonhighered.com/powers.**

Environmental Factors

Environmental factors remain the primary focus for many health-care professionals in treating overweight and obese individuals. Diet and exercise are the two major factors that can be controlled and modified in fighting the obesity epidemic. What you eat, and how much you eat, as well as how much you exercise, are very much within your control.

Understanding what triggers your eating habits is an important first step in weight management. For some people, eating has become a response to emotional stressors, both good and bad. On the one hand, think about how your family celebrates an accomplishment, such as graduation from college, or a milestone,

---

leptin A hormone that appears to depress appetite.

ghrelin A hormone that contributes to feelings of hunger.

STEPS FOR BEHAVIOR CHANGE

What triggers your eating?

Take the following quiz to help assess some of the cues that cause you to eat.

Y N

☐ ☐ I need to have a snack and a beverage nearby when I study.

☐ ☐ I cannot watch television or sit through a movie without a snack in my hand.

☐ ☐ I would order the small portion at a fast food restaurant, but I get more for my money if I order the largest size possible.

☐ ☐ Leaving food on my plate is wasteful.

☐ ☐ I like to have a beverage in my cupholder when I'm driving.

If you answered yes to more than one of these questions, you're likely eating out of habit or because of your environment. This behavior could lead to weight gain.

TIPS TO CURB YOUR CALORIE CONSUMPTION

Tomorrow, you will:

☑ Drink water while studying instead of soda, and if you get hungry, stop for a break and go get a piece of fruit for a snack.

☑ Visit friends or go for a walk in the evening instead of watching television. You'll eat less and work in some physical activity.

Within the next 2 weeks, you will:

☑ Order only small sandwiches and fries when eating fast food, or, better yet, order no fries and a side salad instead.

☑ Not feel obligated to eat your entire plate if you already feel full when eating at home or at a restaurant. Despite what our families may have taught us, clearing your plate is probably leading to your eating long after you're full.

By the end of the semester, you will:

☑ Opt for a reusable water bottle in your car, and use that to stay hydrated during road trips. The calories in sodas and sugar- and milk-laden coffee drinks will quickly add up.

such as a birthday or anniversary. These positive stressors bring people together to celebrate, and food is often at the center of that celebration. On the other hand, when dealing with negative feelings such as depression, loneliness, or boredom, some people turn to food for comfort. Eating habits become ingrained as part of our family practices and may be difficult to change.

Eating habits have also changed as fast food restaurants have proliferated throughout the country. The convenience of these food outlets has made it easy to "grab" a quick sandwich and eat it en route to work, play, or the next event. Convenience, cost, and portion size have made fast food restaurants a contributor to the obesity epidemic. The restaurant industry overall has also increased portion sizes to meet market demand. As portion sizes increase, so do the waistlines of the customers. In fact, serving sizes have increased to the point that the average person does not realize what a normal serving size should be. In the end, most people underestimate the amount of food they eat. Paying attention to how much and what we consume is an important first step in weight management.

Do you know what situations or events affect your eating habits? See the Steps for Behavior Change box above to identify some of your food triggers.

 Assess your eating habits with the *Why Do You Eat?* Take Charge of Your Health! Worksheet online at www.pearsonhighered.com/powers.

LIVE IT! ASSESS YOURSELF

The Concept of Energy Balance

Body fat stores are regulated by two factors: (1) the rate at which fat is ingested or synthesized and stored in fat cells; and (2) the rate at which energy is expended and fat is metabolized (broken down) and used for fuel. In general, fat stores increase when energy intake ("calories in") exceeds energy expenditure ("calories out") and decrease when energy expenditure exceeds energy intake. This concept can be simplified as "calories in versus calories out." If you take in more calories than you expend, you will gain fat weight, and if you expend more calories than you consume, you will lose fat weight [see **Figure 9.1(a)–(b)** on page 231]. An increase in energy intake (calories) in response to increased appetite leads

Weight Gain

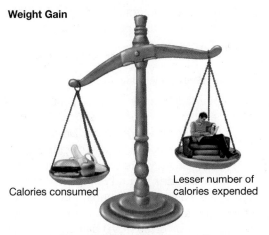

Calories consumed

Lesser number of calories expended

Energy intake > Energy expenditure

(a)

Weight Loss

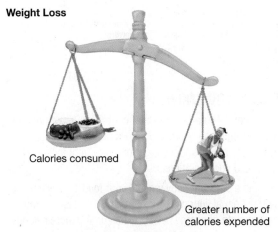

Calories consumed

Greater number of calories expended

Energy intake < Energy expenditure

(b)

Weight Maintenance

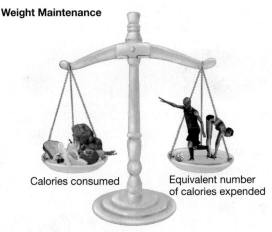

Calories consumed

Equivalent number of calories expended

Energy intake = Energy expenditure

(c)

FIGURE 9.1
The concept of energy balance. An imbalance on either side of the scale will result in a change in body weight **(a and b)**. To maintain body weight, the number of calories you consume must equal the number of calories you expend **(c)**.

to increases in fat synthesis and storage. In contrast, fat stores are reduced when fat is broken down for use as a source of energy for the body.

If you want to maintain a constant body weight, your food energy intake (expressed in calories) must equal your energy expenditure; that is, you must be in **energy balance** [Figure 9.1(c)]. Healthy weight-loss programs include both a reduction in caloric intake and an increase in caloric expenditure achieved through exercise (13–15).

Estimating your daily energy expenditure is a key factor in planning a weight-loss program and adjusting the energy balance equation. The daily expenditure of energy involves both the resting metabolic rate and the exercise metabolic rate.

Resting metabolic rate (RMR) is the amount of energy expended during all sedentary activities. That is, RMR includes the energy required to maintain necessary bodily functions (called the basal metabolic rate) plus the additional energy required to perform such activities as sitting, reading, typing, and digesting food. The RMR is an important component of the energy balance equation because it represents approximately 90% of the total daily energy expenditure in sedentary individuals (16).

Resting metabolic rate is influenced by several factors, including age, gender, and the amount of lean body mass an individual possesses. For example, resting metabolic rate (expressed per pound of body weight) is generally higher in growing children than in adults. Moreover, RMR declines with age, and men have a higher resting metabolic rate than women. Finally, RMR is elevated in people with a low percentage of body fat and a high percentage of lean mass. The explanation for this is that the energy required to maintain muscle tissue is greater than the energy required to maintain fat tissue (13).

Exercise metabolic rate (EMR) represents the energy expenditure during any form of exercise (walking, climbing steps, weight lifting, and so on). In sedentary individuals, EMR constitutes only 10% of the total daily energy expenditure. By comparison, EMR can account for 20%–40% of the total daily energy expenditure in active individuals (16, 17). For example, during heavy exercise, EMR may be 10–20 times greater than

energy balance The state of consuming a number of calories that is equal to the number expended. Over the long term, energy balance results in maintenance of a constant body weight.

resting metabolic rate (RMR) The amount of energy expended during all sedentary activities.

exercise metabolic rate (EMR) The amount of energy expended during any form of exercise.

TABLE 9.1 Estimating Daily Caloric Expenditure

To compute your estimated daily caloric expenditure, multiply your body weight in pounds by the calories per pound corresponding to your activity level.

Activity Level	Description	Calories per Pound of Body Weight Expended during 24-Hour Period
1 Very sedentary	Restricted movement, such as a patient confined to a house	13
2 Sedentary	Light work or office job	14
3 Moderate activity	Some daily activity and weekend recreation	15
4 Very physically active	Vigorous activity at least 3–4 times/week	16
5 Competitive athlete	Daily activity in high energy sport	17–18

RMR (13). Therefore, increased daily exercise increases the EMR and is a key factor in weight-control programs.

One of the simplest ways to estimate your daily caloric expenditure is to determine your activity level and use it to calculate the average number of calories you expend in a 24-hour period (Table 9.1). For example, let's calculate the daily energy expenditure for a moderately active college-aged female who weighs 120 pounds. Using information contained in Table 9.1, this individual would expend 15 calories per pound during a 24-hour period. Therefore, the estimated daily caloric expenditure for this person is calculated by multiplying 120 (her body weight in pounds) by 15 (the calories she expends per pound per day):

$$\text{Daily caloric expenditure} = 120\,\text{pounds} \times 15\,\text{calories/pound/day}$$

$$= 1800\,\text{calories/day}$$

If this woman takes in an average of 2000 calories per day in her meals and snacks, those extra 200 calories put her on the road to weight gain. Do this same calculation for your own daily caloric expenditure. Do you think your daily expenditure is equal to or higher than the amount of calories you take in per day? Now that you know the basic physiological and environmental factors that affect weight management and understand the concept of energy balance, let's discuss the strategies that can lead to safe and effective weight loss.

Assess your dietary habits with the *Out of Control or Overcontrol?* Take Charge of Your Health! Worksheet online at **www.pearsonhighered.com/powers**.

LIVE IT!
ASSESS
YOURSELF

MAKE SURE YOU KNOW...

- Physiological (internal) factors that contribute to overweight and obesity include genetics and hormonal secretions; external factors that affect weight management include diet, exercise, and social settings.

- To maintain a constant body weight, your food energy (caloric) intake must equal your caloric expenditure; that is, you must maintain a state of energy balance. Consuming more calories than you expend results in weight gain, and consuming fewer calories than you expend results in weight loss.

COACHING Corner

How you manage your food intake and calorie expenditure is a matter of personal preference. Consider the following as you develop your weight-management strategy.

- Some find it helpful to have an estimated caloric consumption and caloric expenditure each day. Consider journaling your food choices and using a log of physical activity to estimate your caloric balance for the day. You may also want to try a computer application that offers a similar estimate.

- Small changes in both diet and exercise can yield significant results in relatively short periods of time. Dramatic changes are not usually as successful since they are harder to maintain over time. What are three small steps you can take today in the direction of your goal?

- Practice portion control. You do not have to eat everything on your plate if you are not hungry!

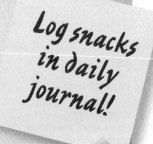

Log snacks in daily journal!

- Daily energy expenditure can be estimated by considering both your resting metabolic rate and your exercise caloric expenditure.

Designing a Successful Weight-Loss Program

The basic strategy for successful weight loss is to expend more calories than you consume. Often this requires changes in both your diet and physical activity lifestyle. Importantly, these diet and lifestyle changes must be sustainable over the long term. The maximum recommended rate for weight loss is 1 to 2 pounds per week. Diets resulting in a weight loss of more than 2 pounds per week are associated with a significant loss of lean body mass (i.e., muscle and body organs) and therefore are not recommended.

The energy deficit required to lose 1 pound per week is approximately 3500 calories. Thus, a negative energy balance of 500 calories per day would theoretically result in a loss of 1 pound of fat per week (3500 calories per week ÷ 7 days per week = 500 calories per day).

The rate of loss during the first several days or weeks of dieting will be greater than later in the dieting period. At the onset of a diet, you lose not only fat, but also carbohydrate and water stores, which also results in some weight loss (13). Further, you may also lose some lean tissue, such as muscle, at the beginning of any diet; therefore, you will often lose more than 1 pound during the first 3500-calorie deficit. However, as the diet continues, you will lose weight at a slower rate. Don't be discouraged if weight loss levels off after the first 2–4 weeks. The weight you lose later will come primarily from fat stores, and sticking with your weight-loss plan for several weeks will result in a significant fat loss.

A CLOSER LOOK

Hot Weight-Loss Topics: Focus on Fructose and Supplements

What Is All the Fuss About Fructose?

It is widely believed that the ingestion of sugars is one of the contributory factors to the obesity epidemic (29–32). Both cane sugar and high-fructose corn syrup contain glucose and fructose. Compared to glucose, fructose has been shown to increase the synthesis of fat, and consumption of fructose does little to suppress appetite. For these reasons, consumption of large amounts of fructose is predicted to increase body fat storage. Even worse, growing evidence suggests that excessive intake of fructose (i.e., >50 grams/day) may be linked to an increased risk of hypertension and diabetes (30, 31, 33).

Fructose is widely available in the American diet since high-fructose corn syrup is used to sweeten many beverages including soft drinks, juices, and sports drinks. Given that soft drink consumption in the U.S. has tripled in recent decades, paralleling the dramatic increase in obesity, this has led to the speculation that consumption of fructose-sweetened soft drinks is a major contributory factor to the rising obesity crisis. Although studies indicate fructose-sweetened soft drinks cause weight gain, it remains unclear if soft drink consumption alone is a major factor in the obesity crisis (32).

Can Dietary Supplements Promote Weight Loss?

Hundreds of weight-loss supplements are available for purchase, and it is estimated that more than 40 million Americans use diet supplements in an effort to lose weight. Unfortunately, the large majority of these "over-the-counter" weight-loss supplements have not been proven to promote weight loss (34, 35). For example, many nutritional supplements called "fat burners" claim to increase fat metabolism to increase weight loss. Often these supplements contain a number of ingredients including caffeine, green tea extracts, chromium, conjugated linoleic acid, and kelp. However, of this list of ingredients, only caffeine and green tea have scientific evidence to back up the claim of increased fat metabolism (36). Further, this increase in fat metabolism is extremely small and would likely be of limited benefit to weight loss (36).

Also, evolving evidence suggests that dietary calcium from supplements or dairy products may play a role in weight management. The proposed mechanism relates to the fact that calcium plays a key role in fat metabolism and fat storage. Specifically, a diet high in calcium from dairy products has been shown to promote fat metabolism, inhibit fat synthesis, and, therefore, increase the loss of body fat. A recent report reviewed the scientific literature and concluded that calcium supplementation generates a small but significant weight loss in overweight and obese individuals (34). Nonetheless, the clinical significance of these findings remains unknown.

In summary, there is limited evidence to support the benefit of most over-the-counter weight-loss products. Also, you should be aware that these dietary supplements are not regulated by the FDA and therefore most products have not undergone quality testing. Further, although some weight-loss products have been reported to promote weight loss, this loss is typically small (i.e., 2–4 pounds), and there is no evidence indicating that these products will be effective for long-term weight loss (35). Therefore, the use of over-the-counter dietary supplements for weight loss is not recommended by nutritional experts (35, 36).

To lose weight and keep it off, you need to implement four basic steps:

1. Establish a realistic goal for weight loss.

2. Assess your diet, and determine how you can modify it to reduce your caloric intake while still consuming all the nutrients you need for health.

3. Decide which physical activities you will begin doing to raise your daily caloric expenditure and increase (or maintain) muscle mass. Choose activities that you enjoy and can perform long-term.

4. Modify your diet and lifestyle to lose the weight you want to lose and prevent future weight gain.

Let's take a closer look at what's involved in each of these steps.

 A new trick for weight loss? Watch *Food Diary Diet Writing* at **www.pearsonhighered.com/powers.**

SEE IT! VIDEOS

Set a Realistic Goal for Weight Loss

The first step in setting a realistic weight loss goal is to decide where your percentage of body fat should fall within the optimal healthy range (8%–19% for men, 21%–32% for women). Many people who are beginning a comprehensive weight-loss program set a long-term weight loss goal that will place them in the middle of the optimal weight range (i.e., 13%–15% body fat for men, 24%–26% body fat for women). After choosing your long-term goal, it is also useful to establish short-term weight-loss goals—usually expressed in the number of pounds lost per week. Keep in mind that 1–2 pounds per week is a realistic weight-loss goal. Establishing a goal of losing 5 pounds in a week is not realistic and will set you up for failure.

If your goal is to lose 1 pound per week, you must establish how you will achieve that. For example, "I will create a daily caloric deficit of 500 calories per day by increasing my daily physical activity (e.g., walking 20–30 minutes each day) and reducing my caloric intake (e.g., no unhealthy snacks between meals and limiting my soda consumption to one 8-ounce glass a day).

Remember, setting realistic goals is an important first step in weight management. Using the optimal healthy range for percent body fat as your guide is healthier and much more realistic than aiming for a tiny dress size or waist measurement. See Laboratory 9.3 for a worksheet you can use to help set your long-term and short-term goals.

Assess and Modify Your Diet

A key to losing weight successfully is to recognize the healthy and less healthy dietary choices you're making on a daily basis. If you're eating fast food regularly, you are likely consuming too many high-fat, high-calorie foods that are impeding your ability to lose weight. Similarly, if you can't remember the last time you ate a fresh fruit or vegetable, you may be getting too few nutrients. A balanced, healthy diet can lead to a caloric deficit and weight loss, and once you know the areas of your diet that could be improved, you can work on making changes that will help you lose weight.

The first step in modifying your diet is to determine how many calories you are consuming each day. Most people tend to underestimate the amount of food they consume. Keeping a food diary for as few as 3 days (Laboratory 8.1, Chapter 8) can determine your total calorie intake and will make you aware of the food choices you are making and allow you to see where you need to make changes in your diet.

When considering a diet for the purpose of losing weight, you should be aware of the following: The diets promoted in books and on websites to promote weight loss often do not provide balanced nutrition and may be difficult diets to sustain (see the Closer Look box on page 235 for more on specific types of weight-loss diets). When you are assessing new diets, a general rule of thumb is to avoid fad diets that promise fast and easy weight loss. If you have concerns about the safety or effectiveness of a published diet, you can either contact your local branch of the Academy of Nutrition and Dietetics for information or approach a dietitian at a hospital or college. Also, if you are considering the use of diet supplements, see A Closer Look on the previous page for more details about these products. After learning the basic nutrition principles contained in this

consider this!

Approximately 90% of fat loss occurs in the body regions with the highest fat storage, generally the thighs and hips in women, and the abdominal region in men.

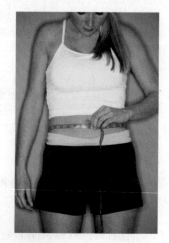

A CLOSER LOOK

Facts and Myths About Popular Diet Plans

Many diet plans exist and more than 1000 diet books are now available. Although some popular diet plans are based on long-standing nutritional and medical advice, others deviate from mainstream nutritional guidelines (37, 38). The most popular diet plans fall into one of four general categories:

1. **Very low-carbohydrate diets:** These diets recommend that carbohydrates make up less than 30% of your total calorie consumption, resulting in a high intake of both proteins and fats. The Atkins diet is the most popular very low-carbohydrate diet plan.

   In general, most such diet plans are structured in 3–4 phases. The first phase limits carbohydrate intake to very low levels (less than 100 calories per day). In subsequent phases, the amounts of carbohydrates consumed typically increase to 20%–30% of your total caloric intake.

   Proponents of these very low-carbohydrate diets argue that they have two major advantages over conventional diet plans. First, eating high-carbohydrate foods reduces the rate of fat metabolism. The evidence to support this claim is that consuming high-carbohydrate foods increases the release of the hormone insulin. High insulin levels can be counterproductive to weight loss because insulin stimulates both fat storage and a reduction in the use of fat as a body fuel (13, 29).

   The second argument is that high-carbohydrate foods are less satiating than foods containing high levels of proteins (29). Therefore, low-carbohydrate diets may promote satiety, reduce overall caloric intake, and assist in achieving a negative caloric balance.

   Based on these assumed advantages of very low-carbohydrate diets, they are often promoted as diets on which "you never feel hungry" and "you will lose weight fast." Both claims can be misleading. Not everyone experiences appetite suppression while on a very low-carbohydrate diet. Further, the initial weight loss is often temporary, due to loss of body water rather than of fat. Consequently, as the individual resumes a normal diet, the body regains the water and the initial weight loss is eliminated (13).

2. **Low-carbohydrate diet:** In general, this class of diets advocates a prescribed ratio of calories from macronutrients (i.e., carbohydrates, proteins, and fats). One of the most popular diets in this category is called the "Zone Diet." This diet program centers on a 40:30:30 ratio of calories obtained from carbohydrates, proteins, and fats. The Zone Diet is a restricted-carbohydrate diet because it limits the consumption of carbohydrates to 40% of the total caloric intake, and it also regulates the types of carbohydrates consumed by limiting the intake of carbohydrates with a high glycemic index.

3. **Low-fat diets:** Low-fat diets limit the number of calories consumed from fats. Some low-fat diets are vegetarian diets, whereas others simply limit protein intake from red meat (red meat contains high levels of fat).

   Advocates of low-fat diets argue that limiting fat intake is an advantage for two major reasons. First, foods rich in fat are also high-calorie foods. Second, consumption of a diet high in fat is often associated with increased risk for cardiovascular disease because high-fat diets often promote elevated blood cholesterol (38–41).

   One of the best-known low-fat diets is the Ornish Diet, a vegetarian plan that concentrates on removing fats and cholesterol from your diet by adding whole grains, legumes, fruits, and vegetables. The Ornish Diet recommends a 70:20:10 ratio of daily calories obtained from carbohydrates, proteins, and fats.

4. **Nutritionally balanced diet with restricted calories:** The Academy of Nutrition and Dietetics recommends that any diet designed to lose weight should be guided by the MyPlate food guidance system (introduced in Chapter 8). This system is based on national nutritional guidelines and, when followed, results in a diet that is low in fat and high in carbohydrates. This weight-loss diet plan is based on long-standing nutritional guidelines and achieves weight loss by restricting caloric intake by limiting food portion sizes.

   Two well-known diets that use this approach are the Weight Watchers Diet and the LEARN diet. The Weight Watchers Diet focuses on eating healthy and smart along with getting more exercise. The LEARN (Lifestyle, Exercise, Attitudes, Relationships, and Nutrition) diet recommends that you consume a 60:30:10 ratio of daily calories obtained from carbohydrates, proteins, and fats. Similar to the Ornish Diet, the LEARN diet is classified as a balanced but low-fat diet.

   So what is the bottom-line recommendation for a weight-loss diet? In short, research indicates that a reduced-calorie diet will result in weight loss regardless of which macronutrient they emphasize (41). Therefore, based on recommendations from the Academy of Nutrition and Dietetics, a nutritionally balanced but reduced-calorie diet is the most desired diet for weight loss. This is because this diet contains a balance of macro- and micronutrients and can be a sustainable diet for the long term.

chapter (and in Chapter 8), you should be able to critically evaluate most diet plans.

Any safe and nutritionally sound diet should adhere to the following guidelines (2, 18, 19).

- The diet should be low in calories but provide all the essential nutrients the body requires. It should be balanced with foods that provide adequate vitamins and minerals on a daily basis.

- The diet should be low in fat (less than 30% of total calories) and high in complex carbohydrates.

- The diet should involve a variety of foods to appeal to your tastes and to prevent hunger between meals, as well as to keep you from getting bored.

- The diet should be compatible with your lifestyle, and the foods should be easily obtainable.

- The diet should be a lifelong diet; that is, it should be one that you can follow for the long term. This will greatly increase your chances of keeping weight off once you've lost it.

COACHING **Corner**

Diet and exercise do NOT have to equal deprivation and pain. Diet does not necessarily mean calorie reduction: The word is used to describe the sum total of the foods we consume. Similarly, the word exercise is often associated with an outdated philosophy of "no pain, no gain." Reframe your conceptualization of the words *diet* and *exercise* by thinking about the following:

- What foods made up your diet today? In what ways did your diet have variety (color, texture, tastes, etc)?

- What improvements might you make in your diet tomorrow?

- What exercises did you do today? What was the most engaging part of your exercise routine?

- What were the intended goals associated with the exercises you chose? In what ways were you successful in your exercise routine?

Eat more vegetables tomorrow

In addition to these diet guidelines, here are some helpful reminders (some of which were covered in Chapter 8) for planning a healthy, balanced diet:

- Avoid high-calorie, low-nutrient foods such as those high in sugar (e.g., candy bars, cookies, soft drinks, and alcohol). Instead, select low-calorie, nutrient-dense foods such as fruits, vegetables, and whole-grain breads.

- Reduce the amount of saturated fat in your diet, and avoid trans fats (which are sometimes found in processed foods and baked goods). High-fat foods are high in calories, and eating too much saturated fat can also increase your risk for heart disease. For example, eat less butter, and choose lean meats such as lean cuts of beef, chicken, and fish. Avoid fried foods; choose nonfat or low-fat dairy products, such as milk, yogurt, and cottage cheese.

- Select fresh fruits and vegetables whenever possible, and avoid fruits that are canned in heavy syrup.

- Limit salt intake. Use herbs and other seasonings instead of salt to flavor foods.

- Drink fewer alcoholic beverages, which are low in nutrients and high in calories.

- Eat to satisfy hunger, not out of boredom or other emotional situations. Remember that a negative energy balance of 500 calories per day will result in a weight loss of approximately 1 pound per week. The key to maintaining a caloric deficit of 500 calories per day is careful planning of meals and accurate calorie counting.

Frozen meals may not be the key to dieting success. Watch *Miscounting Calories* at **www.pearsonhighered.com/powers.**

SEE IT!
VIDEOS

Plan Your Physical Activity

Physical activity and exercise play a key role in weight loss for several reasons (13, 17, 20–23). First, increased physical activity elevates your daily caloric expenditure and therefore helps you expend more calories, and regular cardiorespiratory exercise improves the ability of skeletal muscles to burn fat as energy. Further, regular resistance exercise (such as weight training) can reduce the loss of muscle that occurs during dieting. This is important because your primary goal during weight loss is to lose fat, not muscle mass. Finally, increasing your muscle mass via resistance training increases resting metabolic rate, which further aids in weight loss (22).

What type of exercise is best for losing weight? You should perform both cardiorespiratory training (i.e., running, cycling, swimming, and so on) and strength training while dieting. The combination of these two types of training will maintain cardiorespiratory fitness and reduce muscle loss.

Many people assume aerobic exercise (running, cycling, etc.) must be maintained at a low intensity if fat is to be burned as fuel. It is true that fat is a primary fuel

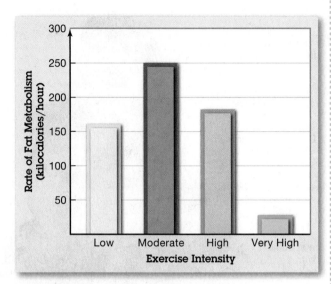

FIGURE 9.2
Illustration of the rates of fat metabolism during low-intensity exercise (20% $\dot{V}O_2$ max), moderate-intensity exercise (50% $\dot{V}O_2$ max), high-intensity exercise (80% $\dot{V}O_2$ max), and very-high-intensity exercise (90% $\dot{V}O_2$ max), While this figure is not intended to promote the "ideal" exercise intensity for all people, it indicates that moderate-intensity exercise is often optimal for maximizing the amount of fat metabolized during physical activity.

Activity	Calories/ Minute/ Kilogram	Calories/ Minute*	METs[†]
Bowling	0.0471	3.2	2.7
Golf	0.0559	3.8	3.2
Walking (17 min per mile)	0.0794	5.4	4.5
Tennis (doubles)	0.0882	6.0	5.1
Cycling (6.4 min per mile)	0.0985	6.7	5.6
Tennis (singles)	0.1029	7.0	5.8
Canoeing (15 min per mile)	0.1029	7.0	5.8
Swimming (50 yards per min)	0.1333	9.1	7.6
Running (10 min per mile)	0.1471	10.0	8.0
Cycling (5 min per mile)	0.1559	10.6	8.5
Handball (singles)	0.1603	10.9	9.1
Running (8 min per mile)	0.1856	12.6	10.0
Running (6 min per mile)	0.2350	16.0	12.8

TABLE 9.2 Calories Expended during Selected Activities

* These values are for a 150-lb (68-kg) person.
[†] 1 MET equals your resting metabolic rate.

Source: From *Physical Fitness: A Way of Life, 5/e* by Bud Getchell, Alan E. Mikesky and Kay Mikesky. Reprinted by permission of Cooper Publishing Group.

source during low-intensity exercise. As illustrated in Figure 9.2, the total amount of fat burned during exercise varies with the intensity of exercise, and for a given exercise duration, more total fat is metabolized during moderate-intensity exercise. Therefore, moderate-intensity exercise (i.e., approximately 50% $\dot{V}O_2$ or 70% maximum heart rate) is typically the optimal intensity of exercise for burning the most fat during an endurance exercise workout. If, however, you are overweight or your fitness level is low, start with a low-intensity workout (i.e., 25% $\dot{V}O_2$ max or 50% maximum heart rate) until you improve your cardiorespiratory fitness level to support higher exercise intensities.

How much exercise must you perform during a weight-loss program? In general, exercise sessions designed to promote weight loss should expend more than 250 calories (13). In this way the negative caloric balance can be shared equally by exercise and diet. For example, an individual who wants to achieve a 500 calorie per day deficit could increase exercise energy expenditure by 250 calories per day (e.g., walking for 45–60 minutes) and decrease caloric intake by 250 calories (i.e., reduce food portions).

While intensity of exercise is an important factor in improving cardiorespiratory fitness, it is the total amounts of energy expended and fat burned that are important in weight loss. Some authors have argued that low-intensity prolonged exercise (such as walking 1–2 miles a day) is better than short-term high-intensity exercise (e.g., sprinting 50 yards) in burning fat calories and promoting weight loss (23). However, evidence clearly demonstrates that both high- and low-intensity exercise can promote

fat loss (13). Nonetheless, for the sedentary or obese individual, low-intensity exercise is the best choice because it can be performed for longer time periods and increases the ability of skeletal muscle to metabolize fat for energy (see the Appreciating Diversity box on page 238) (20).

To determine your caloric expenditure during an activity, simply multiply your body weight in kilograms (2.2 pounds = 1 kilogram) by the calories burned per minute per kilogram, and by the exercise time (see Table 9.2 for calories expended during various activities). For instance, suppose a 70-kilogram (kg) individual plays 20 minutes of handball. How many calories did he expend during the time of play? The total estimated caloric expenditure is computed as follows:

Caloric expenditure = 70 kg × 0.1603 calories–kg–min

× 20 min = 224 calories

If your exercise routine at a fitness club involves using equipment such as stationary bicycles, treadmills, or ellipticals, the exercise apparatus will probably provide a rough estimate of caloric expenditure at the end of your exercise bout.

How can Elena overcome peer pressure and lead a healthy lifestyle? Listen to the online case study at **www.pearsonhighered.com/powers.**

HEAR IT!
CASE STUDY

Focus on Behavior Modification

Research demonstrates that behavior modification plays a key role in both achieving short-term weight loss and maintaining weight loss over the long term (18). Many behaviors are learned and therefore can be modified. For example, many people eat popcorn and candy when they attend a movie at the theater. Similarly, a nightly television habit is often accompanied by snacking on chips, sodas, and other high-calorie, low-nutrition items. The fact that these behaviors are learned means that they can also be unlearned. In regard to weight control, behavior modification is used primarily to reduce or (ideally) eliminate social or environmental stimuli that promote overeating.

The first step in a diet-related behavior modification program is to identify those social or environmental factors that promote overeating. This can be done by keeping a written record of daily activities for 1 or 2 weeks to identify factors associated with consumption of high-calorie meals. Refer to **Figure 9.3** for common social and environmental factors that may contribute to your overeating. How many of these factors occur in your food diary?

After identifying the behaviors that contribute to weight gain, you can design a program to modify those

1. *Activities.* You may find a correlation between specific types of activities, such as watching TV and eating snacks.

2. *Emotional behavior before or during eating.* Many people overeat when they are depressed or under stress.

3. *Location of meals.* Do you eat your meals in front of the television? Do you associate specific rooms with snacking?

4. *Time of day and level of hunger.* Do you eat at specific times of the day? Do you eat even if you are not hungry?

5. *People involved.* Are specific people associated with periods of overeating?

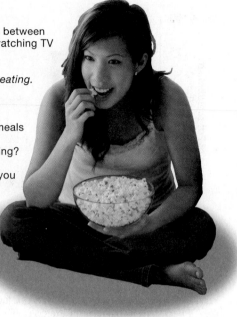

FIGURE 9.3
Do you overeat because of any of these social or environmental influences?

behaviors. The following weight-control techniques will make weight loss easier (18):

- *Make a personal commitment to losing weight.* This is the first step toward behavior modification and weight loss. Establishing realistic short-term and long-term weight-loss goals helps you maintain a lifelong commitment to weight management.

- *Develop healthy low-calorie eating patterns.* Avoid eating when you are not hungry. Learn to eat slowly

Exercise for Obese Individuals

Although it is well established that exercise is an important factor in promoting weight loss, exercise prescriptions for obese individuals require special attention. For example, obese individuals may be limited by the following conditions: heat intolerance, shortness of breath during heavy exercise, lack of flexibility, frequent musculoskeletal injuries, hypertension, and a lack of balance during weight-bearing activities such as walking or running.

Exercise programs for obese individuals should emphasize activities that can be sustained for long periods of time (60–90 minutes), such as walking, swimming, water exercise, or bicycling. Further, obese people should avoid exercise in a hot or humid environment. The initial goal of the exercise program should not be to improve cardiovascular fitness, but rather to increase voluntary energy expenditure and to establish a regular exercise routine. Therefore, the beginning exercise intensity should be below the typical target heart rate range for improving

cardiorespiratory fitness, and the initial duration of exercise should be short (about 5–10 min/day) to reduce the risk of soreness and injury. The duration can be gradually increased in 1-minute increments to achieve an energy expenditure of approximately 300 kcal per workout. As the musculoskeletal system adapts to the exercise regimen, the intensity can gradually be increased as well.

Sources: Fransen, M. Dietary weight loss and exercise for obese adults with knee osteoarthritis: Modest weight loss targets, mild exercise, modest effects. *Arthritis and Rheumatology* 50(5):1366–1369, 2004; Jakicic, J. M. Exercise in the treatment of obesity. *Endocrinology and Metabolic Clinics of North America* 32(4):967–980, 2003; and American College of Sports Medicine. Position stand: The recommended quantity and quality of exercise for developing and maintaining cardiorespiratory and muscular fitness, and flexibility in healthy adults. *Medicine and Science in Sports and Exercise* 30:975–991, 1998.

and only while sitting at the table. Finally, reduce the size of your food portions to keep quantities within your caloric guidelines.

- *Avoid social settings where you are likely to overeat or consume too many liquid calories.* If you go to parties where high-calorie foods are served, don't show up hungry. Eat a low-calorie meal before going. Also, avoid social situations where you are encouraged to drink more than one alcoholic drink. Research shows that alcohol consumed before or after meals tends to increase food intake (24).

- *Exercise daily.* Regular exercise that uses large-muscle groups can play an important role in increasing your daily caloric expenditure and can assist in weight loss and weight management.

- *Reward yourself for successful weight loss with non-food rewards.* Positive feedback is an important part of behavior modification, and it doesn't have to relate to food to be effective. For example, after reaching your first short-term weight-loss goal, do something you like to do but don't get to do often, such as buying a new item of clothing or going to the movies.

- *Think positively.* Positive thinking about your ability to lose weight promotes confidence and maintains the enthusiasm necessary for a lifetime of successful weight management.

MAKE SURE YOU KNOW...

- A safe rate of weight loss is 1 to 2 pounds per week; this equals approximately 3500 fewer calories consumed per week, or 500 fewer calories per day.

- There are four basic steps to designing a successful weight loss program: Set realistic goals, assess and modify your diet, plan regular exercise, and avoid activities that will encourage you to overeat or consume too many liquid calories.

Exercise and Diet Programs to Gain Weight

Thus far, this chapter has focused on how to lose body fat. However, some people may have the opposite problem—being underweight—and they may need to implement a program to gain weight. You can achieve weight gain by creating a positive energy balance, that is, by taking in more calories than you expend. When increasing body weight, however, you'll want to aim to increase muscle mass, rather than fat mass, for the sake of your health. Let's discuss how to do this.

The key to gaining muscle mass is a program of rigorous weight training combined with the increase in caloric and protein intake needed to meet the increased energy expenditure and energy required to synthesize muscle. (Exercise programs designed to improve muscular strength and size are discussed in Chapter 4 and are not addressed here.) Here we focus on the dietary adjustments needed to optimize gains in muscle mass. Again, to gain muscle mass, you need to create a small positive caloric balance to provide the energy required to synthesize new muscle protein. Nonetheless, before we provide dietary guidelines, let's discuss how much energy is expended during weight training and how much energy is required to promote muscle growth.

Energy expenditure during routine weight training is surprisingly small. For instance, a 70-kg man performing a 30-minute weight workout probably burns fewer than 70 calories (13, 19). The reason for this low caloric expenditure is that during 30 minutes in the weight room, the average person spends only 8 to 10 minutes lifting weights because most of the time is spent in recovery periods between sets.

Current estimates are that approximately 2500 calories are needed to synthesize 1 pound of muscle mass, of which about 400 calories (100 grams) must be protein (19). To compute the additional calories required to produce an increase in muscle mass, you must first estimate your rate of muscular growth. This is difficult because the rate of muscular growth during weight training varies among people. Although relatively large muscle mass gains are possible in some individuals, studies have shown that most men and women rarely gain more than 0.25 pound of muscle per week during a 20-week weight-training program (3 days per week, 30 minutes per day). If we assume that the average muscle gain is 0.25 pound per week and that 2500 calories are required to synthesize 1 pound of muscle, a positive caloric balance of fewer than 100 calories per day is needed to promote muscle growth. This estimate was computed as follows:

$$0.25 \text{ pound per week} \times 2500 \text{ calories per pound} = 625 \text{ calories per week}$$

Therefore, 625 calories per week ÷ 7 days per week = 90 calories per day.

You can use the MyPlate food guidance system (presented in Chapter 8) to increase your caloric intake. This will ensure that your diet meets the criteria for healthful living and provides adequate protein for building muscle. Be sure to avoid high-fat foods, and limit your positive caloric balance to approximately 90 calories per day. Increasing your positive caloric balance above this level will not promote a faster rate of muscular growth but will increase body fat. Finally, if you discontinue your weight-training program, be sure to lower your caloric intake to match your daily energy expenditure, as failure to do so will result in fat gain.

MAKE SURE YOU KNOW...

- Weight gain can be achieved by creating a positive caloric balance. Before deciding to gain body weight, you should consider whether your current body composition is within your desired range.

- Gaining muscle mass can be achieved by combining exercise with proper nutrition.

Lifetime Weight Management

Weight loss and weight management are not short-term events. Maintaining a healthy body weight over the long term requires adherence to a healthy diet and regular exercise guidelines. If you diet and exercise for a while to lose weight but then slip into unhealthy habits of overeating or being too sedentary once the weight has come off, you will likely undo your efforts. And you may even gain more weight than you initially lost. This is the reason that short-term, fad diets are typically unsuccessful.

The key factors in long-term weight management are a positive attitude, regular exercise, and a personal commitment to maintaining a desired body composition. Like many other facets of personal or professional life, weight control has its ups and downs. Be prepared for occasional setbacks. For instance, many people gain weight during holiday periods. If this happens to you, avoid self-criticism, quickly reestablish your personal commitment to a short-term weight-loss goal, and develop a new diet and exercise plan to lose the undesired fat. Remember, you can lose any amount of weight you've gained by applying the principles discussed in this chapter.

Finally, the importance of family and friends in lifetime weight management is significant. Their encouragement and support can help you maintain healthy long-term eating habits and sustain a commitment to exercise. Losing weight is much easier if the people close to you try to help you achieve your goals rather than tempt you into unhealthy behaviors. Encourage others to join you as you exercise. Your friends and family members may need a little encouragement to get started, but you may be the role model that they need to make the change. See Table 9.3 for a summary of some myths and facts about weight loss.

Extreme Measures for Weight Loss

Most people can attain a healthy body weight through diet and exercise, but for some extremely obese individuals, these may not be enough. In such cases, surgical procedures or prescription medications may be recommended by a health-care provider.

Surgery

According to the American Society for Bariatric Surgery, surgical procedures may be recommended for weight loss in severely obese individuals. The surgery is considered a last resort for individuals who have tried and failed at losing weight and whose obesity poses a serious health risk. Weight-loss surgery is of two types: restrictive procedures and malabsorptive procedures. Restrictive procedures, such as gastric banding, work by decreasing the amount of food consumed at one time. Reduced stomach capacity, along with behavioral changes, can result in lower caloric intake and consistent weight loss. Malabsorptive procedures alter digestion by bypassing the small intestine, thus limiting the absorption of calories. The most common bariatric surgery is a combination of restrictive and malabsorptive procedures. The combination helps patients lose weight quickly and continue to lose weight for 18–24 months after the surgery (26).

Prescription Medications

Unlike diet pills, which are typically ineffective, prescription medications such as orlistat and Meridia have been scientifically shown to help some people achieve weight loss. Orlistat (also called Xenical) works by preventing about one-third of ingested fat from being

TABLE 9.3 Myths and Facts About Weight Loss	
Weight-Loss Myth	**The Facts**
You can spot-reduce body fat.	There is limited scientific evidence to show that exercising a specific area of the body promotes fat loss in that area. In fact, most evidence suggests that when a caloric deficit exists, fat will be lost from areas where the most fat is stored (13). In contrast, a recent study suggests that exercising a specific body area can assist in spot reduction of adjacent fat stores (25). However, more evidence is required before the concept of spot reduction can be accepted as fact.
Eating before bedtime causes weight gain.	Although eating a late-night meal or snack might not be a good dietary habit, this practice does not result in a greater weight gain than consuming the same meal at another time during the day. The total daily caloric intake determines fat gain, not the timing of the meal.
Cellulite is a special form of fat.	Although many people believe that cellulite is different from other body fat, this is not true. Cellulite is just plain fat, not a special type of fat. The "dimpled" appearance comes from accumulation of fat in small clusters beneath the skin. Many products, from special creams and lotions to massage appliances, are advertised as helping reduce cellulite, but no scientific evidence exists to support these claims. The only way to lose fat is to reduce calorie intake and increase exercise. Weight training helps tighten the skin over the muscle and eliminates space between the skin and muscle for fat pockets.
Saunas, steambaths, and rubber suits can aid in weight loss.	These methods do result in body water loss due to sweating. However, the weight is regained as soon as body water is restored to normal levels. Using saunas or steambaths and exercising while wearing a rubber suit may increase body temperature well above normal, which puts additional stress on the heart and circulatory system and could increase the risk of cardiac problems for older individuals or anyone with heart problems.

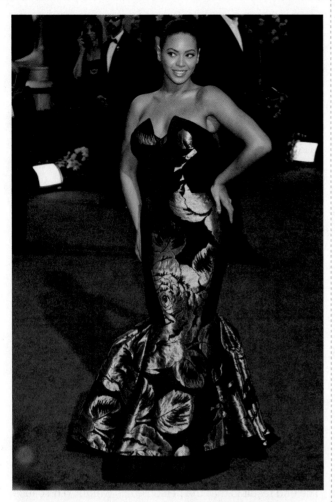

Some celebrities have undergone liquid diets, in which they only drink certain liquids for a set number of days to quickly lose weight. These diets may be nutritionally inadequate and have particular side effects.

absorbed in the digestive tract. The undigested fat is eliminated in bowel movement; hence, one side effect may be an oily stool. Orlistat is the only FDA-approved weight-loss drug that acts to block fat absorption.

The prescription drug Meridia suppresses appetite by increasing serotonin levels in the brain. Meridia and Xenical are the only two weight-loss medications approved for longer-term use in significantly obese people; however, their safety and long-term effectiveness remain unclear.

 Do weight loss drugs work? Watch *Diet Dream Drug* at **www.pearsonhighered.com/powers.**

SEE IT!
VIDEOS

What Is Disordered Eating?

Although attaining a healthy body weight is a highly desirable goal, for some people the social pressures to be thin and/or muscular can lead to a negative body image and an unhealthy relationship with food. Women may feel like they need to emulate the often unattainably thin figures of popular actresses and models, or men may wish to achieve the bulked-up look of professional athletes, in the pursuit of a more "perfect" body. When these desires lead to unhealthy behaviors, such as bouts of self-starvation, binging, and/or purging, the individual may develop a pattern of disordered eating.

Three common forms of disordered eating that affect young adults are anorexia nervosa, bulimia nervosa, and binge eating. Let's discuss the symptoms and health consequences of these conditions.

Anorexia Nervosa

Anorexia nervosa is an eating disorder in which the individual severely limits caloric intake, eventually resulting in a state of starvation. As the condition advances, the individual becomes emaciated. The psychological cause of anorexia nervosa is unclear, but it seems to be linked to an unfounded fear of fatness that may be related to familial or societal pressures to be thin (13).

Although the condition occurs in both men and women, rates of anorexia nervosa are particularly high among adolescent girls, and as many as 1 of every 100 adolescent girls may suffer from this condition. Anorexia nervosa affects approximately 1% of the female adolescent population, with an average age of onset between 14 and 18 years (27, 28). Upper-middle-class young women who are extremely self-critical have the highest probability of developing anorexia nervosa.

consider this!

The average "female" store mannequin is 6 feet tall and has a 23-inch waist, whereas the average woman is 5 feet, 4 inches tall and has a 30-inch waist.

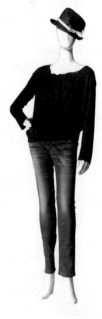

anorexia nervosa An eating disorder in which a person severely restricts caloric intake because of an intense fear of gaining weight.

People suffering from anorexia nervosa may use a variety of techniques to remain thin, including starvation, excessive exercise, and laxatives. The effects of anorexia nervosa include excessive weight loss, cessation of menstruation, and, in extreme cases, death. Because the condition is a serious mental and physical disorder, medical treatment by a team of professionals (physician, psychologist, and nutritionist) is needed to correct the problem. Treatment may require long-term psychological counseling and nutritional guidance.

The first step in seeking treatment for anorexia nervosa is recognizing that a problem exists. The following common symptoms may indicate that someone is exhibiting anorexia nervosa:

- An intense fear of gaining weight or becoming obese
- The feeling that one is fat even at normal or below-normal body fatness because of a highly distorted body image
- In women, the absence of three or more menstrual cycles
- The possible development of odd behaviors concerning food; for example, preparing elaborate meals for others but only a few low-calorie foods for one's own consumption

Bulimia Nervosa

About 50% of people with anorexia nervosa eventually suffer from **bulimia nervosa**, which is characterized by cycles of binging and purging. People with bulimia nervosa may repeatedly ingest large quantities of food and then force themselves to vomit to prevent weight gain. The frequent vomiting associated with bulimia nervosa may result in damage to the teeth and the esophagus due to exposure to stomach acids. Like anorexia nervosa, bulimia nervosa is most common in young women, has a psychological origin, and requires professional treatment

---

bulimia nervosa An eating disorder that involves overeating (called *binge eating*) followed by vomiting (called *purging*).

binge eating disorder The compulsive need to gorge on food without purging.

---

when diagnosed. Bulimia affects approximately 1%–3% of adolescents in the United States. The illness usually begins in late adolescence or early adult life (28).

People with bulimia nervosa may look "normal" and be of normal weight. However, even when their bodies are slender, their stomachs may protrude because they have been stretched by frequent eating binges. Other common symptoms of bulimia nervosa include the following:

- Recurrent binge eating
- A lack of control over eating behavior
- Regular self-induced vomiting and/or use of diuretics or laxatives
- Strict fasting or use of vigorous exercise to prevent weight gain
- Averaging two or more binge eating episodes per week during a 2- to 3-month period
- Excessive concern with body shape and weight

Binge Eating Disorder

A disordered eating pattern that has recently begun to attract attention from the medical community is **binge eating disorder**, a condition in which an individual consumes mass quantities of food but, unlike people with bulimia nervosa, does not purge after binging. The person may feel embarrassed and ashamed about gorging and resolve to stop doing it, but the compulsion continues. The end result is that the person gains weight. The cause of binge eating is unknown, and only a very small percentage of overweight and obese individuals engage in it.

Although maintaining an optimal body composition is a primary health goal, eating disorders are not appropriate means of weight loss. If you or any of your friends exhibit one or more of the symptoms cited here, please seek professional advice and treatment.

MAKE SURE YOU KNOW...

- Eating disorders such as anorexia nervosa, bulimia nervosa, and binge eating disorder involve patterns of severe calorie restriction, binging, and/or purging.
- Severe and prolonged eating disorders can result in an unhealthy body weight, leading to poor health and possibly death.

SUMMARY

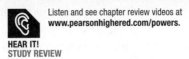

Listen and see chapter review videos at www.pearsonhighered.com/powers.

HEAR IT! STUDY REVIEW

1. Factors that can affect weight management include genetic, dietary, and lifestyle factors. Genetic disorders cause extreme obesity in about 1% of the population. For the rest, however, research indicates that environmental and lifestyle factors are more likely than genetics to affect body weight.
2. Energy balance is achieved when the number of calories you take in through food and beverages equals the number of calories you expend through physical activity and normal body processes.
3. Total daily energy expenditure is the sum of resting metabolic rate and exercise metabolic rate.
4. Losing 1 to 2 pounds per week is considered a safe rate of weight loss. Body fat will be lost first in the areas of the body that store the most fat, such as the thighs and hips in women, and the abdominal region in men.
5. The four basic components of a comprehensive weight-control program are setting realistic goals for weight loss, assessing and modifying your diet, planning physical activity, and modifying your behaviors that contribute to weight gain.
6. Weight-loss goals should include both short-term and long-term goals.
7. Research indicates that a reduced calorie diet will result in weight loss regardless of which macronutrient they emphasize. Therefore, a low-carbohydrate or low-fat diet is not superior to any other diet that results in a similar caloric deficit.
8. It is currently believed that a nutritionally balanced but reduced calorie diet is the most desired diet for weight loss because this diet contains a balance of nutrients and can be sustainable for the long-term.
9. People seeking to gain weight need to take in more calories than they expend. They should seek to gain muscle mass rather than fat by engaging in an appropriate strength-training program.
10. The eating disorders anorexia nervosa, bulimia nervosa, and binge eating disorder are serious medical conditions that require professional treatment.

STUDY QUESTIONS

Find more review questions online at www.pearsonhighered.com/powers.

REVIEW IT! QUIZZES

1. The optimal percentage of body fat for men and women is
   a. 5%–15% for men and 10%–20% for women.
   b. 8%–19% for men and 21%–32% for women.
   c. 15%–25% for men and 20%–30% for women.
   d. 20%–30% for men and 25%–35% for women.
2. Hormones that play a role in appetite include which of the following?
   a. insulin
   b. ghrelin
   c. leptin
   d. estrogen
   e. both (a) and (d) are correct
   f. both (b) and (c) are correct
3. Identify the true statement regarding energy balance:
   a. Caloric intake should equal caloric expenditure.
   b. Weight gain occurs when caloric intake exceeds caloric expenditure.
   c. Weight loss occurs when caloric expenditure exceeds caloric intake.
   d. All of the above statements are true.
4. The two forms of exercise that are most beneficial in helping you lose and maintain weight are
   a. flexibility and Pilates training.
   b. yoga and anaerobic exercise.
   c. strength training and cardiorespiratory endurance training.
   d. Exercise is not helpful for weight loss.
5. Disordered eating includes all of the following except
   a. anorexia nervosa.
   b. bulimia nervosa.
   c. binge eating.
   d. using MyPlate to plan a healthy diet.
6. What is optimal body weight, and how is it calculated?
7. Explain the roles of resting metabolic rate and exercise metabolic rate in determining total caloric expenditure. Which is more important in total daily caloric expenditure in a sedentary individual?
8. Outline a simple method for computing your daily caloric expenditure. Give an example.

9. List the four major components of a weight-loss program.

10. Discuss the role of behavior modification in weight loss.

11. Compare and contrast the symptoms of anorexia nervosa, bulimia nervosa, and binge eating disorder.

12. Define the following terms:
    energy balance
    resting metabolic rate
    fad diet

13. Compare exercise metabolic rate with resting metabolic rate.

14. List the four major categories of weight loss diets. Which of these diet plans is recommended by the Academy of Nutrition and Dietetics for weight loss?

HELPFUL WEBLINKS

**DO IT!
WEBLINKS**

For links to the organizations and websites listed, visit **www.pearsonhighered.com/powers.**

Academy of Nutrition and Dietetics
Contains articles about nutrition and fad diets.
www.eatright.org

Centers for Disease Control: Obesity at a glance 2011
Discusses the obesity epidemic and the health consequences of obesity. www.cdc.gov/chronicdisease/resources/publications/aag/obesity.htm

ChooseMyPlate.gov
Walks you through the advice illustrated in the MyPlate food guidance system. www.choosemyplate.gov

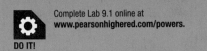
Name _____ Date _____

Determining Ideal Body Weight Using Percent Body Fat and the Body Mass Index

There are several different ways to compute an ideal body weight. Method A of this laboratory enables you to compute and record your ideal body weight using skinfold measurements. (In Chapter 6 we discussed body fat percentage estimated from skinfold measurements.) Method B enables you to calculate and record your ideal body weight using the body mass index (BMI) procedure (Chapter 6). Choose one of these techniques, and complete the appropriate section.

METHOD A: COMPUTING IDEAL BODY WEIGHT USING PERCENT BODY FAT

STEP 1: Calculate fat-free weight

100% − your percent body fat estimated from skinfold measurement = _____ % fat-free weight

Therefore,

_____ % fat-free weight expressed as a decimal × _____ your body weight in pounds

= _____ pounds of fat-free weight

STEP 2: Calculate optimal weight

Remember: Optimal body fat ranges are 8%–19% for men and 21%–32% for women. Optimal weight = fat-free weight ÷ (1.00 − optimal % fat), with optimal % fat expressed as a decimal. Therefore, the low and high optimal weight ranges for your gender are as follows:

For low %fat : Optimal weight _____ pounds

For high %fat : Optimal weight _____ pounds

METHOD B: COMPUTING IDEAL BODY WEIGHT USING BODY MASS INDEX (BMI)

The BMI uses the metric system. Therefore, you must express your weight in kilograms (1 kilogram = 2.2 pounds) and your height in meters (1 inch = 0.0254 meter).

STEP 1: Compute your BMI

$$BMI = body\ weight\ (kg) \div (height\ in\ meters)^2$$

Your BMI = _____

STEP 2: Calculate your ideal body weight based on BMI

The ideal BMI is 21.9 to 22.4 for men and 21.3 to 22.1 for women. The formula for computing ideal body weight using BMI is

$$Ideal\ body\ weight\ (kilograms) = Desired\ BMI \times (height\ in\ meters)^2$$

Consider the following example as an illustration of the computation of ideal body weight. A man who weighs 60 kilograms and is 1.5 meters tall computes his BMI to be 26.7. His ideal BMI is between 21.9 and 22.4; therefore, his ideal body weight range is as follows:

Low end range : 21.9 × 2.25 = 49.3 kilograms

High end of range: 22.4 × 2.25 = 50.4 kilograms

Now complete this calculation using your values for BMI.

My ideal body weight range using the BMI method is _____ to _____ kilograms.

Note: BMI may not be a good method to determine ideal body weight for a highly muscled individual.

LABORATORY 9.2

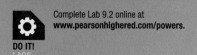

Name _____ **Date** _____

Estimating Daily Caloric Expenditure and the Caloric Deficit Required to Lose 1 Pound of Fat per Week

PART A: ESTIMATING YOUR DAILY CALORIC EXPENDITURE

Using the table below, compute your estimated daily caloric expenditure.

Estimated daily caloric expenditure = _____ calories/day.

Note: For you to maintain current body weight, your caloric intake should equal your daily caloric expenditure.

To compute your estimated daily caloric expenditure, multiply your body weight in pounds by the calories per pound corresponding to your activity level.

Activity Level	Description	Calories per Pound of Body Weight Expended during 24-Hour Period
1 Very sedentary	Restricted movement, such as a patient confined to a house	13
2 Sedentary	Light work or office job	14
3 Moderate activity	Some daily activity and weekend recreation	15
4 Very physically active	Vigorous activity at least 3–4 times/week	16
5 Competitive athlete	Daily activity in high energy sport	17–18

PART B: CALCULATING CALORIC INTAKE REQUIRED TO PROMOTE 1 POUND PER WEEK OF WEIGHT LOSS

Recall that 1 pound of fat contains approximately 3500 calories. Therefore, a negative caloric balance of 500 calories per day will result in a weight loss of 1 pound per week. Use the following formula to compute your daily caloric intake to result in a daily caloric deficit of 500 calories.

Estimated daily caloric expenditure − 500 calories (deficit) = Daily caloric intake needed to produce a 500-calorie deficit

In the space provided, compute your daily caloric intake needed to produce 1 pound per week of weight loss.

_____ (estimated caloric expenditure) − 500 (caloric deficit) = _____ (target daily caloric intake)

Note: To increase body weight by 1–2 pounds per week, increase daily caloric intake by 90–180 calories per day.

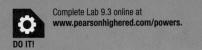
Name _____ **Date** _____

Weight-Loss Goals and Progress Report

In the spaces provided, record your short-term and long-term weight-loss goals. Then keep a record of your progress on the chart.

Ideal body weight (range): _____

Short-term weight loss goal: ___1–2___ (pounds/week)

Long-term weight loss goal: _____ pounds

Week No.	Body Weight	Date	Weight Loss
1			
2			
3			
4			
5			
6			
7			
8			
9			
10			
11			
12			
13			
14			
15			

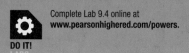
Name _____ **Date** _____

Assessing Body Image

Respond to the questions below to assess your body image.

1. Where do you get your ideas about the "ideal body"? If more than one applies, how do they rank?

    a. TV/movies _____

    b. friends (including partners) _____

    c. parents and family _____

    d. professional athletes _____

2. What other sources contribute to your image of the "ideal body"?

    _____

    _____

Fill in the blanks to complete the following statements about your body image. Use extra paper if needed.

3. The thing I like most about my body is

    _____

    _____

4. The thing I like least about my body is

    _____

    _____

5. When I eat a big meal, I feel

    _____

    _____

6. When I look in the mirror, I see

    _____

    _____

7. I like/dislike (choose one) shopping for clothes because

    _____

    _____

8. I feel self-conscious when

    _____

    _____

9. Compared to others, I feel my body is

    _____

    _____

10. In the presence of someone I find attractive, I feel

    _____

    _____

11. I feel that my appearance is

    _____

    _____

12. One word to describe my body is

    _____

INTERPRETATION

Now review your answers to the previous questions and think about whether they are positive or negative. To improve a negative body image, keep the following strategies in mind:

- Focus on good physical health. Engage in physical activities that you enjoy.
- Remember that your self-worth is not dependent on how you look.
- Avoid chronic, restrained dieting.
- Recognize that there is much more to you than your body. Think about the qualities that you like best about yourself, and be sure to appreciate them.

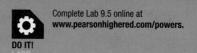
Name _____ Date _____

What Triggers Your Eating?

There are many things that cause us to eat. Usually, just by identifying the triggers that cause you to eat, you can develop a strategy to counter those habits. Use the questions below to determine your motivation for eating. For each statement, check yes or no.

EMOTIONAL TRIGGERS

Yes   No

____   ____   I cannot lose weight and keep it off.

____   ____   My eating is out of control.

____   ____   Even if I'm not hungry, I eat.

____   ____   I eat when I am stressed or upset.

____   ____   Food gives me great pleasure and I use it as a reward.

____   ____   Eating is usually on my mind.

____   ____   My eating causes problems with weight management.

____   ____   I go on eating "binges" or find myself eating constantly.

____   ____   My eating habits cause me embarrassment.

____   ____   I use food to help me cope with feelings.

SOCIAL TRIGGERS

Yes   No

____   ____   I eat whenever others around me are eating.

____   ____   If anyone offers food, I take it.

____   ____   Whenever I am in a stressful social situation, I want to eat.

____   ____   Whenever I am in a relaxed social situation, I want to eat.

____   ____   I eat more in a social setting than I do at home.

____   ____   I eat less when others are around to see me.

____   ____   In a social setting, the amount of food I eat depends on the group of people.

____   ____   I eat different foods in a social setting than I do at home.

ENVIRONMENTAL TRIGGERS

Yes   No

____   ____   I eat more at restaurants than I do at home.

____   ____   I eat less at restaurants than I do at home.

____   ____   If I smell or see food, I can't resist the urge to eat.

____   ____   If I walk by a restaurant or bakery, I can't resist the urge to eat.

____   ____   I like to eat while reading or watching TV.

____   ____   I find food comforting in different environmental conditions, such as on a rainy day or in cold weather.

____   ____   I find food comforting when I am in unfamiliar surroundings.

____   ____   If I am outdoors, I feel like I can eat more.

INTERPRETATION

Insignificant influence: If you answered "yes" to one question within a section or fewer than six questions total, weight management is probably relatively easy for you.

Some influence: If you answered "yes" to two questions within a section or six to nine questions total, there are issues complicating your weight management. It might help to talk with a health-care professional while developing a weight-management plan.

Significant influence: If you answered "yes" to three questions within a section or 10–13 questions total, there are several issues affecting your weight-management plan. Speaking with a health-care professional or counselor can help you deal with issues that trigger your eating.

Severe influence: If you answered "yes" to four or more questions within a section or 14 or more questions total, there are many issues that complicate your weight management. Counseling and speaking with a health-care professional will help you to develop a weight-management plan.

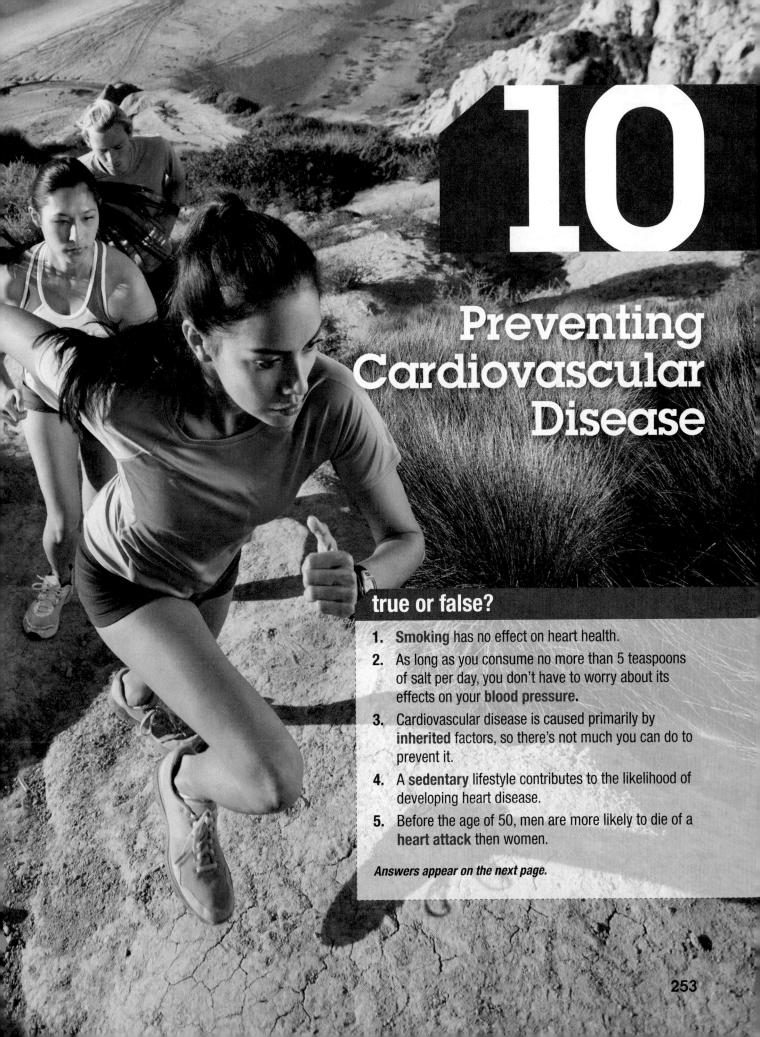

10
Preventing Cardiovascular Disease

true or false?

1. **Smoking** has no effect on heart health.
2. As long as you consume no more than 5 teaspoons of salt per day, you don't have to worry about its effects on your **blood pressure.**
3. Cardiovascular disease is caused primarily by **inherited** factors, so there's not much you can do to prevent it.
4. A **sedentary** lifestyle contributes to the likelihood of developing heart disease.
5. Before the age of 50, men are more likely to die of a **heart attack** then women.

Answers appear on the next page.

Have you ever known someone who's been the victim of a heart attack or stroke? If so, perhaps you're familiar with the symptoms that occur during a heart attack or with the weeks and months of rehabilitation necessary for heart attack and/or stroke survivors to return to a "normal" life. Every year, millions of people worldwide die and/or are permanently injured from heart attack and stroke. Although genetics plays a role in cardiovascular disease in some people, most people can reduce their risk by adopting healthy diet and lifestyle habits. In this chapter, we'll explore the factors that increase your risk of developing cardiovascular disease. We'll also focus on lifestyle changes (e.g., exercise and diet) that can reduce your risk of cardiovascular disease.

What Is Cardiovascular Disease and How Prevalent Is It?

Cardiovascular disease (CVD) is a major health problem around the world, but its greatest incidence occurs in industrialized countries, and the United States has one of the world's highest CVD death rates (1, 2). Although it is impossible to place a dollar value on human life, the economic cost of cardiovascular disease in the United States is great. Estimates of lost wages, medical expenses, and other related costs exceeded $444 billion in 2010 (3). Further, as the U.S. population ages, the economic burden of cardiovascular disease on our nation's health-care system will become even greater. For example, it estimated that during the next 20 years, more than 40% of the U.S. population will have some form of cardiovascular disease, and this will triple the medical costs of managing heart disease during this period **(Figure 10.1)**. Developing a national strategy to reduce the risk of cardiovascular disease is thus a major health priority. Let's begin our discussion with an overview of cardiovascular disease in the United States.

Cardiovascular Disease in the United States

Although public awareness is often more focused on diseases such as cancer, cardiovascular disease remains the number-one cause of death in the United States, accounting for nearly one of every two deaths. More than 83 million adults have one or more forms of CVD, and over 1 million people die annually from cardiovascular disorders (1). CVD is the leading cause of death in men between the ages of 35 and 44, and its incidence among women is rising (1).

SEE IT! VIDEOS
What can you do to detect heart disease? Watch *Heart Disease in America* at **www.pearsonhighered.com/powers.**

answers

1. **FALSE** Smoking is a major risk factor for the development of cardiovascular disease.
2. **FALSE** For salt-sensitive people, consuming high levels of salt (which contains sodium) may increase blood pressure.
3. **FALSE** Heredity is only one of several major risk factors for heart disease. There are several other major risk factors you can modify by changing your behavior (e.g., stop smoking, be more active).
4. **TRUE** Inactivity is a major risk factor for developing heart disease.
5. **TRUE** Throughout their younger years, men are at greater risk of dying of a heart attack than women. However, after age 65, the risk of dying from heart disease increases markedly in women.

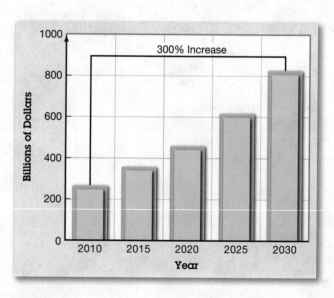

FIGURE 10.1
Projections of the increase in health-care cost of cardiovascular disease in the United States from 2010 to 2030.

Source: Data from Trogdon, P., O. Khavjou, J. Butler, K. Dracup, M. Ezekowitz, et al. Forecasting the future of cardiovascular disease in the United States: A policy statement from the American Heart Association. *Circulation* 123:933–944, 2011.

Types of Cardiovascular Disease

There are hundreds of diseases that can impair normal cardiovascular function. The four most common are arteriosclerosis, coronary heart disease, stroke, and hypertension. Let's look at each of these in more depth.

Arteriosclerosis Arteriosclerosis is a group of diseases characterized by a narrowing, or "hardening," of the arteries. The end result of any form of arteriosclerosis is a progressive blockage of the artery, which eventually impedes blood flow to vital organs. **Athero-sclerosis** is a special type of arteriosclerosis that results in arterial blockage due to buildup of a fatty deposit inside the blood vessel (**Figure 10.2**). This plaque deposit is typically composed of cholesterol, cellular debris, fibrin (a clotting material in the blood), and calcium. Atherosclerosis is a progressive disease that begins in childhood, with symptoms appearing later in life. The disease occurs in varying degrees, with some arteries exhibiting little blockage and others exhibiting major obstruction. Development of severe atherosclerosis within arteries that supply blood to the heart is the cause of almost all heart attacks.

Coronary Heart Disease **Coronary heart disease (CHD)** is the result of atherosclerotic plaque blocking one or more of the blood vessels that supply the heart. When a major coronary artery becomes more than 75% blocked, the restriction of blood flow to the heart muscle causes chest pain. This type of chest pain, called *angina pectoris,* occurs most frequently during exercise or emotional stress, when the heart rate increases and the heart works harder than normal (4). The elevated work requires an increase in blood flow to the heart muscle to provide both oxygen and nutrients. Blockage of coronary blood vessels by atherosclerotic

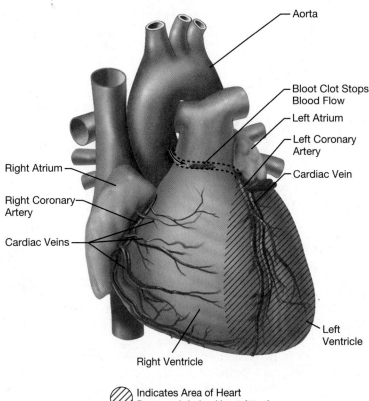

FIGURE 10.3
If the coronary arteries become blocked, the lack of oxygen due to restricted blood flow will lead to damaged muscle tissue.

Source: Johnson, Michael D., *Human Biology: Concepts and Current Issues, 4th Ed.,* © 2008. Reprinted and Electronically reproduced by permission of Pearson Education, Inc., Upper Saddle River, New Jersey.

plaque prevents the necessary increase in blood flow to the heart, and pain results.

If coronary arteries are severely blocked, a blood clot can form around the layer of plaque. If the resulting blockage completely impedes blood flow to the heart, a **heart attack** can occur (**Figure 10.3**). A heart attack results in the death of heart muscle cells in the left ventricle,

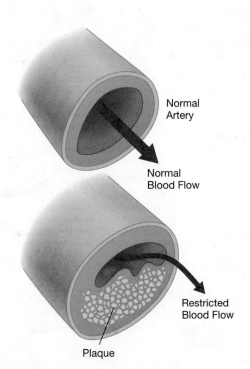

FIGURE 10.2
As plaque builds up in an artery, blood flow is restricted.

Source: Blake, Joan Salge, *Nutrition and You, 1st Ed.,* © 2008. Reprinted and Electronically reproduced by permission of Pearson Education Inc., Upper Saddle River, New Jersey.

cardiovascular disease (CVD) Any disease that affects the heart or blood vessels.

arteriosclerosis A group of diseases characterized by a narrowing, or "hardening," of the arteries.

atherosclerosis A special type of arteriosclerosis that results in arterial blockage due to buildup of a fatty deposit (called *atherosclerotic plaque*) inside the blood vessel.

coronary heart disease (CHD) Also called *coronary artery disease*; the result of atherosclerotic plaque blocking one or more coronary arteries (the blood vessels that supply the heart).

heart attack Stoppage of blood flow to the heart resulting in the death of heart cells; also called *myocardial infarction.*

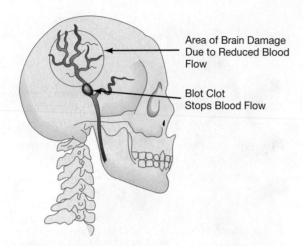

FIGURE 10.4
A blocked artery in the brain can result in a stroke.

and the severity of the heart attack is judged by how many heart muscle cells are damaged (5). A "mild" heart attack may damage only a small portion of the heart, whereas a "major" heart attack may destroy a large number of cells. Because the number of cells destroyed during a heart attack determines the patient's chances of recovery, recognizing the symptoms of a heart attack and getting prompt medical attention are crucial (see the Closer Look below).

Stroke Each year, an estimated 790,000 Americans suffer a **stroke** (1), during which the blood supply to the brain is reduced for a prolonged period of time. A common cause of stroke is blockage (due to atherosclerosis) of arteries leading to the brain (**Figure 10.4**). However, strokes can also occur when a blood vessel in the brain ruptures and disturbs normal blood flow to that region of the brain.

Similar to a heart attack, which results in death of heart cells, a stroke results in death of brain cells. The severity of the stroke may vary from slight to severe, depending on the location and the number of brain cells damaged. Minor strokes may involve a loss of memory, speech problems, disturbed vision, and/or mild paralysis in the extremities. Severe strokes may result in major paralysis and/or death.

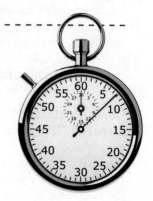

consider this!
40% of heart attack victims die within the first hour.

Hypertension **Hypertension** is abnormally high blood pressure. Your blood pressure is the force blood exerts against the artery walls. When the heart contracts, blood pressure increases, and it decreases when the heart relaxes. Blood pressure is measured in millimeters of mercury (mm Hg) and is expressed with two numbers: the systolic blood pressure (pressure when your heart contracts) and the diastolic blood pressure (pressure when your heart relaxes). Normal resting systolic blood pressure is typically 120 mm Hg, and normal

A CLOSER LOOK

During a Heart Attack, Every Second Counts

If you ever witness someone having a heart attack, or have one yourself, recognizing the symptoms and taking appropriate emergency action could mean the difference between life and death. Here are the common signs of a heart attack (4):

- Mild to moderate pain in the chest that may spread to the shoulders, neck, or arms
- Uncomfortable pressure or sensation of fullness in the chest
- Severe pain in the chest
- Dizziness, fainting, sweating, nausea, or shortness of breath

Note that not all of these symptoms occur in every heart attack. Therefore, if you or someone you're with experiences

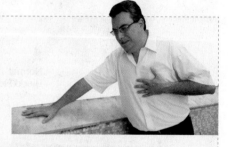

any one of these symptoms for 2 minutes or more, call the emergency medical service or get to the nearest hospital that offers emergency cardiac care. If you are trained in cardiopulmonary resuscitation (CPR) and the patient is not breathing or does not have a pulse, call 911 or the emergency medical service in your area, and then start CPR immediately. In any cardiac emergency, rapid action is essential.

diastolic is 80 mm Hg. Clinically, hypertension is defined as a resting blood pressure over 140 mm Hg systolic or 90 mm Hg diastolic (4).

Your blood pressure will increase during exercise (walking or running). This increase in blood pressure is short-term and does not cause damage to the heart or blood vessels. However, longer-term, chronic hypertension can be a significant health problem. High blood pressure increases the workload on the heart, which may eventually damage the heart muscle's ability to pump blood effectively throughout the body (4). Chronic high blood pressure can also damage the lining of arteries, resulting in atherosclerosis and increasing the risk of CHD and stroke (4).

Several factors can increase your risk of hypertension, including lack of regular exercise, a high-salt diet, obesity, chronic stress, family history of hypertension, gender (men have a greater risk than women), and race (blacks have a greater risk than whites). Note that you can control some of these factors, but you cannot control others (more on this later in the chapter).

The prevalence of hypertension in the United States is remarkably high (**Figure 10.5**). The American Heart Association estimates that approximately one of every three people suffers from hypertension (1). Unfortunately, the symptoms of hypertension, such as severe headaches or dizziness, don't show up in everyone, and many people are unaware that they are hypertensive. In fact, without annual medical checkups or blood pressure screenings, hypertension may go undiagnosed

for years. For this reason, hypertension is often called the "silent killer."

MAKE SURE YOU KNOW...

- Cardiovascular disease remains the number-one cause of death in the United States.
- The term *cardiovascular disease* refers to any disease that affects the heart or blood vessels.
- The four major cardiovascular diseases are arteriosclerosis, coronary heart disease, stroke, and hypertension.

What Are the Risk Factors Associated with Coronary Heart Disease?

Because CHD is the leading contributor to heart attacks, researchers are focused on reducing its occurrence and understanding its causes. They have identified a number of major and contributory risk factors that increase the chance of developing both CHD and stroke. Major risk factors (also called *primary risk factors*) are directly related to the development of CHD and stroke. In contrast, contributory risk factors (or *secondary risk factors*) are those that increase the risk of CHD but their direct contribution to the disease process has not been precisely determined.

Major Risk Factors

Each year the American Heart Association publishes new information concerning the major risk factors associated with the development of CHD and stroke. The most recent list includes tobacco smoking, hypertension, high blood cholesterol levels, physical inactivity, obesity and being overweight, diabetes mellitus, heredity, gender, and increasing age (1). The greater the number of CHD risk factors an individual has, the greater the likelihood that he or she will develop CHD (see **Figure 10.6** on page 258).

Assess your cardiovascular disease risk with the *Cardiovascular Risk Assessment* Take Charge of Your Health! Worksheet online at **www.pearsonhighered.com/powers.**

LIVE IT!
ASSESS
YOURSELF

Smoking   A smoker's risk of developing CHD is more than twice that of a nonsmoker (1). Smoking is also considered the biggest risk factor for sudden death

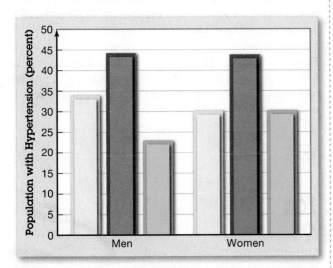

Key

White

African American

Mexican American

FIGURE 10.5
One in three Americans will develop hypertension.

Source: Heart disease and stroke statistics—2009 update. *Circulation* 119:e21–e181, 2009.

stroke Brain damage that occurs when the blood supply to the brain is reduced for a prolonged period of time.

hypertension High blood pressure.

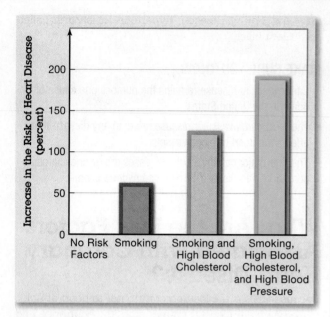

FIGURE 10.6
Your risk of developing CHD increases as the number of risk factors increases.

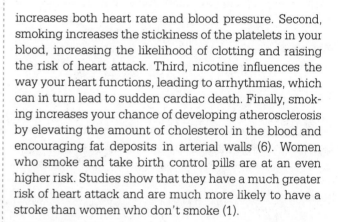

due to cardiac arrest, a heart attack, or irregular heartbeats (**arrhythmias**). In addition, smoking promotes the development of atherosclerosis in peripheral blood vessels (such as in the arms or legs), which can lead to hypertension and increased risk of stroke. Finally, smokers who have a heart attack are more likely to die suddenly (within an hour after the attack) than are nonsmokers. Studies have also concluded that passive inhalation of cigarette smoke (second-hand smoke) can increase the risk of both cardiovascular and lung disease (6). In fact, both the American Heart Association and the American Cancer Society report that breathing second-hand smoke can be as dangerous to your health as direct inhalation.

Cigarette smoking can influence your risk of CHD in at least four ways. First, the nicotine in the smoke increases both heart rate and blood pressure. Second, smoking increases the stickiness of the platelets in your blood, increasing the likelihood of clotting and raising the risk of heart attack. Third, nicotine influences the way your heart functions, leading to arrhythmias, which can in turn lead to sudden cardiac death. Finally, smoking increases your chance of developing atherosclerosis by elevating the amount of cholesterol in the blood and encouraging fat deposits in arterial walls (6). Women who smoke and take birth control pills are at an even higher risk. Studies show that they have a much greater risk of heart attack and are much more likely to have a stroke than women who don't smoke (1).

Hypertension Hypertension is unique because it is both a disease in its own right and a risk factor for stroke and CHD. It contributes to CHD by accelerating the rate of atherosclerosis development (4, 7).

APPRECIATING DIVERSITY

Who Is at Greatest Risk for Cardiovascular Disease?

Ethnicity, gender, age, and socioeconomic status can all affect an individual's risk of developing cardiovascular disease, and these factors explain why CVD is more prevalent in certain segments of the U.S. population. African Americans, for example, are at greater risk of developing hypertension (one form of cardiovascular disease) compared to the U.S. population as a whole. Similarly, Native Americans and people of Latino heritage have higher prevalence of diabetes, an important contributory risk factor for cardiovascular disease. Between the ages of 20 and 50, men are at greater risk than women for developing cardiovascular disease. Finally, individuals who earn low incomes experience higher incidences of both heart disease and obesity (a contributory risk factor for heart disease).

A diet high in sodium (such as from processed foods and/or table salt) increases the risk of developing hypertension. High plasma levels of sodium expand the blood volume and thereby increase blood pressure. Although sodium is a required micronutrient, the daily requirement for most people is small (less than ¼ teaspoon, or 400 mg). Some individuals are more sensitive to sodium than others, and sodium-sensitive individuals with hypertension can often lower their blood pressure by reducing their salt intake. For example, people who ingest less than ½ teaspoon of sodium each day typically do not develop hypertension. In contrast, sodium-sensitive people who consume more than 1 teaspoon of salt per day are at risk for developing hypertension.

Even athletes or laborers who lose large amounts of water and electrolytes via sweat rarely require more than 1.5 teaspoons (3000 mg) of salt per day. Currently, many U.S. citizens consume more than 6 teaspoons (12,000 mg) of salt per day; clearly, this level of sodium intake is beyond the amount needed for normal body function.

The key to lowering your sodium intake is avoiding foods that are high in salt. Table 10.1 lists some common foods that are high in sodium. Take the time to learn which foods contain a lot of sodium, and limit your intake to less than 1 teaspoon per day (8). Because of the link between hypertension and salt intake, the National Institutes of Health has developed a Dietary Approach to Stop Hypertension (called DASH). This DASH eating plan is recognized as an excellent approach to prevent and lower hypertension.

High Blood Cholesterol Levels Cholesterol is a type of lipid that can either be consumed in foods or be synthesized in the body, and it is a primary risk factor for CHD (as discussed in Chapter 8). The risk of CHD increases as blood cholesterol increases.

Because cholesterol is not soluble in blood, it is combined with proteins in the liver so it can be transported in the bloodstream. This combination of cholesterol and protein results in two major forms of cholesterol: **low-density lipoproteins (LDL)** and **high-density lipoproteins (HDL)**. The association between elevated blood cholesterol and CHD is due primarily to LDL. Individuals with high blood LDL levels have an increased risk of CHD, whereas those with high levels of HDL have a decreased risk of CHD (1, 4, 9, 10). Because of these relationships, LDL has been called "bad cholesterol," whereas HDL has been called "good cholesterol."

Even though the risk of developing CHD is best predicted from LDL and HDL levels in the blood, measurement of total blood cholesterol (the sum of all types of cholesterol) also provides a good indication of CHD risk (1, 4, 10). A total blood cholesterol concentration of less than 200 mg/dl (milligrams per deciliter) indicates a low risk of developing CHD, whereas a concentration greater

TABLE 10.1	Sodium Content of Selected Foods	
Food	**Serving Size**	**Sodium Content (mg)**
Bologna	2 oz	700
Cheese		
American	1 oz	305
Cheddar	1 oz	165
Parmesan	1 oz	525
Frankfurter	1	495
Hamburger patty	1 small	550
Pickle (dill)	1 medium	900
Pizza (cheese)	1 slice (14-inch diameter)	600
Potato chips	20	300
Pretzels	1 oz	890
Canned soup		
Chicken noodle	1 cup	1010
Vegetable beef	1 cup	1046
Soy sauce	1 tablespoon	1320

than 240 mg/dl indicates a high CHD risk (4, 10). Unfortunately, because of high-fat diets and lack of exercise, more than 34 million people in the United States have total blood cholesterol levels above 240 mg/dl (1).

The National Institutes of Health released new guidelines for assessing CHD risks using blood levels of LDL and HDL. For a brief overview of these guidelines, see the Closer Look box on page 260.

Is good cholesterol even better than we thought? Watch *Tips to Raise Good Cholesterol* at **www.pearsonhighered.com/powers**.

SEE IT! VIDEOS

Physical Inactivity The first evidence that physical activity reduces the risk of heart disease emerged

arrhythmia An irregular heartbeat.

low-density lipoproteins (LDL) A combination of protein, fat, and cholesterol in the blood, composed of relatively large amounts of cholesterol. LDLs promote the fatty plaque accumulation in the coronary arteries that leads to heart disease; also called "bad" cholesterol.

high-density lipoproteins (HDL) A combination of protein, fat, and cholesterol in the blood, composed of relatively large amounts of protein. Protects against the fatty plaque accumulation in the coronary arteries that leads to heart disease; also called "good" cholesterol.

COACHING corner

Lack of exercise, poor diet, and smoking rank high as factors that contribute to heart disease. Each of us usually has room for improvement in at least one of these behavioral aspects. Consider the following as you evaluate your heart disease risk and which areas you might be able to improve.

- Engage in activity daily. Physical activity doesn't just mean exercise. Increasing levels of physical activity through actions like taking the stairs can also have a positive effect.

- Plan your meals so you are less likely to indulge in fast foods.

- Avoid places where smoking is allowed. If you are a smoker, find a program to help you reduce or eliminate tobacco products.

- Reduce your stress levels by practicing a stress management technique daily or several times per week.

Take the stairs!

more than 50 years ago in a study that compared the rates of CHD between bus conductors (i.e., ticket collectors) and bus drivers in London, England (11). Whereas the conductors spent their days walking up and down the stairs of "double-decker" London buses collecting tickets, the bus drivers remained seated and sedentary throughout the workday. This study found that the rate of CHD was much higher in the sedentary drivers than in the more physically active conductors.

Since this initial study, numerous investigations have consistently reported that regular physical activity reduces the risk of developing CHD (10, 12–16).

Although it is well known that exercise reduces the risk of CHD, the mechanism by which this works is unclear. Possible explanations include improvements in body weight, blood pressure, and blood lipid profile, and the reduced risk of diabetes (8, 16–19), all of which are associated with regular exercise. Collectively, these

A CLOSER LOOK

Blood Cholesterol Guidelines from the National Institutes of Health

In response to studies conclusively showing that lowering blood LDL ("bad cholesterol") levels can reduce the risk of heart disease by 40% (9), the National Institutes of Health (NIH) has released guidelines for optimal blood levels of LDL and HDL. Even though the major focus of the guidelines is recommendations for managing blood LDL levels, NIH included recommendations for blood levels of HDL ("good cholesterol") because HDL can carry cholesterol away from arteries and back to the liver. The guidelines are summarized in the table.

In short, the guidelines consider LDL levels of 100 mg/dl or lower to be optimal for reducing the risk of developing CHD, whereas LDL levels above 190 mg/dl are considered indicative of a high risk for CHD. Because the presence of HDL can lower LDL levels, low blood levels of HDL can indicate an increased risk of developing CHD. Accordingly, the guidelines consider blood HDL levels below 40 mg/dl to be low and undesirable in terms of CHD risk.

Cholesterol Concentration (mg/dl)	Classification
LDL	
<100	Optimal
100–129	Near optimal
130–159	Borderline high
160–189	High
>190	Very high
HDL	
<40	Low (undesirable)
>60	High (very desirable)

changes can greatly reduce the overall risk of developing CHD.

Diabetes Mellitus Diabetes is a disease that results in elevated blood sugar levels due to the body's inability to use blood sugar properly (as discussed in Chapter 1). Diabetes occurs most often in middle age and is common in people who are overweight. The link between diabetes and CHD is well established, as approximately 75% of all individuals with diabetes die from some form of cardiovascular disease. The role that diabetes plays in increasing the risk of CHD could be linked to the fact that people with diabetes are often inactive, have elevated blood cholesterol levels, and suffer from hypertension (13).

Obesity and Overweight Compared to individuals who maintain their ideal body weight, overweight and obese individuals are more likely to develop CHD, even if they have no other major risk factors (20). However, obese individuals more commonly will exhibit multiple major risk factors for CHD such as elevated blood cholesterol levels and hypertension (13).

Of particular interest is the fact that a person's fat distribution pattern affects the risk of CHD. Waist-to-hip circumference ratios greater than 1.0 for men and 0.8 for women indicate a significant risk for development of CHD. The physiological reason for the link between CHD and regional fat distribution may be that people with high waist-to-hip circumference ratios often eat high-fat diets, which elevate blood cholesterol levels.

Possible causes of hypertension in obese individuals include high sodium intake, which elevates blood pressure, and increased vascular resistance, which results in the need for higher pressure to pump blood to the tissues (4).

Heredity Children of parents with CHD are more likely to develop CHD than are children of parents who do not have CHD (1, 4). Evidence suggests that the familial risk for CHD may be linked to factors such as high blood cholesterol, hypertension, diabetes, and obesity. People with a family history of CHD are not doomed to develop this disease, but to reduce their risk for CHD they will have to work harder to develop a healthy lifestyle.

Gender Up to age 55, men have a greater risk of developing CHD and stroke than do women. Much of the protection against CHD in women is linked to the female sex hormone estrogen, which may elevate HDL cholesterol. Although the risk of CHD increases markedly in women after menopause, it never becomes as great as for men (4).

Increasing Age As you get older, your risk for developing CHD will increase. This is partly due to the fact that the buildup of arterial plaque is an ongoing process; the longer one lives, the greater the buildup. In fact, more than 80% of people who die of CHD are age 65 or older (13). Increasing age also increases your risk of stroke. Most people who have strokes are over 55, and the risk of stroke increases with age (21).

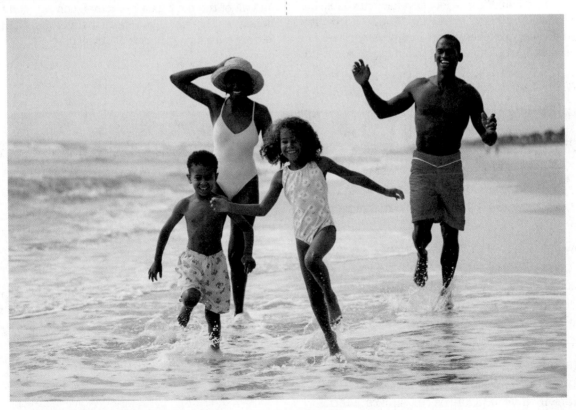

People who engage in regular physical activity are at lower risk for developing heart disease.

Contributory Risk Factors

Contributory risk factors are those that increase your risk of developing a major risk factor. The American Heart Association recognizes stress, alcohol, and diet and nutrition as contributory risk factors for CHD.

Stress Stress contributes to the development of several major CHD risk factors. For example, stress may be linked to smoking habits. People under stress may start smoking in an effort to relax, or stress could influence smokers to smoke more than they normally would. Further, stress increases the risk of developing both hypertension and elevated blood cholesterol. The physiological connection between stress and hypertension appears to be the stress-induced release of hormones that elevate blood pressure.

Alcohol Consumption Although there is some evidence that moderate alcohol consumption (one drink per day for women and two drinks per day for men) may lower risk for heart disease, drinking too much alcohol raises risk. People who drink too much alcohol are more likely to suffer high blood pressure, heart failure, and stroke. Excessive alcohol consumption can also contribute to high triglycerides, cancer, and other diseases. The American Heart Association recommends that nondrinkers continue to abstain from alcohol and that moderate drinkers not increase their intake (13).

Diet and Nutrition A healthy diet can reduce your risk of developing cardiovascular disease. The food you eat (and the amount) can affect several controllable risk factors including blood cholesterol levels, blood pressure, diabetes, and overweight and obesity. Therefore (as discussed in Chapter 8), consuming nutrient-rich foods that are rich in vitamins, minerals, fiber, and other nutrients but are lower in calories and fat can reduce your risk of developing major risk factors for cardiovascular diseases.

MAKE SURE YOU KNOW...

- Researchers have identified several major and contributory risk factors that increase the chance of developing both coronary heart disease (CHD) and stroke.

- Major risk factors for CHD and stroke include smoking, hypertension, high blood cholesterol levels, physical inactivity, diabetes mellitus, obesity and overweight, heredity, gender, and increasing age.

- Contributory risk factors for CHD and stroke include stress, consumption of too much alcohol, and a high fat diet.

 Assess your heart I.Q. with the *Healthy Heart I.Q.* Take Charge of Your Health! Worksheet online at **www.pearsonhighered.com/powers.**

LIVE IT! ASSESS YOURSELF

How Can You Reduce Your Risk of Heart Disease?

Although cardiovascular disease remains the number-one killer in the United States, incidence of the disease has declined in recent years (1). This drop has occurred primarily because people have reduced their risk factors for CHD. Note that six of the nine major risk factors, and all of the contributory factors, can be modified by behavior. Therefore, you can modify 70% of CHD risk factors to reduce your risk of developing cardiovascular disease.

COACHING Corner

Heart disease is our nation's greatest threat to life expectancy. Consider the following questions as you evaluate your cardiovascular disease risk:

- How has the "normal" activity level changed for an average American over the last 100 years? Can you find specific information about the normal amount of activity or an average diet then versus now?

- What lifestyle practices do you have in common with your parents, grandparents, or guardians? Which lifestyle practices are different? If your patterns are similar, what are some of the outcomes that you might experience as a result?

- Interview your family. At what ages did your parents, grandparents, or guardians begin to develop symptoms associated with cardiovascular disease? Do some have symptoms without a formal diagnosis, based on what you've learned here?

Ask Mom about heart disease

Reduce Blood Cholesterol Levels

High blood cholesterol levels are a key factor in risk of CHD, and the best way to reduce blood cholesterol is diet and exercise. Decreasing your intake of saturated fats and cholesterol may significantly reduce your blood cholesterol levels. Saturated fats stimulate cholesterol synthesis in the liver and therefore contribute to elevated blood cholesterol. Saturated fats are found mostly in meats and dairy products, so avoiding high intake of these foods can reduce your blood cholesterol levels. Table 10.2 lists the cholesterol content of selected foods. If diet and exercise are not effective in lowering blood lipid levels to a desirable range, cholesterol-lowering drugs (called statins) are available (see the Closer Look box on page 264).

Be Physically Active

Regular exercise has been shown to improve blood lipid profiles in most people. Even modest levels of exercise (e.g., 30 minutes of walking performed 3 to 5 times per week) have been shown to reduce the risk of developing CHD due to physical inactivity (1, 4, 12–14). In addition, regular aerobic exercise has been shown to modify other CHD risk factors by positively influencing blood pressure, body composition, insulin resistance, and blood cholesterol levels.

Even small amounts of exercise can provide some protection against CHD, but studies reveal that the risk of death from CHD decreases as the total physical activity energy expenditure increases from 500 to 3500 kilocalories per week (16). Further, while total energy expenditure from exercise is important in preventing CHD, the intensity of exercise is also important. A study of Harvard alumni reported that individuals engaged in

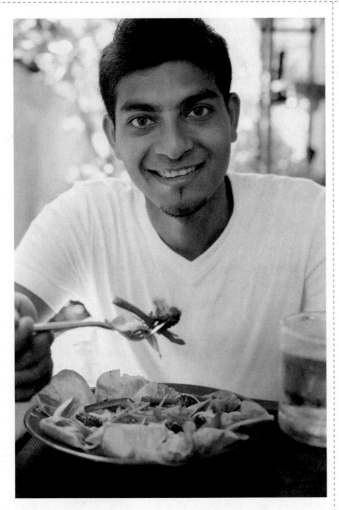

Eating a healthy diet, particularly one that's low in sodium, saturated fat, and cholesterol, can reduce your risk for heart disease.

The more risk factors you avoid or eliminate, the less your risk for developing CHD. Let's discuss the actions you can take today to eliminate these risk factors.

Don't Smoke

As soon as a smoker quits smoking, CHD risk drops. If you don't currently smoke, the best advice is not to start. If you do smoke, you need to stop. Unfortunately, for most people, smoking is a difficult habit to break. Major behavior modification is needed to stop smoking and to remain smoke-free for the rest of your life.

Lower Your Blood Pressure

Hypertension can be combated in several ways. In some instances, medication may be required to control high blood pressure. However, in many cases of hypertension, exercise, and a healthy diet low in sodium can assist in lowering blood pressure. Because stress can also contribute to hypertension, maintaining low levels of daily stress is also important. (Chapter 11 discusses approaches to stress management in detail.)

TABLE 10.2	Cholesterol and Saturated Fat Content of Selected Foods		
Food	Serving Size	Cholesterol (mg)	Saturated Fat (g)
Bacon	2 slices	30	0.7
Beef (lean)	8 oz	150	12
Butter	1 tablespoon	32	0.4
Cheese (American)	1 oz	27	5.4
Cheese (cheddar)	1 oz	30	5.9
Egg	1 (boiled)	113	2.8
Frankfurter	1	30	5.2
Hamburger	1 small patty	68	5.9
Milk (whole)	1 cup	33	5
Milkshake	10 oz	54	8.2
Pizza (meat)	1 slice (14" diameter)	31	8
Sausage	3 oz	42	8.6

A CLOSER LOOK

Frequently Asked Questions about Exercise, Diet, and Heart Disease

What if diet and exercise aren't enough to lower my cholesterol to desirable levels?

When diet and exercise alone are not successful in lowering blood cholesterol, drug therapy may help. The most effective and widely tested cholesterol drugs are a class of drugs called *statins*. These drugs work by preventing the formation of cholesterol in the liver and also help remove cholesterol from the blood. Statins can reduce the "bad cholesterol" (i.e., LDL) level by 20%–45% depending on the drug used and the dosage (26, 27). Although statins have been shown to reduce the risk of atherosclerosis in many people, they can produce some potentially serious side effects (26). If diet and exercise alone cannot successfully lower your cholesterol, you and your physician can decide together whether a statin drug is right for you. For more information on the treatment for high cholesterol, consult the National Cholesterol Education Program online at www.nhlbi.nih.gov/about/ncep/index.htm.

Some doctors recommend aspirin to reduce the risk of heart attack. How does aspirin reduce the risk of heart attack?

Extensive research indicates that taking aspirin daily (80–325 mg/day) can help prevent heart attacks by preventing

blood platelets from sticking together, thereby reducing the likelihood of blood clots.

However, taking aspirin daily is not risk free. For example, people with bleeding disorders, liver disease, kidney disease, or peptic ulcers, and individuals who are allergic to aspirin should not take it. Note, however, that for middle-aged and older people without these disorders, the benefits of aspirin are likely to outweigh the risks (28).

Are some people at risk for sudden cardiac death during exercise?

Yes. Although regular physical activity reduces the risk of developing coronary heart disease, vigorous exercise can acutely increase the risk of both sudden cardiac death and heart attacks in susceptible persons (29). For example, people with advanced heart disease might have an increased risk for sudden death during exercise because of blockage in a major coronary artery. Further, individuals with hereditary cardiac abnormalities may also be at risk during exercise (29). A medical exam can usually identify whether the person is at risk for sudden cardiac death during exercise. Specifically, a medical history and a physical exam from a qualified physician can detect hidden heart disease that could pose a risk for participating in regular exercise.

regular vigorous exercise (50% $\dot{V}O_2$ max or higher) were better protected against CHD than people exercising at much lower levels (22). Other studies have also reported a strong link between exercise intensity and reduction in death from CHD (16).

Remember, "regular" endurance exercise (3 or more days per week) is the key. Sporadic bouts of exercise (3–4 days per month) will not reduce the risk of CHD. Moreover, cessation of exercise will result in a loss of exercise-induced protection from heart disease (23–25). So make a commitment to a consistent and lifelong exercise program today. Your heart will love you for it!

Reduce Your Stress Level

Relaxation techniques (discussed in Chapter 11) can help counteract the effects of a stressful lifestyle and thereby reduce the risk of developing CHD. Every lifestyle contains stressful elements. For example, college students are often posed with "school stress" related to such factors as studying for exams and completing course assignments. If you are stressed about

school-related issues, try exercising (e.g., going for a run) at the end of the day to reduce tension. If you find yourself getting angry or hostile easily, consider scheduling counseling sessions with a school counselor trained in anger management.

MAKE SURE YOU KNOW...

- Although heart disease remains the number-one killer in the United States, the incidence of heart disease has declined in recent years. This reduction in CHD has occurred because people have modified their behavior to reduce their risk factors for CHD.

- You can reduce your risk of developing CHD by not smoking, by controlling your blood pressure, by eating a healthy diet, by being physically active, and by reducing your stress level.

HEAR IT!
CASE STUDY

How can Keisha reduce her risk of heart disease? Listen to the online case study at **www.pearsonhighered.com/powers.**

STEPS FOR ▶ BEHAVIOR CHANGE

What's your risk for cardiovascular disease?

Although you may not be able to imagine the day when you'll have high blood pressure or diabetes, you do have a chance of developing one or more of these conditions during your lifetime. Take this quiz to determine whether your current habits put you at higher risk for developing CVD.

Y N

☐ ☐ Do you get up and move around often enough to accumulate 30 minutes of physical activity per day?

☐ ☐ Do you usually avoid eating high-fat foods?

☐ ☐ Do you watch your sodium intake and refrain from using too much salt during cooking and at the table?

☐ ☐ Do you monitor your stress level and practice stress management when necessary?

☐ ☐ Do you avoid smoking cigarettes and using other tobacco products?

If you answered yes to three or more of these questions, congratulations! You are on your way to developing a lifetime of healthy habits. If you answered no to most of these questions, you may already be at increased risk for CVD.

TIPS TO LOWER YOUR CVD RISK

Tomorrow, you will:

☑ Start an exercise program. Even a half hour per day a few days a week will go a long way in improving heart health. And you'll look and feel better, too.

Within the next 2 weeks, you will:

☑ Watch your diet. Although the occasional fast food meal isn't the end of the world, in general, you should eat whole foods, such as fruits, vegetables, and whole grains, and avoid deep-fried or other high-fat foods.

☑ Eat less salt. Sodium is an essential nutrient for several body processes, but you actually need very little of it to be healthy, and too much sodium has been linked to high blood pressure. To lower your sodium intake, use pepper at the table instead of salt, and use spices to flavor foods during cooking.

By the end of the semester, you will:

☑ De-stress. Too much stress is linked not only to increased risk of CVD, but also to high blood pressure. (Try some of the techniques in Chapter 11 to manage your stress level.)

☑ Establish a plan to quit smoking. Tobacco use leads to numerous health problems. For the sake of your heart, your lungs, your breath, and those around you, you should avoid smoking. If you don't smoke, don't start; and if you do, stop.

SUMMARY

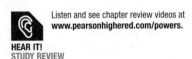

Listen and see chapter review videos at
www.pearsonhighered.com/powers.

HEAR IT!
STUDY REVIEW

1. Heart disease is the number-one cause of death in the United States, and the incidence of cardiovascular disease in the U.S. is expected to rise as the baby boomer generation grows older.

2. Cardiovascular disease refers to any disease that affects the heart and blood vessels. Common cardiovascular diseases include atherosclerosis, coronary heart disease, stroke, and hypertension.

3. CHD risk factors are classified as either major or contributory. Major risk factors are those that directly increase the risk of coronary heart disease. Contributory risk factors may increase your chance of developing coronary heart disease by promoting the development of a major risk factor.

4. Major risk factors for developing coronary heart disease include smoking, hypertension, high blood cholesterol, physical inactivity, diabetes mellitus, obesity and overweight, heredity, gender, and increasing age.

5. Contributory risk factors for the development of coronary heart disease include stress and alcohol.

6. You can reduce your risk of developing coronary heart disease by not smoking, by eating a healthy diet (particularly by avoiding saturated fat and dietary cholesterol in foods), by being physically active, by maintaining a healthy body weight, and by reducing stress.

STUDY QUESTIONS

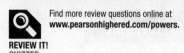

Find more review questions online at
www.pearsonhighered.com/powers.

REVIEW IT!
QUIZZES

1. Which of the following is NOT a major risk factor for CHD?
   a. smoking
   b. hypertension
   c. high blood cholesterol
   d. resting pulse rate

2. Which of the following blood pressure measurements would be considered hypertension?
   a. 100/80
   b. 110/80
   c. 130/80
   d. 140/90

3. Cholesterol exists in several forms in your blood. The form of blood cholesterol that is classified as "good cholesterol" is called
   a. total cholesterol
   b. HDL cholesterol
   c. LDL cholesterol
   d. EDL cholesterol

4. The leading cause of death in the United States is
   a. AIDS.
   b. cancer.
   c. cardiovascular disease.
   d. accidents.

5. Which of the following risk factors for CHD cannot be modified by a change in behavior?
   a. obesity   b. heredity
   c. hypertension   d. stress

6. Define the following terms:
   cardiovascular disease
   coronary heart disease
   coronary artery disease
   hypertension

7. What are the major and contributory risk factors for developing CHD?

8. Discuss the difference between major and contributory risk factors for developing coronary heart disease.

9. Why are high-density lipoproteins known as "good" cholesterol? Conversely, why are low-density lipoproteins labeled "bad" cholesterol?

10. Which major coronary heart disease risk factors can be modified?

11. Which contributory coronary heart disease risk factors can be modified?

12. How does a high-sodium diet contribute to hypertension?

13. What is the link between diet and blood cholesterol?

14. How does smoking increase your risk of developing cardiovascular disease?

15. How are arteriosclerosis and atherosclerosis related?

HELPFUL WEBLINKS

For links to the organizations and
websites listed, visit
www.pearsonhighered.com/powers.

DO IT!
WEBLINKS

American Heart Association
Contains information about a variety of topics related to both heart disease and stroke. www.heart.org

American Medical Association
Offers many sources of information about a wide variety of medical problems, including heart disease. www.ama-assn.org

Lowering Your Blood Pressure with DASH
A guide to the DASH eating plan from the National Heart Lung and Blood Institute. www.nhlbi.nih.gov/health/public/heart/hbp/dash/new_dash.pdf

Mayo Clinic
Contains wide-ranging information about diet, fitness, and health. www.mayoclinic.org

WebMD
Presents information about a wide variety of diseases and medical problems, including heart disease. www.webmd.com

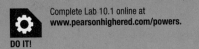
Name _____   Date _____

Finding Your Cholesterol Plan

The following two-step program will guide you through the National Cholesterol Education Program's treatment guidelines. The first step helps you establish your overall coronary risk; the second uses that information to determine your LDL treatment goals and how to reach them. You'll need to know your blood pressure, your total LDL and HDL cholesterol levels, and your triglyceride and fasting glucose levels. If you're not sure of those numbers, ask your doctor and, if necessary, schedule an exam to get them. (Everyone should have a complete lipid profile every 5 years, starting at age 20.)

STEP 1: TAKE THE HEART-ATTACK RISK TEST

This test will identify your chance of having a heart attack or dying of coronary disease in the next 10 years. (People with previously diagnosed coronary disease, diabetes, aortic aneurysm, or symptomatic carotid artery disease or peripheral artery disease already face more than a 20% risk; they can skip the test and go straight to step 2.) The test uses data from the Framingham Heart Study, the world's longest-running study of cardiovascular risk factors. The test is limited to established, major factors that are easily measured. Circle (or select) the point value for each of the risk factors shown.

AGE

Years	Women	Men
20–34	−7	−9
35–39	−3	−4
40–44	0	0
45–49	3	3
50–54	6	6
55–59	8	8
60–64	10	10
65–69	12	11
70–74	14	12
75–79	16	13

TOTAL CHOLESTEROL

mg/dL	Age 20–39 Women	Age 20–39 Men	Age 40–49 Women	Age 40–49 Men	Age 50–59 Women	Age 50–59 Men	Age 60–69 Women	Age 60–69 Men	Age 70–79 Women	Age 70–79 Men
<160	0	0	0	0	0	0	0	0	0	0
160–199	4	4	3	3	2	2	1	1	1	0
200–239	8	7	6	5	4	3	2	1	1	0
240–279	11	9	8	6	5	4	3	2	2	1
280+	13	11	10	8	7	5	4	3	2	1

HIGH-DENSITY LIPOPROTEIN (HDL) CHOLESTEROL

mg/dL	Women and Men
60+	−1
50–59	0
40–49	1
>40	2

SYSTOLIC BLOOD PRESSURE (THE HIGHER NUMBER)

Mm/Hg	Treated		Untreated	
	Women	Men	Women	Men
<120	0	0	0	0
120–129	1	0	3	1
130–139	2	1	4	2
140–159	3	1	5	2
>159	4	2	6	3

Smoking

Age 20–39		Age 40–49		Age 50–59		Age 60–69		Age 70–79	
Women	Men	Women	Men	Women	Men	Women	Men	Women	Men
9	8	7	5	4	3	2	1	1	1

Total Your Points _____

Now find your total point score in the men's or women's column to locate your 10-year risk (the far-right column).

TEN-YEAR RISK FOR HEART DISEASE

Women's Score	Men's Score	Your 10-Year Risk
<20	<12	<10%
20–22	12–15	10–20%
>22	>15	>20%

STEP 2: FIND YOUR LOW-DENSITY LIPOPROTEIN (LDL) TREATMENT PLAN

Consult the table to learn whether your overall CHD risk indicates that you need to lower your LDL cholesterol level and, if you do, by how much. First, locate your CHD risk in the left column. (That's based on the 10-year heart attack risk that you just calculated, as well as your CHD risk factors and any heart-threatening diseases you may have.) Then look across that row to see whether you should make lifestyle changes and take cholesterol-lowering medication, based on your current LDL level.

LDL TREATMENT PLAN

CHD Risk Group	Start lifestyle changes if your LDL level is ...*	Add drugs if your LDL level is ...
Very High 1. Ten-year heart attack risk of 20% or more *or* 2. History of coronary heart disease, diabetes, peripheral artery disease, carotid artery disease, or aortic aneurysm.	100 mg/dl or higher. (Aim for an LDL under 100.) Get retested after 3 months.	130 or higher. (Drugs are optional if your LDL is between 100 and 130.)
High 1. Ten-year heart attack risk of 10% to 20% *and* 2. Two or more major coronary risk factors.[†]	130 or higher. (Aim for an LDL under 130.) Get retested after 3 months.	130 or higher and lifestyle changes don't achieve your LDL goal in 3 months.
Moderately High 1. Ten-year heart attack risk under 10% *and* 2. Two or more major coronary risk factors.[†]	Same as above.	160 or higher, and lifestyle changes don't achieve your LDL goal in 3 months.[‡]
Low to Moderate 1. One or no major coronary risk factors.[†§]	160 or higher. (Aim for an LDL under 160.) Get retested after 3 months.	190 or higher, and lifestyle changes don't achieve your LDL goal in 3 months. (Drugs are optional if your LDL is between 160 and 189.)

*People who have the metabolic syndrome should make lifestyle changes even if their LDL level alone doesn't warrant it. You have the metabolic syndrome if you have three or more of these risk factors: HDL under 40 in men, 50 in women; systolic blood pressure of 130 or more or diastolic pressure of 85 or more; fasting glucose level of 110 to 125; triglycerides level of 150 or more; and waist circumference over 40 inches in men, 35 inches in women. People with the syndrome should limit their carbohydrate intake, get up to 30 to 35 percent of their calories from total fat (more than usually recommended), and make the other lifestyle changes, including restriction of saturated fat.

[†]The major coronary risk factors are cigarette smoking; coronary disease in a father or brother before age 55 or a mother or sister before age 65; systolic blood pressure of 140 or more, a diastolic pressure of 90 or more, or being on drugs for hypertension; and an HDL level under 40. If your HDL is 60 or more, subtract one risk factor. (High LDL is a major factor, of course, but it's already figured into the table.)

[‡]Although the goal is to get LDL under 130, the use of drugs in these people usually isn't worthwhile, even if lifestyle steps fail to achieve that goal.

[§]People in this group usually have a 10-year risk of less than 10%. Those who have higher risk should ask their doctor whether they need more aggressive treatment than shown here.

Source: Donatelle, Rebecca J., *Access to Health, 8th Ed.*, © 2004. Reprinted and Electronically reproduced by permission of Pearson Education, Inc., Upper Saddle River, New Jersey.

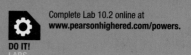
Name _____   Date _____

Understanding Your Risk for Cardiovascular Disease

Each of us has a unique level of risk for various diseases. You can take action to change some of these risks; others are risks that you need to consider as you plan a lifelong strategy for overall risk reduction. Complete each of the following questions, and total your points in each section. If you score between 1 and 5 in any section, consider your risk: The higher the number, the greater your risk. If you answered "Don't know" to any question, talk to your parents or other family members as soon as possible to find out whether you have any unknown risks.

PART I: ASSESS YOUR FAMILY RISK FOR CVD

1. Do any of your primary relatives (mother, father, grandparents, siblings) have a history of heart disease or stroke?

    Yes _____ (1 point)   No _____ (0 points)   Don't know _____

2. Do any of your primary relatives (mother, father, grandparents, siblings) have diabetes?

    Yes _____ (1 point)   No _____ (0 points)   Don't know _____

3. Do any of your primary relatives (mother, father, grandparents, siblings) have high blood pressure?

    Yes _____ (1 point)   No _____ (0 points)   Don't know _____

4. Do any of your primary relatives (mother, father, grandparents, siblings) have a history of high cholesterol?

    Yes _____ (1 point)   No _____ (0 points)   Don't know _____

5. Would you say that your family consumed a high-fat diet (lots of red meat, dairy products, butter or margarine) during your time spent at home?

    Yes _____ (1 point)   No _____ (0 points)   Don't know _____

Total points _____

PART II: ASSESS YOUR LIFESTYLE RISK FOR CVD

1. Is your total cholesterol level higher than it should be?

    Yes _____ (1 point)   No _____ (0 points)   Don't know _____

2. Do you have high blood pressure?

    Yes _____ (1 point)   No _____ (0 points)   Don't know _____

3. Have you been diagnosed as pre-diabetic or diabetic?

    Yes _____ (1 point)   No _____ (0 points)   Don't know _____

4. Do you smoke?

    Yes _____ (1 point)   No _____ (0 points)   Don't know _____

5. Would you describe your life as being highly stressful?

    Yes _____ (1 point)   No _____ (0 points)   Don't know _____

Total points _____

PART III: ASSESS YOUR ADDITIONAL RISKS FOR CVD

1. How would you best describe your current weight?

    a. Lower than what it should be for my height and weight. (0 points)

    b. About what it should be for my height and weight. (0 points)

    c. Higher than it should be for my height and weight. (1 point)

2. How would you describe the level of exercise that you get each day?

    a. Less than what I should be exercising each day. (1 point)

    b. About what I should be exercising each day. (0 points)

    c. More than what I should be each day. (0 points)

3. How would you describe your dietary behaviors?

    a. Eating only the recommended number of calories per day. (0 points)

    b. Eating less than the recommended number of calories each day. (0 points)

    c. Eating more than the recommended number of calories each day. (1 point)

4. Which of the following best describes your typical dietary behavior?

    a. I eat from the major food groups, trying hard to get the recommended fruits and vegetables. (0 points)

    b. I eat mostly red meat and consume high amounts of saturated fat from meats and dairy products each day. (1 point)

    c. Whenever possible, I try to substitute olive oil or canola oil for other forms of dietary fat. (0 points)

5. Do you have a history of *Chlamydia* infection?

    a. Yes. (1 point)

    b. No. (0 points)

Total points _____

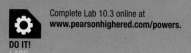
Name _____ **Date** _____

Assessing Your Genetic Predisposition for Cardiovascular Disease

The following is a family tree that allows you to fill in risk factors and conditions for heart disease in your family members. Remember that heart disease has a genetic component, so examining your relatives' health and lifestyles will provide insight into your future susceptibility to heart disease. Write in risk factors directly related to heart disease. Examples include hypertension, high blood cholesterol, diabetes, stroke, obesity, and heart attack.

Your Family History of Heart Disease

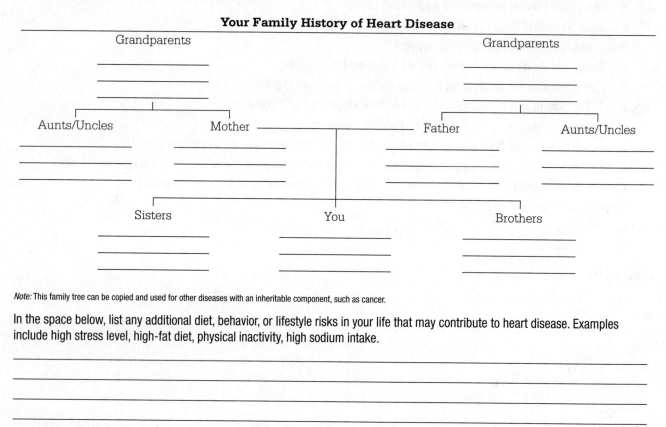

Note: This family tree can be copied and used for other diseases with an inheritable component, such as cancer.

In the space below, list any additional diet, behavior, or lifestyle risks in your life that may contribute to heart disease. Examples include high stress level, high-fat diet, physical inactivity, high sodium intake.

_____

_____

_____

_____

INTERPRETATION

Inherited traits can increase your risk of cardiovascular disease. The good news is that you are not destined to develop heart disease or any of the conditions present in your relatives. Lifestyle changes that include moderate exercise and proper diet can reduce your risk of developing cardiovascular disease. Being aware of health concerns and problems within your family that may be passed on genetically will make you a more informed, health-conscious individual.

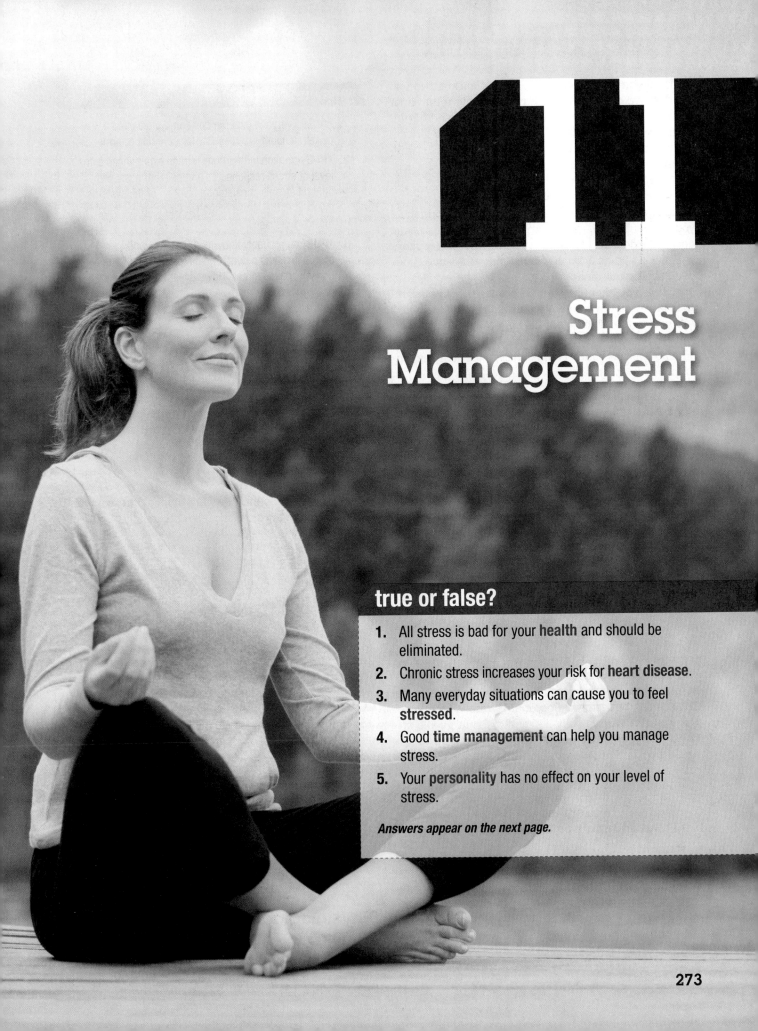

11
Stress Management

true or false?

1. All stress is bad for your **health** and should be eliminated.
2. Chronic stress increases your risk for **heart disease**.
3. Many everyday situations can cause you to feel **stressed**.
4. Good **time management** can help you manage stress.
5. Your **personality** has no effect on your level of stress.

Answers appear on the next page.

Do you tend to get sick during finals, or do you have difficulty sleeping when a big term paper is due? Does a fight with your boyfriend or girlfriend leave you unfocused? Do you feel muscle tension while sitting frustrated in rush-hour traffic? These familiar, everyday situations often lead to stress and the negative physical symptoms associated with stress. On the other hand, you may have noticed that if you do not feel some stress before a test, competition, or performance, you do not do your best. A certain amount of stress is good. The goal is not to eliminate all stress, but to manage it well so it does not have a negative impact on your health and performance.

Have you thought about the specific physical responses your body undergoes during a period of stress? Are you aware of the potential long-term effects stress can have on your health? We will discuss these topics and more in this chapter as we analyze the complex topics of stress and stress management.

What Are Stress and the Stress Response?

Most people are familiar with the term *stress,* but few are aware of its precise definition. Let's find out how scientists define the term.

Defining Stress

During **stress,** the body is in a state of mental and physical tension, and the balance (homeostasis) of the body's systems is disrupted. Stress is caused by one or more **stressors,** which can be physical (such as an injury) or mental (such as emotional distress resulting from a personal relationship). Regardless of the nature of the stressor, the body's physiological and mental responses usually include feelings of strain, tension, and anxiety. Our bodies' reactions to stress, called the **stress response,** prepare us to deal with stressors so balance can be restored. People are stressed by numerous stressors during daily life, and different people are stressed by different things. For example, you might find a long commute to work stressful, but someone else might enjoy the alone time.

stress A state of physical and mental tension in response to a situation that is perceived as a threat or challenge.

stressor A factor that produces stress.

stress response The physiological and behavioral changes that take place when a person is presented with a stressor.

eustress A stress level that results in improved performance; also called *positive stress.*

distress Negative stress that is harmful to performance.

answers

1. **FALSE** Everyone experiences some stress and a certain amount is necessary for optimal performance.

2. **TRUE** A person with chronic stress experiences some level of stress response on a consistent basis with little relief. This consistent activation of the systems involved in the stress response can increase the risk for heart disease.

3. **TRUE** You probably know that certain significant events, such as a death, finals, or the end of a relationship, cause stress. However, a number of everyday annoyances, such as rush-hour traffic, waiting in line, or being late, can also be a significant source of stress for some people.

4. **TRUE** Good time management skills can help you use time more effectively and reduce the stress of deadlines, being late, and procrastination.

5. **FALSE** Personality characteristics influence the way we perceive situations and the way we respond to stressful situations. Our past experiences and gender also impact our level of stress.

There are different classifications of stressors, and each can affect our behaviors, health, and life. Stressors can be acute (such as the death of a loved one), cumulative (such as a series of events that lead to a breakup with a boyfriend or girlfriend), or chronic (such as daily job- or school-related pressures). Although it is clear that chronic or extreme stress is unhealthy, some degree of stress is required to maximize performance. For any type of "performance" activity there is an optimal level of stress that pushes us to perform and excel. This level is specific to each individual, and it is motivating and energizing. Stress that is positive and that is associated with improved performance is called **eustress.**

Some level of stress is desirable and beneficial, but too much stress or poorly managed stress can have a negative impact on health and lead to poor performance and decisions. Negative stress is called **distress.** For example, regular exercise can be described as a positive stressor. However, regular exercise at very high frequency or intensity increases the risk of injury and emotional tension, and it can be considered a negative stressor because performance often suffers. Stress that results from negative situations is also considered distress, as when your computer crashes before you saved the final version of your senior project.

Physiological Changes of the Stress Response

You are driving home, and another driver runs a stop sign and barely misses hitting your car. Your body will

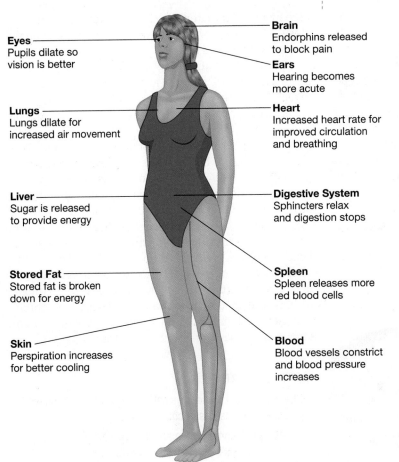

Eyes
Pupils dilate so vision is better

Lungs
Lungs dilate for increased air movement

Liver
Sugar is released to provide energy

Stored Fat
Stored fat is broken down for energy

Skin
Perspiration increases for better cooling

Brain
Endorphins released to block pain

Ears
Hearing becomes more acute

Heart
Increased heart rate for improved circulation and breathing

Digestive System
Sphincters relax and digestion stops

Spleen
Spleen releases more red blood cells

Blood
Blood vessels constrict and blood pressure increases

FIGURE 11.1
The body's physiological responses to stress.

have a set of predictable reactions to this acute stressor: Your heart rate increases, your senses heighten, and **endorphins** are released, to name a few of the changes that take place. These reactions are part of the stress response. The body's responses to stress are mediated by an area in the brain called the *hypothalamus* and are initiated when the hormones **epinephrine, norepinephrine,** and **cortisol** are released into the bloodstream. The hormones cause a number of physiological changes, some of which are illustrated in Figure 11.1. Hence the two body systems primarily responsible for the changes that occur during the stress response are the *nervous system* and the **endocrine system.**

Your nervous system controls both your voluntary movements (such as your raising your hand in class) and your involuntary bodily processes (such as your heart beating and digestion). The involuntary actions are controlled by the **autonomic nervous system,** of which there are two branches: the **parasympathetic branch** and the **sympathetic branch.** The parasympathetic branch is in control of body processes and functions when you are relaxed or resting. Maintaining your resting heart rate and blood pressure, growth, digestion, and storing energy are examples of processes under the control of the parasympathetic nervous system.

The sympathetic branch is the excitatory part of the autonomic nervous system. This branch is activated when you need to react and produce energy. The increase in heart rate, faster breathing, perspiration, and initial release of epinephrine are some of the changes produced by activation of the sympathetic division.

As part of the stress response, the sympathetic nervous system activates the endocrine system, which in turn releases hormones. The main stress hormone released by the system is cortisol, which is more predominant during distress and prolonged stress situations. Cortisol helps make glucose and break down fat for energy, increase the production of epinephrine and norepinephrine, and suppress an immune response.

The Fight-or-Flight Response

Together the responses of the autonomic nervous system and the endocrine system make up the **fight-or-flight response.** This initial response to stress was first

endorphins A group of hormones (endogenous opioids, or "painkillers") released during the stress response.

epinephrine A hormone secreted by the inner core (medulla) of the adrenal gland; also called *adrenaline.*

norepinephrine A hormone secreted by the inner core (medulla) of the adrenal gland.

cortisol A hormone secreted by the outer layer (cortex) of the adrenal gland.

endocrine system A series of glands and tissues in the body that secrete hormones to regulate bodily processes.

autonomic nervous system The branch of the nervous system that controls basic bodily functions that do not require conscious thought; includes the parasympathetic and sympathetic branches.

parasympathetic branch The division of the autonomic nervous system that is dominant at rest and controls the energy conservation and restoration processes.

sympathetic branch The division of the autonomic nervous system that is in control when we need to react or respond to challenges; the excitatory branch.

fight-or-flight response A series of physiological reactions by the body to prepare to combat a real or perceived threat.

discovered by Harvard physiologist Walter Canon (1) and later elaborated on by the biologist Hans Selye (2). Canon described the stress response as an inborn, automatic, and primitive response designed to prepare individuals to face (fight) or run away from (flight) any type of perceived threat or challenge to survival. According to Canon, once a person perceives a threat, the brain initiates a sequence of physiological and physical changes that ready the body for action. The challenge does not have to be a matter of life or death; the stressors we are presented with in everyday life can also evoke the fight-or-flight response.

----

consider this!

In one survey, 33% of students experienced stress to the point that their academic performance was negatively affected.

Imagine you are at home asleep and the telephone rings. You answer the phone and hear your professor's voice asking why you did not take the final exam. You look at your clock and realize you overslept and missed class! Suddenly your heart is racing, you are sweating profusely, your blood pressure rises, and your hands become cold and clammy. These responses prepare you to deal with the threatening or stressful situation. Do you try to explain the situation to your professor (fight) or quickly hang up and never return to school again (flight)?

Your body has "activation" responses to enable you to fight or flee (Figure 11.1). In addition to the changes already mentioned, blood is directed away from the digestive tract and into the muscles to provide extra energy for fighting or fleeing. You will have an increased awareness of your surroundings, quickened impulses, and diminished pain perception. Your body physically and mentally prepares to "battle" the stressor. After you successfully cope with your stressor or no longer

perceive it as threatening, the body returns to homeostasis. However, if the situation is not resolved, you will stay in this aroused state.

During the fight-or-flight response, people are in an "attack mode" and are focused on short-term "survival." Primitive people were required to exert physical activity while fighting or fleeing from wild animals, and the physical exertion of fighting or fleeing would rid the body of excess levels of stress hormones, allowing it to return to homeostasis. However, today's modern stressors, such as congested roads, too few parking spaces, missing an exam, bouncing a check, or having an argument with your significant other, do not typically require physical exertion. People living highly stressful lives can experience chronic stress, meaning that they have some level of arousal from stress almost constantly. There is often no release from these stressors in the form of physical exertion, and over time the stress hormones accumulate in the body, causing illness and chronic disease. We'll discuss the relationship between chronic stress and disease later in the chapter.

MAKE SURE YOU KNOW...

- Stress is a mental and physical response to situations we perceive as pressures or challenges.

- Stressors can come from many sources, and they can be positive (eustress) or negative (distress). Some degree of stress is required to maximize performance.

- The autonomic nervous system and the endocrine system are responsible for the changes that occur during the stress response. The parasympathetic branch of the autonomic nervous system is in control at rest, and the sympathetic branch is activated when you need to react. Cortisol is the main stress hormone produced by the endocrine system.

- The changes in the body that occur during the stress response prepare our bodies to fight or flee the stressful situation. These responses are collectively referred to as the fight-or-flight response.

What Factors Affect Your Stress Level?

Although everyone feels stress, life events and situations do not affect everyone the same way. Our personalities, past experiences, and gender are three influences on the way we perceive situations and cope with stress. For example, your grandmother who recently recovered from a hip fracture might experience stress when she enters a setting with a lot of stairs and uneven terrain. However, as a healthy young adult, you do not find that environment threatening. You might have a tendency to freak out during finals, whereas your roommate remains calm. We will discuss some of the factors that impact your ability to handle stressful situations next.

Personality Behavior Patterns

People's different reactions to the same stressful situation can be due to personality differences and how they have learned to respond.

There are many different ways to describe personalities and behavior patterns. Note that although there is no one specific (or completely reliable) way of identifying stress-prone personality patterns, one of the most common, and easily interpreted, classification groupings describes individuals as having characteristics that fit into one of four behavior pattern categories: Type A, Type B, Type C, and Type D (Table 11.1). This classification system describes the four most common behavior patterns.

People who exhibit Type A behavior pattern (TABP) are highly motivated, time-conscious, hard-driving, impatient, and sometimes hostile, cynical, and angry. They have a heightened response to stress, and their hostility and anger, especially if repressed, place them at greater risk for heart disease (3, 4). Individuals with Type B behavior pattern are easygoing, nonaggressive, and patient, and they are not prone to hostile episodes like their TABP counterparts. People with Type B behavior pattern are less likely to perceive everyday annoyances as significant stressors and are at low risk for heart disease from stress.

Most people have heard of TABP and Type B behavior pattern, but you might not be familiar with the other behavior patterns. People with Type C behavior pattern have many of the positive qualities of TABP. They are confident, highly motivated, and competitive. However, individuals with Type C behavior pattern typically do not express the hostility and anger seen with TABP, and they use their personality characteristics to maintain a constant level of emotional control and to channel their ambition into creative directions. Because people with Type C behavior pattern do not express negative emotions and feelings in the same manner as those with TABP, they experience the same low risk for stress-related heart disease as do those with Type B behavior pattern. However, a person with Type C behavior pattern, keeping emotions in and not expressing them, can face a higher risk for heart disease.

Individuals with Type D behavior pattern also are considered to be at greater risk for stress-related disease. These individuals are prone to worry and anxiety and also tend to be inhibited and uneasy when interacting with others. Their social clumsiness results in a chronic state of anxiety, which places them at greater risk for heart disease (5, 6).

Past Experiences

Discovering aspects of one's personality can be interesting and entertaining, but we must keep in mind that ultimately it is our perception of a stressor and the way we react to it that will determine any resulting health effects. We learn from our experiences, and what we learn can help us respond more positively in future situations. For example, finals time is a common stressor. You would expect a person with TABP to be extremely stressed during the time leading up to finals. But a person with TABP who has learned that too much stress leads to unfocused study time and poor grades might plan to manage and structure study time weeks in advance to avoid the last-minute stress. Likewise, a student with Type B behavior who performed poorly in the past because she was too relaxed and did not prepare well might learn to prepare more diligently for future finals to improve her performance.

Gender

Gender is another factor that impacts the way we react to stressors. There are no sex differences in the physiological responses to stress, but gender might affect the way we perceive situations and how we react to

TABLE 11.1	**Personality Behavior Patterns and Their Risks for Heart Disease**	
Personality Behavior Pattern	**Qualities**	**Risk for Heart Disease**
A	Impatient, competitive, aggressive, highly motivated, and sometimes hostile	High
B	Patient, with low aggression, and easygoing	Low
C	Competitive, highly motivated, high level of confidence, and constant level of emotional control	Low
D	Negative, anxious, worried, and socially inhibited	High

stressors. For example, our society has traditionally deemed it more acceptable for women to express their emotions openly. Thus, a woman might feel more comfortable discussing stressors and be better able to cope with them than a man who has been socialized to "keep his feelings in." Conversely, a woman might have been taught that certain responses, such as explosive anger, are not "ladylike" and will therefore refrain from expressing her anger, leading to greater stress. Participating in activities outside traditional gender roles also might produce stress. A man who decides to be a stay-at-home dad or work from home so his wife can pursue her career, for example, might experience higher levels of stress because his choice does not fit with societal norms. Gender-related reactions to stress also might vary across different cultures.

Regardless of your personality characteristics, past experiences, and gender, you can learn ways to deal with the stress in your life, and the first step is to examine your stress level. A convenient way to do this is to complete a questionnaire designed to evaluate your stress level, such as Laboratory 11.1 at the end of this chapter. If the results suggest that you are under unhealthy levels of stress, you should implement stress management and stress reduction techniques.

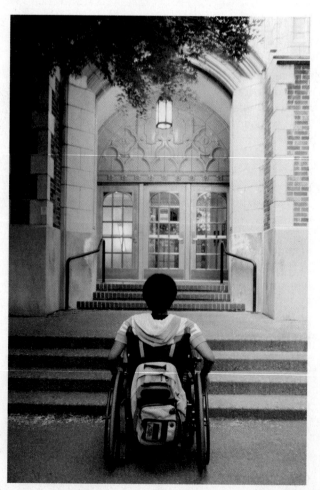

College life comes with stressors from many sources.

**HEAR IT!
CASE STUDY**

Hector is a typical procrastinator. Listen to the online case study to determine how he can better manage his time at **www.pearsonhighered.com/powers**.

Common Causes of Stress

Recognizing the everyday life situations that contribute to your stress level is important in managing stress. The pressure of performing well in your classes, along with competing deadlines for papers, projects, and tests, can be a source of stress, especially if you do not have strong time-management skills. Choosing a major and planning for your future after graduation are also stressful processes. Making use of career services and talking with your professors and faculty advisors can help you find the best options for your strengths and interests.

Interpersonal relationships often change when you enter college. If you move to attend college, getting connected within the college community and developing new relationships can be a source of stress. Leaving family and friends also can be a challenge. If you did not have to move, your existing relationships still might be affected as you balance your time with schoolwork, new friends, and other responsibilities of college life.

---

consider this!
About 15% of college students say their academic performance has been impaired because of Internet use or computer games.

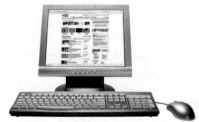

Financial responsibilities can be a source of stress in many stages of life. Costs associated with college tuition, fees, and books are high, and you may have to rely on student loans to assist with college expenses. Work-study and other college programs can relieve some of the financial burden, but they place additional demands on your already limited time. Maybe you are among the many students who have to work during the school year and summers to make money for school. Work demands can be a significant source of stress, because they affect relationships, time, and schoolwork. Also, when selecting your major, you have to consider the job opportunities and earning potential of the career paths that interest you. The need to attend graduate school or take low-paying or nonpaying internships can further add to financial strain and stress. Budgeting and planning for expenses are important skills to develop. Avoiding credit card debt also reduces the stress of the financial burden of college.

Other common college stressors include traffic, parking on campus, and adjusting to college life. (See the Closer Look box on page 282 for a discussion of road rage, one common source of traffic stress.) Students who are married with families have the combined stresses of balancing home and family responsibilities with the demands of school. Nontraditional students—for example, people who have returned to school after several years—may feel out of place and experience additional stress related to those feelings. In addition to balancing the demands of school, work, and relationships, some students engage in leisure activities, such as spending time on the Internet, which affect productivity and, in turn, may lead to stress. Students with disabilities are likely to face stressors in learning to navigate a college campus that might not adequately accommodate their specific disabilities.

SEE IT! VIDEOS
Put down that cell phone! Watch *The Multi-Tasking Myth* at **www.pearsonhighered.com/powers** to understand why doing multiple things at once might not be the best idea.

MAKE SURE YOU KNOW...

- Personality can impact the way we perceive situations and respond to stress. Type A and Type D behavior patterns are associated with higher risk for heart disease.

- Past experiences and gender also influence our reactions to situations we perceive as stressful.

- College life can present many stressors. Some of the most common include academic responsibilities, poor time management, the demands of relationships, and finances.

SEE IT! VIDEOS
Can stress be deadly? Watch *Stress at Work and Home* at **www.pearsonhighered.com/powers** to understand how stress can be hazardous to your health.

Stress and Health

Chronic (persistent) stress is related to some of the most significant health problems in the United States. Heart disease, depression, and migraines are all associated with stress and have significant direct and indirect health care costs. Stress is a risk factor for depression and anxiety, and up to 25% of the U.S. adult population suffers from these and other mental health problems every year (7). Approximately 75%–90% of all physician visits are for stress-related complaints, and millions of people take medication for stress-related illnesses (8). From a medical standpoint, stress can affect both emotional and physical

COACHING Corner

Stress is omnipresent in college. As you become aware of how you respond to demands placed on you, managing your stress becomes more practical. Each time you have an emotional or stressful reaction to a demand placed on you, ask yourself the following questions:

- Before making a hasty decision in a stressful situation, think: Are my perceptions of this situation correct or do I need more information to make a decision or plan of action? Many times we think and rethink a situation when in fact we do not have enough information to make a great decision. When in doubt seek more information.

- Is there room to negotiate the time line or due dates that are causing increased

stress? Although most people will not accommodate procrastination, many people are open to negotiate due dates if up-front communication occurs. The key is to be honest and ask well before a deadline is looming.

- Will this matter to me tomorrow, 2 weeks from now, or a year from now? In many cases you can "reduce" anxiety or stress simply by evaluating the long-term impact of a situation. If it won't matter beyond the 2-week mark it may not be that big a situation.

Will this stressor matter later?

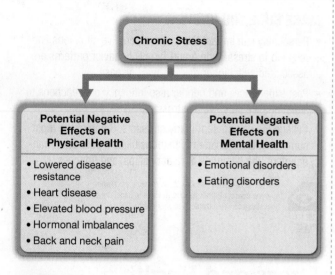

FIGURE 11.2
Chronic stress can have negative effects on both physical and mental health.

health. Chronic stress has been linked to elevated blood pressure, heart disease, hormonal imbalances, reduced resistance to disease, and emotional disorders (9, 10, 11) **(Figure 11.2)**.

Stress-related problems cost both businesses and government billions of dollars every year in the form of employee absenteeism and health care costs. Stress can suppress the immune system, making a person more susceptible to illness. Acute stress can also impact productivity. Headaches and tension might cause a person to miss work or class or be less focused. Therefore, stress is a major health problem that affects individual lives and the economy as a whole.

Hans Selye developed one of the earliest scientific theories to explain the relationship between stress and disease. Selye proposed that humans adapt to stress in a response he termed the **general adaptation syndrome,** which involves three stages: an alarm stage, a resistance stage, and an exhaustion stage (2).

During the alarm stage, the fight-or-flight response, discussed earlier, occurs. Stress hormones are released, and their effects on the body can cause anxiety, headaches, and disrupted patterns of sleeping and eating (2). During this phase, the body is more susceptible to disease and more prone to injury.

With continued exposure to stress, the individual reaches the resistance stage. During this stage, the body's resistance to stress is higher than normal, and mechanisms are activated that allow the body to resist disease effectively. In short, the resistance stage represents an improved ability to cope with stress (2).

Selye proposed that when the stress persists, the individual reaches the exhaustion stage. Note that

"exhaustion" in this sense refers to a depletion of the physical and psychological resources to cope with stress that occurs with chronic exposure to stress. Selye suggested that the body is vulnerable to disease during this stage because of this depletion of resources. During this phase, physical symptoms that appeared in the alarm stage can reappear, but they now are more serious and can sometimes compromise health.

Although Selye's model of adaptation to stress is still viewed as an important contribution to our understanding of the stress response, newer research findings have improved our understanding of the relationship between stress and disease. We now know that the underlying cause of many stress-related diseases is the body's inability to respond to stress in the normal way, and that the body's resources to respond to stress are not depleted with long-term exposure to stress. Instead, repeated and/or prolonged response to stress results in the continual activation of the nervous, endocrine, and immune systems, which includes the continual release of stress hormones, including cortisol.

The concepts of **allostasis** and **allostatic load** are better explanations of the relationship between stress and disease. Allostasis refers to the body's ability to change and adapt in stressful situations. Under long-term stress, we do not adapt as well. The allostatic load is the point at which there is too much stress, which taxes the system's stress response (12). The constant level of activation or repeated activation causes the stress response to become inefficient.

One's risk of developing a stress-related illness increases because, over time, high levels of cortisol in the blood impair the immune system's ability to fight infections (12, 13, 14). As you have realized by now, prolonged stress places an individual at greater risk for illness and other associated problems. As a result, understanding and implementing stress management skills are important for maintaining a high level of wellness.

 Assess what irritates you with the *Stress Tolerance Test* Take Charge of Your Health! Worksheet online at **www.pearsonhighered.com/powers.**

**LIVE IT!
ASSESS
YOURSELF**

MAKE SURE YOU KNOW...

- Depression and anxiety have a significant impact on the U.S. adult population, and stress is a risk factor for both conditions.

- General adaptation syndrome, which includes alarm, resistance, and exhaustion stages, was one of the first theories proposed about the relationship between stress and disease.

- The concept of the allostatic load is that long-term and repeated exposure to stress and the continual activation of the stress response compromise health.

STEPS FOR BEHAVIOR CHANGE

How well do you manage your time?

Take the quiz below to find out whether you are a good time manager.

Y N

☐ ☐ Do you procrastinate?

☐ ☐ Do you take on more responsibilities than you can handle?

☐ ☐ Are you consistently late for class, appointments, or work?

☐ ☐ Do you need more hours in the day to accomplish all of your daily tasks?

☐ ☐ Do you have little time for fun with friends or family?

If you answered yes to most or all of these questions, you can probably use some tips for better time management.

TIPS TO IMPROVE YOUR TIME MANAGEMENT SKILLS, REDUCE STRESS, AND INCREASE PRODUCTIVITY

Tomorrow, you will:

☑ Plan ahead. Plan your day by using your cell phone or daily planner to organize tasks. Make a schedule you are able to implement, and allow time for unscheduled events and delays.

☑ Evaluate how you spend your time. Determine how you can make adjustments in your day to increase or better use your free time (e.g., cut back or eliminate time spent watching TV, texting, or using social network sites).

Within the next 2 weeks, you will:

☑ Establish goals. Establish a list of goals you plan to accomplish. Include short- and long-term SMART goals.

☑ Prioritize. List your tasks in order of their importance (high priority to low priority), and then follow that list. Establish a daily goal of accomplishing the three most important tasks on your priority list.

☑ Schedule time for you. Find time each day to relax and do something you enjoy. Regularly evaluate your ratio of work time to home and leisure time, and make sure you maintain balance.

By the end of the semester, you will:

☑ Delegate responsibility. If you are involved with clubs or group projects, share and delegate responsibility to lower stress. Also, learn to say no to activities that prevent you from achieving your goals. Before accepting a new responsibility, complete your current task or eliminate an unnecessary project.

☑ Re-evaluate your progress and goals to make any necessary adjustments.

How Can You Manage Stress?

Once you know your stress level, you can cope with the stress by using stress management techniques. There are two general steps to managing stress: Reduce the amount of stress in your life, and cope with stress by improving your ability to relax (15). Let's discuss each of these steps individually. You can also use the sample program for stress management on pages 288–289.

Manage Stressors

People who experience chronic stress or very high levels of stress and its associated feelings of anxiety can experience **burnout** (16). The first significant way to lower the impact of stress on your life is to reduce the number of stressors you encounter. Although you will not be able to avoid all sources of stress, you can eliminate many "unnecessary" forms. The first step is to recognize those

general adaptation syndrome A pattern of responses to stress that consists of an alarm stage, a resistance stage, and an exhaustion stage.

allostasis The ability to maintain homeostasis through change.

allostatic load The inability to respond appropriately to stress; leads to compromised health.

burnout The loss of physical, emotional, and mental energy, which, if ignored, can lead to emotional exhaustion and withdrawal.

A CLOSER LOOK

Road Rage

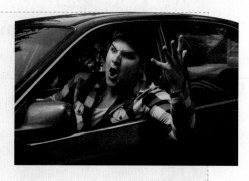

What is Road Rage?

Road rage refers to extreme acts of aggression resulting from disagreements between drivers. Typical road rage behaviors include tailgating, headlight flashing, obscene gestures, deliberately blocking other vehicles, verbal abuse, and its most extreme form—physical assault. According to estimates, aggressive driving injures or kills at least 1500 people each year. Road rage is a serious problem and a criminal offense.

What Causes Road Rage?

For many of us, driving is our most stressful daily activity. Roadways are crowded, and we must deal with all levels of drivers—good and bad. Everyone makes traffic mistakes at times, whether intentionally or unintentionally. Often, road rage starts as a simple misunderstanding between drivers and then escalates into a more serious situation. Usually, the driving incident is not the immediate cause of anger. For some, mounting professional or personal troubles, plus frustration over another driver's "stupid" mistakes, is enough to cause them to erupt in anger. Drivers in a "bad mood" before they get behind the wheel are more likely to have strong reactions to the actions of other drivers. Researchers believe that some personality characteristics make one more prone to aggressive driving.

If you drive aggressively, the following tips can help you reduce your traffic stress:

- Avoid driving during times of heaviest congestion.
- Allow yourself plenty of time so you do not have to speed, run traffic lights, or roll through stop signs.
- Drive in comfort. Use your air conditioner, get a comfortable seat cover, and listen to classical music during your drive. Do not listen to emotionally stimulating radio talk shows. Enjoy audio books.
- Do not drive when you are angry or upset.
- When in traffic, concentrate on being relaxed. Practice breathing for relaxation.

---

factors that produce daily stress. Use Laboratory 11.1 to assess your stressors and to help determine which ones you can most readily work to eliminate, avoid, or better manage. Getting adequate amounts of rest and sleep and exercising regularly are also important factors in managing your stress levels.

One example of a stressor that you can eliminate is overcommitment, a frequent cause of stress in college students. If you plan your time carefully and prioritize your activities, you can avoid feeling overwhelmed by having too much to do and not enough time to do it. You can plan a daily schedule that allows you to accomplish the things you need to without being distracted by less important activities. Be aware of activities that steal your time. The increase in the number of social networking websites available can use more of your time than you realize (see the Closer Look box on page 283). The Steps for Behavior Change box on page 281 can help you determine how well you manage your time.

Another common stressor that you may be able to better manage is financial pressure. You cannot eliminate the high costs associated with paying tuition, rent (or room and board), or buying course materials, but you can prioritize your spending and make sure you budget for the essential expenses. For example, you can choose to wait to get a manicure or purchase the newest smart phone until after buying your books. Then reward yourself if you can do so without using a credit card, or save until you have the money. Working to minimize the amount of debt you accrue as a student, particularly credit card debt, can reduce both present and future financial stress. Avoiding overuse of credit cards and developing a budget are two very important strategies for preventing excessive debt. Look for ways to reduce your everyday costs, and do not buy expensive clothes or gadgets if you do not have the money to pay for them now, no matter how popular they may be. If you do have your eye on trendy new boots or the latest smart phone, make a saving plan and purchase the item when you do not have to put it on a credit card.

Assess your time management with the *Time Management Self-Test* Take Charge of Your Health! Worksheet online at www.pearsonhighered.com/powers.

LIVE IT!
ASSESS
YOURSELF

Rest and Sleep

One of the most effective means of reducing stress and tension is to get adequate rest and sleep. How much sleep do you need? Although individual needs vary greatly, adults typically need 7 to 9 hours of restful sleep per night. Because of the body's natural hormonal rhythms, you should also try to go to bed at approximately the same time every night. See the Steps for

A CLOSER LOOK

How Many "Friends" Do You Have?

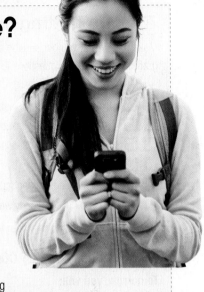

Having a strong or large support network is typically associated with better stress management and mental health. But what is the effect if the social network is an online network? As more social networking websites have been developed, more and more adolescents and young adults are developing large online and text social networks. Does having a network of 500 or more "friends" really mean one has a stronger support network? Texting and the use of social networks are not necessarily problematic, but they can be for some. People use sites differently and for different reasons. How and why you choose to use these sites can affect the impact that use has on social relationships and health. It appears that extraverts use social network sites to enhance their social relationships and interactions, whereas introverts use them for social compensation. Studies also have shown that more time spent using social network sites is associated with depression, psychological distress, and lower self-esteem. Furthermore, some might experience increases in anxiety when the use of social networking sites is limited or stopped. So how do you know whether your texting or use of social network sites is problematic? If you have multiple "yes" answers to the following questions, you might want to re-evaluate your use of online social networking and texting.

- Do you spend less time in face-to-face interactions than you do in online interactions? Or have your online "friends" replaced people in your life?
- Do you experience symptoms of stress or anxiety when you are unable to text, update your status, or interact using a social network site?
- Do you frequently text or use social network sites at times that are considered inappropriate (e.g., class, work, church, or on a date)?

- Do you compare your life to the lives of those in your network? Do you feel bad or inadequate when you make comparisons?
- Have your texting and social network habits had a negative impact on your relationships, grades, work performance, or any other aspect of your life?
- Does the time spent texting and using social network sites impact your time management?

Sources: Chou, H. T., and N. Edge. "They are happier and having better lives than I am": The impact of using Facebook on perceptions of others' lives. *Cyberpsychology, Behavior and Social Networking* 15(2):117–121, 2012; Durocher, J. J., Lufkin, K. M., M. E. King, and J. R. Carter. Social technology restriction alters state-anxiety but not autonomic activity in humans. *American Journal of Physiology: Regulatory, Integrative and Comparative Physiology* 301(6):R1773–1778, 2011; Kujath, C. L. Facebook and MySpace: Complement or substitute for face-to-face interaction? *Cyberpsychology, Behavior and Social Networking* 14(1–2):75–78, 2011; Kuss, D. J., and M. D. Griffiths. Online social networking and addiction: A review of the psychological literature. *International Journal of Environmental Research and Public Health* 8(9):3528–3552, 2011; Mango, A. M., T. Taylor, and P. M. Greenfield. Me and my 400 friends: The anatomy of college students' Facebook networks, their communication patterns, and well-being. *Developmental Psychology* 48(2):369–390, 2012; O'Dea, B., and A. Campbell. Online social networking amongst teens: Friend or foe? *Studies in Health Technology and Informatics* 167:133–138, 2011; Wilson, K., S. Fornasier, and K. M. White. Psychological predictors of young adults' use of social networking site. *Cyberpsychology, Behavior and Social Networking* 13(2):173–177, 2010.

Behavior Change box on page 284 to help determine whether you're getting enough sleep.

In addition to a good night's sleep, 15 to 30 minutes of rest during the day can help reduce stress. You can do this by simply putting your feet up on a desk or table and closing your eyes. A well-rested body is the best protection against stress and fatigue.

HEAR IT!
CASE STUDY
Are you like Meena, struggling to find time to sleep in your freshman year? Listen to the online case study at **www.pearsonhighered.com/powers.**

LIVE IT!
ASSESS YOURSELF
Assess your sleep with the *Sleep Inventory* Take Charge of Your Health! Worksheet online at **www.pearsonhighered.com/powers.**

Exercise

Light to moderate exercise can reduce many types of stress and anxiety. Even if you are not an experienced exerciser, you can benefit from the calm feeling that comes after an exercise session. The recommended types of exercise for optimal stress reduction are low- to moderate-intensity aerobic exercises, such as brisk walking, swimming, and cycling. (The guidelines for this type of exercise prescription are presented in Chapter 3.) Yoga, tai-chi, and Pilates are other popular types of exercise that help you relax and reduce stress. Many gyms and health clubs offer classes in these forms of exercise.

STEPS FOR ▶ BEHAVIOR CHANGE

Are you getting enough sleep?

Making sure that you get enough sleep will help you effectively deal with your daily stressors and may also help improve your grades. Answer these questions to find out whether you are getting enough sleep.

Y   N

☐ ☐   Do you fall asleep as soon as your head hits the pillow?

☐ ☐   Do you find yourself dozing in class or at other inappropriate times of the day?

☐ ☐   Do you frequently take naps during the day?

☐ ☐   Do you have an irregular bedtime?

☐ ☐   Do you "binge" sleep on the weekend?

☐ ☐   Do you have difficulty waking in the morning?

If you answered yes to more than two of the above questions, you may not be getting enough sleep at night.

TIPS TO HELP YOU GET CONSISTENT, RESTFUL SLEEP

Tomorrow, you will:

☑ Establish a bedtime and a set time to wake up that can be maintained on a regular schedule.

☑ Sleep in a comfortable environment. A cool, dark room with little noise is recommended for a good night of sleep.

☑ Use bright light in the morning to help you wake up.

Within the next 2 weeks, you will:

☑ Discontinue drinking caffeinated beverages after 4:00 P.M.

☑ Avoid stimulating reading or television/movies in the evening. Instead, try meditating or listening to soothing music to help you unwind and relax.

By the end of the semester, you will:

☑ Avoid disrupting your regular sleep pattern. Long naps during the day and using the weekend to play "catch up" on sleep missed during the week can disrupt sleep patterns.

☑ Be well rested and ready for finals!

Studies have shown that exercise is very effective for stress reduction (17, 18, 19). **Figure 11.3** compares the effects of a 30-minute session of exercise (running) to other common forms of stress reduction: rest, reading, and meditation. In this study, meditation provided the greatest stress reduction, with exercise finishing a close second (17). Other studies have shown that exercise reduces stress about as much as other types of relaxation techniques (20). Also, the relaxing effects of exercise can last for hours after an exercise session (16).

Although we consistently see that people feel more relaxed after exercise, we do not know exactly how exercise reduces stress. Several ideas have been proposed. It has not been proven, but one theory is that exercise causes the brain to release several natural tranquilizers (endorphins), which can produce a calming effect (21). Another theory is that exercise may be a diversion or break from your stressors and the worries of

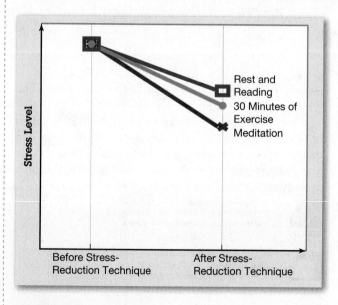

FIGURE 11.3
Rest, exercise, and meditation are all techniques you can use to reduce your stress level.

life. The improved physical fitness and self-image that you enjoy as a result of regular exercise also increase your resistance to stress. A final possibility is that all of these factors may contribute to the beneficial effects of exercise on stress management. The next time you feel stressed, try exercising; you will feel and look better as a result.

Use Relaxation Techniques to Cope with Stress

Stress management techniques can help reduce the potentially harmful effects of stress. Most of these techniques are designed to relax you and thereby reduce your stress level. When trying to relax, ask yourself two questions: (a) What prevents me from relaxing? and (b) What am I not doing that could help me relax? (9).

Your answers can help you determine how and where to focus your efforts to manage your stress. Lowering your levels of stress and practicing effective stress management techniques will increase your overall level of wellness (14). The following are some of the more common approaches used in stress management.

Progressive Relaxation   Progressive relaxation is a stress reduction technique that uses exercises to reduce muscle tension. (Muscle tension is a common symptom of stress.) You practice the technique while sitting quietly or lying down. First you contract muscle groups, and then you relax them, one at a time, beginning with your feet and then moving up your body to your hands and neck, until you achieve a complete state of muscle relaxation. You can find specific directions for one progressive relaxation exercise in the Closer Look box below.

A CLOSER LOOK

Progressive Relaxation Training

There are many types of progressive relaxation training methods, and over 200 different exercises have been described. The basic technique involves contracting and relaxing muscle groups, starting in your lower body and moving toward your upper body. The following technique is one of the many forms that you can use.

1. Find a quiet, comfortable, and private place. Remove your shoes. Wear loose, comfortable clothing, or loosen any tight clothing. The first few times you can expect emerging thoughts and emotions to distract you from your attempts to relax. After some practice, you will be able to block distractions. Listening to soothing music during your relaxation sessions is one way to help you relax and filter distractions; there are many commercial relaxation music CDs and MP3s available. You may also read the instructions into a recorder and use them to guide you through your relaxation session. This strategy will avoid having to remember the steps involved.

2. Assume a relaxed position (either sitting or lying down). Close your eyes, and begin by focusing on your breathing. Become aware of how it feels to breathe in and breathe out. Breathe deeply and slowly through your nose, and imagine that you are breathing in good, healing air and breathing out stress and muscle tension. While developing your breathing you may find it useful to inhale to a count of 7—1-2-3-4-5-6-7—and exhale to the same count. Breathe this way for several minutes before starting your progressive relaxation exercise.

3. Without speaking, focus on relaxing each part of your body. You are consciously "telling" each part of your body to relax.

Contracting the muscles in each body part first and then relaxing them can help you to feel the difference, because sometimes we are not aware of tension we carry in our muscles. Do not move on to the next area until you have relaxed the part you are focusing on.

Proceed by relaxing your body in the following order:

a. Toes of left foot	m. Chest
b. Toes of right foot	n. Left shoulder
c. Left foot	o. Right shoulder
d. Right foot	p. Left arm
e. Left ankle	q. Left hand
f. Right ankle	r. Left fingers
g. Lower left leg	s. Right arm
h. Lower right leg	t. Right hand
i. Left thigh	u. Right fingers
j. Right thigh	v. Neck
k. Buttocks	w. Face
l. Abdomen	

4. Now you should be completely relaxed. Continue breathing for the next few minutes. Try not to let your mind wander—remain in this relaxed state.

5. At the end of your session, take yourself out of your relaxed state should feel renewed and refresh

Visuali
agery use
is to create a
mountain settin

The proponents of progressive relaxation techniques argue that relaxing the muscles in this manner will also relax the mind and thereby relieve stress. The theory behind this concept is that an anxious (stressed) mind cannot exist in a relaxed body.

Breathing Exercises Breathing exercises can also help you relax. The following is a sample step-by-step breathing exercise for reducing stress:

1. Assume a comfortable position, sitting or lying down, with your eyes closed.

2. Begin to slowly inhale and exhale. Count from 1 to 3 during each inhalation and each exhalation to maintain a slow and regular breathing pattern.

3. Next, combine stretching and breathing to provide greater relaxation and stress reduction. For example, stretch your arms toward the ceiling as you inhale, then lower your arms as you exhale.

Try this exercise for 5 to 15 minutes in a quiet room.

Meditation **Meditation** has been practiced for ages to help people relax and achieve inner peace. There are many types of meditation, and there is no scientific evidence that one form is superior to another. Most types of meditation have the same common elements: sitting quietly for 15 to 20 minutes twice a day, concentrating on a single word or image, and breathing slowly and regularly. The goal is to achieve a complete state of physical and mental relaxation.

Although beginning a successful program may require the help of an experienced instructor, the following is a brief overview of how to practice meditation:

1. First, choose a word or sound, called a *mantra*, to repeat during the meditation. The idea of using a mantra is that this word or sound should become your symbol of complete relaxation. Choose a mantra that has little emotional significance for you, such as the word *red*.

2. Next, find a quiet area and sit comfortably with your eyes closed. Take several deep breaths and concentrate on relaxing; let your body go limp.

3. Concentrate on your mantra. This means that you should not hear or think about anything else. Repeat your mantra over and over again in your mind, and relax. Avoid distracting thoughts, and focus only on the mantra.

4. After 15 to 20 minutes of concentration on the mantra, open your eyes, and begin to move your thoughts away from the mantra. End the session by making a fist with both hands and saying to yourself that you are alert and refreshed.

Visualization Visualization (sometimes called *imagery*) uses mental pictures to reduce stress. The idea is to create an appealing mental image (such as a quiet mountain setting) that promotes relaxation and reduces

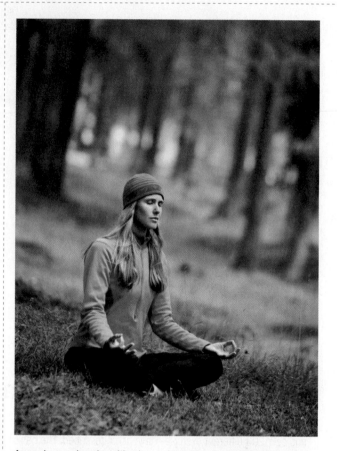

Assuming a relaxed position in a quiet setting is central to several relaxation techniques.

stress. To practice visualization, follow the instructions presented for meditation, but substitute a relaxing mental scene for the mantra. If you fail to reach a complete state of relaxation after your first several sessions, do not be discouraged. Achieving complete relaxation with this technique may require numerous practice sessions.

Develop Spiritual Wellness

Spiritual wellness is associated with better recovery from illness and improved mental health (as we discussed in Chapter 1). Spiritual wellness can provide a sense of peace. People who report high levels of spiritual wellness often practice behaviors such as prayer, meditation, or enjoying the beauty of nature to reduce stress and anxiety.

 Assess your spiritual growth with the *Developing Your Spirituality* Take Charge of Your Health! Worksheet online at **www.pearsonhighered.com/powers**.

LIVE IT!
ASSESS
YOURSELF

Develop a Support Network

Having a network of friends and family to help you cope with stressors can help to reduce or eliminate stress. Sometimes just talking through your stressful situation can help you think more clearly about the situation and develop an effective plan to address your stressors.

COACHING Corner

Guided meditation has long been supported as a way to begin learning to manage your stress. Consider using the Internet to find a short guided meditation, or find a meditation professional to share a guided journey with you. The value of meditation occurs after repeated experience. Consider the following to help you develop a meditation schedule.

- Commit to clearing your mind for at least 5 minutes each day.

- Try a meditation before you get out of bed in the morning or just before you go to sleep at night.

- Take a 5–10 minute break in your day to daydream about your surroundings.

- Take a break and look at a piece of art. Maintain your focus on the piece for as long as you can.

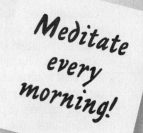

Meditate every morning!

Others who have your best interest as a concern will likely help you with a plan for stress management. When you are dealing with stressors that cannot be eliminated, your network will be there for support while you work through your period of stress.

Avoid Counterproductive Behaviors

Some people choose poor health behaviors, such as smoking cigarettes or drinking alcohol, in an attempt to manage stress. However, these behaviors are counterproductive and can lead to more cumulative stress in the long term.

Using Tobacco Many people say that they smoke cigarettes "to relax," but the nicotine in cigarettes and other tobacco products is actually a stimulant that produces responses similar to the fight-or-flight response. Additionally, nicotine is an addictive substance that has serious long-term effects. Smoking is the leading cause of preventable death, increasing the risk for lung and other types of cancer and for heart disease. Smoking and tobacco also are very costly habits.

Using Alcohol or Other Drugs Using alcohol or other substances might make you briefly forget about problems or stressors, but these behaviors do not eliminate or reduce the stressor. In some cases they might add to your level of stress. Alcohol (especially binge drinking) or drug use can affect your sleep patterns and productivity. Using alcohol or other substances to solve or cope with your problems can lead to abuse. Even legal substances, such as caffeine, can cause problems instead of solving them.

Disordered Eating Patterns *Disordered eating patterns* are eating patterns that are not healthy, but that do not meet the clinical definitions for eating disorders. These patterns can lead to the development of an eating disorder. Undereating or overeating can be disordered eating. Skipping meals will result in lack of nutrients and energy, which can affect how well you can focus and cope with stressors. Overeating, binge eating, or using "comfort foods" to cope with stress can lead to weight gain and health problems. Also, blood glucose levels can be affected, resulting in fluctuations in your energy level and decreased ability to focus on managing your stress.

MAKE SURE YOU KNOW...

- The two general steps involved in stress management are reducing the sources of stress and using relaxation techniques to help you cope with stress.

- The ideal way to lessen the effects of stress on your life is to reduce the sources of stress.

- Getting more rest and sleep; engaging in exercise; and practicing progressive muscle relaxation, breathing exercises, meditation, and visualization are some of the many relaxation techniques that can help you cope with stress.

- Developing your spiritual and social wellness can be very important in managing stress.

- Adopting unhealthy behaviors, such as smoking or drinking alcohol, to relax will lead to higher levels of stress in the long term.

meditation A method of relaxation that involves sitting quietly, focusing on a word or image, and breathing slowly.

visualization A relaxation technique that uses appealing mental images to promote relaxation and reduce stress; also called *imagery*.

Can Nutritional Supplements Reduce Emotional Stress?

Currently, there is no scientific evidence that any specific nutritional supplement, including megadoses of vitamins, will reduce emotional stress. According to researchers at the University of Texas Southwestern Medical Center at Dallas, most "stress formulas" contain B vitamins, such as niacin and riboflavin, which are meant to aid in recovery from physical stress (e.g., injuries), not emotional stress. The B vitamins are sometimes used to supplement the diets of people recovering from surgery. However, emotional stress does not increase the body's energy or nutrient needs, so taking vitamins will not calm us down.

Getting plenty of rest and exercising regularly, combined with a healthy diet, are the best ways to deal with emotional stress. Combining healthy lifestyle practices with stress management techniques such as those offered in this chapter can help you deal with life's stressors.

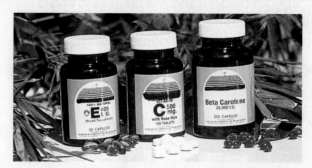

Although numerous nutritional products are marketed as stress relievers, none have been proven effective for stress reduction.

Sample Program for Stress Management

Scan to plan your individualized program for stress management. ▶

It is important to find a stress management technique that works for you. Some of the strategies discussed in this chapter require practice and regular use for you to become proficient and to maximize the benefits. The plan below suggests multiple techniques. It might take trial and error to find the technique that works best for you. Also, remember that most individuals report feeling more relaxed after moderate-intensity aerobic exercise, so your regular exercise is a great way to relax after a stressful event or day.

Every night, try to sleep for 6–8 hours. Try yoga, meditation, or progressive muscle relaxation for your relaxation techniques. On a daily basis, strive to reduce activities that waste time, such as excessive TV, video games, social networking sites, and texting.

	Stress Management Technique	Monday	Tuesday	Wednesday	Thursday	Friday	Saturday	Sunday
Week 1	**Sleep**	6–8 hours	6–8 hours	6–8 hours	6–8 hours	6–8 hours	6–8 hours	6–8 hours
	Relaxation (yoga, meditation, or progressive muscle relaxation)	15 min		15 min		15 min		15 min
	Time management	Schedule activities, work, and study time for the week. Reduce time spent in activities that waste time	Reduce time spent in activities that waste time	Reduce time spent in activities that waste time	Reduce time spent in activities that waste time	Reduce time spent in activities that waste time	Plan a social activity. Reduce time spent in activities that waste time	Plan a social activity. Assess time management during the previous week. Reduce time spent in activities that waste time
Week 2	**Sleep**	6–8 hours	6–8 hours	6–8 hours	6–8 hours	6–8 hours	6–8 hours	6–8 hours
	Relaxation (yoga, meditation, or progressive muscle relaxation)	15–20 min	15–20 min		15–20 min		15–20 min	15–20 min
	Time management	Schedule activities, work, and study time for the week. Reduce time spent in activities that waste time	Reduce time spent in activities that waste time	Reduce time spent in activities that waste time	Reduce time spent in activities that waste time	Reduce time spent in activities that waste time	Plan a social activity. Reduce time spent in activities that waste time	Plan a social activity. Assess time management during the previous week. Reduce time spent in activities that waste time
Week 3	**Sleep**	6–8 hours	6–8 hours	6–8 hours	6–8 hours	6–8 hours	6–8 hours	6–8 hours
	Relaxation (yoga, meditation, or progressive muscle relaxation)	20–30 min	20–30 min	20–30 min	20–30 min	20–30 min	20–30 min	20–30 min
	Time management	Schedule activities, work, and study time for the week. Reduce time spent in activities that waste time	Reduce time spent in activities that waste time	Reduce time spent in activities that waste time	Reduce time spent in activities that waste time	Reduce time spent in activities that waste time	Plan a social activity. Reduce time spent in activities that waste time	Plan a social activity. Assess time management during the previous week. Reduce time spent in activities that waste time

SUMMARY

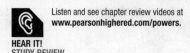

Listen and see chapter review videos at
www.pearsonhighered.com/powers.

HEAR IT!
STUDY REVIEW

1. Stress is defined as a physiological and mental response to things in our environment that we perceive as threatening. Any factor that produces stress is called a stressor.
2. Excessive stress or poorly managed stress can lead to headaches, digestive problems, heart disease, and mental health problems.
3. The autonomic nervous system consists of the para sympathetic and sympathetic branches and works with the endocrine system to produce the stress response. The combined physiological responses of these systems result in the fight-or-flight response, which prepares the body to fight or flee.
4. Personality factors, past experiences, and gender can affect the way we perceive situations and behave in response to stressors.
5. Common stressors include academic and financial responsibilities, managing interpersonal relationships, and everyday life hassles.
6. Two steps in managing stress are to reduce stressors in your life and to learn to cope with stress by improving your ability to relax.
7. Common relaxation techniques to reduce stress include rest and sleep, exercise, progressive relaxation, breathing exercises, meditation, and visualization. Developing spiritual wellness and a social network can also help you better manage stress. Avoiding unhealthy habits is key to maintaining manageable stress levels.

STUDY QUESTIONS

Find more review questions online at
www.pearsonhighered.com/powers.

REVIEW IT!
QUIZZES

1. Which of the following is a physical symptom of stress?
   a. muscle tension
   b. headaches
   c. anxiety
   d. all of the above
2. Positive stress that is associated with optimal performance is called _____.
   a. distress
   b. visualization
   c. eustress
   d. productive stress
3. Which of the following is not a hormone that is part of the stress response?
   a. dopamine   b. cortisol
   c. epinephrine   d. norepinephrine
4. Common stressors include _____.
   a. financial responsibilities
   b. interpersonal relationship problems
   c. academic pressures
   d. all of the above
5. Which of the following is not a healthy way to cope with stress?
   a. exercise
   b. alcohol
   c. meditation
   d. progressive muscle relaxation
6. Define *stress*. Define *stressor*, and name common stressors.
7. Why is stress management important to health?
8. List the steps in stress management. Identify some common stress management (relaxation) techniques.
9. Discuss the concept of eustress.
10. Explain potential ways exercise is useful in reducing stress.
11. List the key guidelines for the development of a time management program.

HELPFUL WEBLINKS

DO IT!
WEBLINKS

For links to the organizations and websites listed, visit **www.pearsonhighered.com/powers.**

American College Counseling Association
Offers information related to counseling and college students. www.collegecounseling.org

American College Health Association (ACHA)
Offers health-related information for college students. www.acha.org

American Psychological Association
Provides information on stress management and psychological disorders. www.apa.org

Mayo Clinic
Contains wide-ranging information about stress, diet, fitness, and mental health. www.mayoclinic.org

National Institute of Mental Health
Working to improve mental health through biomedical research on mind, brain, and behavior. www.nimh.nih.gov/index.shtml

WebMD: Stress Management Health Center
Contains information about stress management and stress and health. www.webmd.com/balance/stress-management/default.htm

Weil Lifestyle
Provides a wide range of wellness information. www.drweil.com

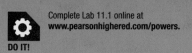
Name _____ Date _____

Stress Index Questionnaire

The purpose of this stress index questionnaire is to increase your awareness of stress in your life. Select either yes or no to answer each of the following questions.

Yes   No   1. I have frequent arguments.

Yes   No   2. I often get upset at work.

Yes   No   3. I often have neck and/or shoulder pains due to anxiety/stress.

Yes   No   4. I often get upset when I stand in long lines.

Yes   No   5. I often get angry when I listen to the local, national, or world news or read the newspaper.

Yes   No   6. I do not have enough money for my needs.

Yes   No   7. I often get upset when driving.

Yes   No   8. At the end of a workday I often feel stress-related fatigue.

Yes   No   9. I have at least one constant source of stress/anxiety in my life (e.g., conflict with boss, neighbor, mother-in-law).

Yes   No   10. I often have stress-related headaches.

Yes   No   11. I do not practice stress management techniques.

Yes   No   12. I rarely take time for myself.

Yes   No   13. I have difficulty in keeping my feelings of anger and hostility under control.

Yes   No   14. I have difficulty in managing time wisely.

Yes   No   15. I often have difficulty sleeping.

Yes   No   16. I am generally in a hurry.

Yes   No   17. I usually feel that there is not enough time in the day to accomplish what I need to do.

Yes   No   18. I often feel that I am being mistreated by friends or associates.

Yes   No   19. I do not regularly perform physical activity.

Yes   No   20. I rarely get 7 to 9 hours of sleep per night..

SCORING AND INTERPRETATION

Answering yes to any of the questions means that you need to use some form of stress management techniques (see the text for details). Total your yes answers, and use the following scale to evaluate the level of stress in your life.

Number of Yes Answers	Stress Category
6–20	High stress
3–5	Average stress
0–2	Low stress

1. Are you satisfied with your score? If not, name the areas you could target to reduce your level of stress.

    _____

    _____

    _____

2. If you named areas you want to target in the previous question or you are in the high-stress category, what techniques will you employ to help lower your stress level? Write out a specific plan for how you will attempt to use at least of one of the stress management strategies for a specific stressor that you face.

    _____

    _____

    _____

    _____

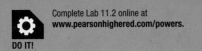
Name _____   Date _____

Keeping a Stress Diary

For this exercise, you will need seven copies of this worksheet. Keep a daily stress diary for one week. Indicate the time of day the stressor occurred, your perceived level of stress (10 is the worst stress you have ever felt), any symptoms you experienced, and your response to the symptoms. A response can include, for example, practicing a relaxation technique, getting angry, or doing nothing. At the end of 7 days, analyze your stress diary to determine the greatest sources of stress and the times that they occur. Once you have done this, you will be ready to practice effective stress management techniques.

Date: _____

Time	Level of Perceived Stress (0 to 10)	Cause of Stress	Symptoms of Stress	Your Response
7:00 A.M.				
8:00				
9:00				
10:00				
11:00				
12:00 P.M.				
1:00				
2:00				
3:00				
4:00				
5:00				
6:00				
7:00				
8:00				

1. What are the greatest sources of stress in your life, and when do they occur?

    _____

    _____

    _____

2. What are some specific steps you can take to eliminate or minimize these stressors?

    _____

    _____

    _____

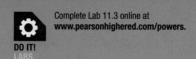
Name _____   Date _____

Managing Time and Establishing Priorities

Often people feel that there are not enough hours in the day. They feel that at some future point, such as "when I graduate," they will have more time to focus on priorities. Delaying things until the future results in lack of completion. Use the following time management tool to help you budget your time and organize your priorities.

STEP 1: ESTABLISH PRIORITIES

Rank each priority that applies to you in the list below. Use 1 for the highest priority, 2 for the second highest, and so on. You may add priorities as necessary.

Priority	Rank	Priority	Rank
More time with family		More time for exercise and physical activity	
More time with friends		More time to relax	
More time for work and professional pursuits		More time to study	
More time for leisure and recreation		More time for myself	
More time with boyfriend/girlfriend/spouse		Other: _____	

STEP 2: MONITOR YOUR CURRENT TIME USE

Pick one day of the week, and track what you do each hour of the day.

Time	Activity
5:00 A.M.	
6:00	
7:00	
8:00	
9:00	
10:00	
11:00	
12:00 P.M.	
1:00	
2:00	
3:00	
4:00	
5:00	
6:00	
7:00	
8:00	
9:00	
10:00	
11:00	
12:00 A.M.	

STEP 3: ANALYZE YOUR CURRENT TIME USE

1. In what activity can you spend less time? For example, did you watch TV for 3 hours? How much time did you spend texting or using social networking sties?

    _____

    _____

2. What can you do to spend less time in these activities? How can you replace those activities with ones on your prioritized list?

    _____

    _____

3. During which hours can you spend time doing activities that are important to you?

    _____

    _____

STEP 4: MAKE A SCHEDULE

Write in your planned activities for the next day, and try to stick closely to this schedule.

Time	Activity
5:00 A.M.	
6:00	
7:00	
8:00	
9:00	
10:00	
11:00	
12:00 P.M.	
1:00	
2:00	
3:00	
4:00	
5:00	
6:00	
7:00	
8:00	
9:00	
10:00	
11:00	
12:00 A.M.	

Were you able to modify your schedule to find time for your priorities? If not, state how you will modify your plan to accommodate your priority activities.

_____

_____

_____

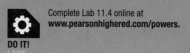
Name _____   Date _____

Assessing Your Personality Behavior Pattern

Select the position that you feel best reflects your typical behavior in the situations described. Behaviors exhibited by extreme Type A behavior pattern fall to the left, and those exhibited by extreme Type B behavior pattern fall to the right.

Extreme Type A Behavior Pattern	1	2	3	4	5	Extreme Type B Behavior Pattern
Fast at doing things	1	2	3	4	5	Slow at doing things (eating, talking, walking)
Unable to wait patiently	1	2	3	4	5	Able to wait patiently
Never late	1	2	3	4	5	Unconcerned about being on time
Very competitive	1	2	3	4	5	Not competitive
Poor listener (I finish other people's sentences for them)	1	2	3	4	5	Good listener
Always in a hurry	1	2	3	4	5	Never in a hurry
Always do two or more things at once	1	2	3	4	5	Take one thing at a time
Speak quickly and forcefully	1	2	3	4	5	Speak slowly and deliberately
Need recognition from others	1	2	3	4	5	Don't worry about what others think
Push myself (and others) hard	1	2	3	4	5	Easygoing
Don't express feelings	1	2	3	4	5	Good at expressing feelings
Few interests outside school or work	1	2	3	4	5	Many hobbies and interests
Very ambitious	1	2	3	4	5	Not ambitious
Eager to get things done	1	2	3	4	5	Deadlines don't bother me

INTERPRETATION

- If the majority of your responses are 1s, then you fall in the **Extreme Type A Behavior Pattern.** This personality behavior pattern is described as extremely competitive, highly committed to work, with an extreme sense of time urgency. Such individuals are extremely goal oriented, and can become hostile if someone gets between them and a goal they have established.

- If the majority of your responses are 2s with a few 1s, then you fall in the **Type A Behavior Pattern.** Type A behavior pattern is characterized by the traits listed for Extreme Type A behavior pattern, but they are moderated somewhat. People who exhibit this behavior pattern are ambitious, competitive, and goal oriented, with a sense of time urgency.

- If your responses are a mixture of the behavior patterns, you are described as a **Balanced Personality.** People with this type of personality get things done, but not at all costs. They can compete but do not feel they have to. They are more laid-back and inclined to give people the benefit of the doubt. They balance leisure time and work time.

- If the majority of your responses are 4s with some 5s, then you fall in the **Type B Behavior Pattern.** People with Type B behavior pattern are easygoing and lack a strong sense of time urgency. They don't like to compete and won't let deadlines interfere with vacation or leisure time. It is not that they are less ambitious than those with Type A behavior pattern; they are just more relaxed.

- If the majority of your responses are 5s, then you fall in the **Extreme Type B Behavior Pattern.** This personality behavior pattern is very relaxed, with no sense of time urgency. In fact, Extreme Type Bs typically don't wear a watch. They try to avoid competition at all costs and never mix leisure time and work time.

Remember: This inventory is only one aspect of your personality. If your responses indicate Type A tendencies, you may want to assess your lifestyle and address some of the more stressful areas.

Appendix A

Chapter 1

1. c. Physical activity is any type of occupational, leisure, or lifestyle-related physical movement. Exercise is one example of leisure physical activity.

2. a. Although exercise is not a component of wellness, it can help you achieve physical health, which is one of the components of total wellness.

3. c. Agility may be important for sport performance, but it is not linked to improved overall health and therefore is not considered a major component of health-related physical fitness.

4. d. Reduced risk for osteoporosis and heart disease, as well as improved mental health, are all benefits of regular physical activity.

5. e. *Healthy People 2020* is the current health goals for the nation. The objectives address a broad range of health behaviors and outcomes needed to improve the health of the nation. See www.healthypeople.gov for a comprehensive list of the *Healthy People 2020* objectives.

6. b. An individual in the action stage of change has been participating in a new health behavior for 6 months or less, but once this individual has moved beyond 6 months, she will be in the maintenance stage of change.

7. d. Developing a plan, getting the support of friends and family, and seeking outside help from others are all important actions to take in initiating a health behavior change.

8. d. Assessing your current behavior—including number and effort of behaviors you want to change, your motive for behavior change, and current behaviors patterns—is an important step to take when planning a change.

9. c. For goals to be successful, it is important that they be specific and that the outcome can be measured to determine whether the goal was reached. It is also important to have a plan of action for meeting the goal. Goals should be challenging but realistic. Setting a time frame to achieve the goal provides direction and helps you maintain focus.

Chapter 2

1. d. Supercompensation is not one of the five key principles of exercise training.

2. c. Current guidelines indicate that a minimum of 30 minutes of moderate exercise each day can produce numerous health benefits.

3. a. A few minutes of low-intensity exercise (a warm-up) at the beginning of an exercise training session benefits the body by increasing both muscle temperature and blood flow to active muscles.

Chapter 3

1. c. Aerobic exercises include activities that promote cardiorespiratory fitness, such as jogging, swimming, and cycling.

2. a. Activities that promote muscle strength and endurance, such as wrestling, utilize the anaerobic energy pathway to create ATP and provide energy to muscles.

3. b. As an individual's cardiorespiratory fitness level increases, resting heart rate will decrease because the heart becomes more efficient at pumping blood throughout the body. This allows the heart to beat fewer times per minute to pump the same amount of blood.

4. c. You should exercise at a level of at least 50% of your heart rate reserve in order to improve health-related physical fitness and cardiorespiratory endurance.

5. d. Increases in heart rate, cardiac output, and breathing are normal physical changes you will experience during cardiorespiratory exercise.

6. a. Arteries are the blood vessels that move oxygen-rich blood away from your heart. Veins return oxygen-depleted blood back to the heart.

Chapter 4

1. b. Eccentric contractions are an important aspect of the adaptation to training. The eccentric contraction phase is responsible for muscle damage with overload/overtraining (DOMS).

2. a. The slow-twitch fiber is recruited first during low-intensity activities. Slow fibers are also the most fatigue resistant.

3. b. Maximal strength is determined by the cross-sectional area of the muscle and number of motor units activated, as well as the biomechanical aspects of the muscle/joint in question.

4. a. Strength training is specific to the muscle being used during the training. Lower back pains are often

associated with weak and shortened back muscles. After strength training the back muscles, the incidence of lower back pain may be reduced.

5. d. Muscle overload (high resistance) is necessary to see strength gains. With high resistance, the number of repetitions due to the overload is limited. Therefore, high resistance lifting necessitates low repetitions.

Chapter 5

1. d. The shape of the bones and tight skin and tendons can all affect one's flexibility at a joint. Bone length is typically not a factor.

2. e. The two types of proprioceptors are Golgi organs and muscle spindles; they are found in tendons and muscles, respectively. Motor units are not a type of proprioceptor.

3. b. False. Most people, including athletes and nonathletes, would benefit from the improved flexibility that results from regular static stretching.

4. b. A few minutes of light exercise before stretching will minimize your risk of injury. Where and when you stretch is not likely to affect your risk. Stretching to the point of pain is more likely to result in injury than stretching to the point of mild discomfort.

5. d. An imbalance in muscle strength caused by weak hamstrings or abdominal muscles (or a combination of the two) can result in a forward curve (or hyperextension) of the lower back, resulting in back pain. Stretching and strengthening these muscles are important for avoiding LBP.

Chapter 6

1. b. Essential fat, necessary fat the body requires to maintain certain functions, should be at least 3% of total body weight in men and 12% in women.

2. True. Excess fat stored in the abdomen or waist increases the risk of heart disease and diabetes.

3. d. Anemia is not a health consequence of overweight or obesity.

4. d. Type I diabetes does not result from being underweight or from most eating disorders.

5. a. While air displacement, underwater weighing, and bioelectrical impendence analysis are reliable methods for assessing body composition, the waist-to-hip ratio is the technique used to determine disease risk associated with body fat distribution.

6. c. A BMI of 30 kg/m^2 or greater is considered obese. A healthy BMI is less than 25 for men and less than 27 for women.

7. b. A skinfold test is an easy measure to obtain and can provide good estimates when done properly.

8. a. True. Your BMI is a good estimate of your weight status; however, BMI does not give you a direct measure of percent fat. The method can over- or underestimate body fatness.

Chapter 7

1. c. Establishing goals is the first and most important step in establishing a successful personal fitness plan.

2. c. Most cardiorespiratory health benefits occur with 120–150 minutes per week of moderate-intensity aerobic exercise.

3. a. Exercise training to improve muscular strength should be performed 2–3 times per week.

4. b. Stretching should be performed at least 2 times per week.

5. d. Environmental health is an important aspect of wellness. Leading a lifestyle that respects the environment and reduces harm to it is critical in supporting health and wellness.

6. c. Establishing your goals is necessary before pursuing the other steps of the plan. You can't select the concepts related to your plan, plan behavior changes, or monitor your progress until you have established what goals you intend to pursue.

7. b. Understanding your health insurance coverage is important in knowing how best to manage your health in case of injury/sickness.

8. a. Use of a support network and finding friends who can help you with accountability are critically important in losing weight. A behavior change contract may be useful in establishing a support network.

9. d. Too rigid a schedule makes it much more difficult to stay on track with your plan. Being flexible with your scheduling can ease the implementation of your plan.

Chapter 8

1. b. Carbohydrates provide the main source of fuel for your brain and are the main source of energy during exercise.

2. c. Protein is used by the body to build muscle, skin, connective tissues, and other structural body tissues.

3. c. While water doesn't provide energy or build bone or protein, it is involved in numerous metabolic and other body processes, including blood formation.

4. d. A well-balanced diet consists of 58% carbohydrates, 30% fats, and 12% protein.

5. c. Antioxidants neutralize free radicals in the body, preventing them from causing damage to cells.

Chapter 9

1. b. Optimal body fat percentages for health and fitness in men range from 8% to 19%, and from 21% to 32% in women.

2. f. Leptin and ghrelin are hormones that play a role in appetite. Leptin depresses appetite, while ghrelin contributes to appetite.

3. d. Energy balance occurs when the amount of calories you consume is equal to the amount of calories you burn, and therefore your weight will not change. If you consume more calories than you burn, you will gain weight. If you consume fewer calories than you burn, you will lose weight.

4. c. Physical activity that uses large muscle groups, such as cardiovascular and strength training is best to achieve weight loss. While flexibility training, yoga, and Pilates can be part of a physical fitness program, cardiovascular training improves muscles' ability to burn fat as energy, resulting in weight loss.

5. d. Using the MyPlate plan is a healthy way to eat for nutrition and overall health. Drastic measures for weight loss such as anorexia, bulimia, or using diet pills can be harmful to your health; these practices constitute disordered eating.

Chapter 10

1. d. Smoking, hypertension, and high blood cholesterol are major risk factors for cardiovascular disease. Resting pulse rate is not a risk factor.

2. d. Normal blood pressure is 120/80 mm/Hg, so a blood pressure reading of 140/90 would be considered high blood pressure, or hypertension.

3. b. HDL is "good" cholesterol and LDL is "bad" cholesterol. When your LDL is high you are at increased risk for CHD, but if your HDL is high, your risk for developing CHD decreases.

4. c. Cardiovascular disease is the leading cause of death in the United States for all ages.

5. b. Obesity, hypertension, and stress can all be modified by healthy lifestyle changes; however, heredity—the genes you are born with—cannot be changed.

Chapter 11

1. d. There are a variety of physical symptoms associated with stress, including headaches, anxiety, and muscle tension.

2. c. Eustress is positive stress that motivates and energizes us. Distress is the type of stress that can have a negative impact on our mental and physical health.

3. a. Epinephrine, cortisol, and norepinephrine are hormones released into the bloodstream during the stress response. Dopamine does not play a role in the body's response to stress.

4. d. Everyday life situations can contribute to our stress levels. These situations can include financial responsibilities, interpersonal relationship problems, and academic pressures.

5. b. Alcohol is not an effective way to cope with stress. Using alcohol to cope may eventually increase your stress level by affecting your ability to sleep and be productive, and may even lead to alcohol abuse.

Appendix B
NUTRITIVE VALUE OF SELECTED FOODS AND FAST FOODS

The following table of nutrient values presents nutritional information about a wide array of foods, including many fast foods. Values are given for calories, protein, carbohydrates, fiber, fat, saturated fat, and cholesterol for common foods and serving sizes. Use this information to assess your diet and make improvements. This is only a selection of common foods. See the MyDietAnalysis database for an extensive list of foods. When using the software, the foods identified here can be quickly found by entering the MyDietAnalysis code in the search field.

Values are obtained from the USDA Nutrient Database for Standard Reference, Release 21.

A "0" displayed in any given field indicates that nutrient value is determined to be zero; a blank space indicates that nutrient information is not available.

Ener = energy (kilocalories); *Prot* = protein; *Carb* = carbohydrate; *Fiber* = dietary fiber; *Fat* = total fat; *Sat* = saturated fat; *Chol* = cholesterol.

Index:

MDA Code	Food Name	Amt	Wt (g)	Ener (kcal)	Prot (g)	Carb (g)	Fiber (g)	Fat (g)	Sat (g)	Chol (mg)
	BEVERAGES									
	Alcoholic									
22831	Beer	12 fl-oz	360	157	1	13		0	0	0
34067	Beer, dark	12 fl-oz	355.5	150	1	13		0	0	0
34053	Beer, light	12 fl-oz	352.9	105	1	5	0	0	0	0
22849	Beer, pale ale	12 fl-oz	360.2	179	2	17		0	0	0
22545	Daiquiri, frozen, from concentrate mix	1 ea	36	101	0	26	0	0	0	0
22514	Gin, 80 proof	1 fl-oz	27.8	64	0	0	0	0	0	0
22544	Liqueur, coffee, 63 proof	1 fl-oz	34.8	107	0	11	0	0	0	0
34085	Martini, prepared from recipe	1 fl-oz	28.2	69	0	1	0	0	0	0
22593	Rum, 80 proof	1 fl-oz	27.8	64	0	0	0	0	0	0
22515	Tequila, 80 proof	1 fl-oz	27.8	64	0	0	0	0	0	0
22594	Vodka, 80 proof	1 fl-oz	27.8	64	0	0	0	0	0	0
22670	Whiskey, 80 proof	1 fl-oz	27.8	64	0	0	0	0	0	0
22884	Wine, red	1 fl-oz	29	24	0	1		0	0	
22861	Wine, white	1 fl-oz	29.3	24	0	1		0	0	
	Coffee									
20012	Coffee, brewed w/tap water	1 cup	237	2	0	0	0	0	0	0
20686	Coffee, decaffeinated, brewed w/tap water	1 cup	236.8	0	0	0	0	0	0	0
20439	Coffee, espresso, restaurant prepared	1 cup	237	5	0	0	0	0	0.2	0
20023	Coffee, instant, prepared w/water	1 cup	238.4	5	0	1	0	0	0	0
21210	Coffee, instant, vanilla, sugar free, cafe style	1 Tbs	6	30	0	2	0	2	2	0
	Dairy Mixed Drinks and Mixes									
85	Chocolate milk, prepared w/syrup, whole milk	1 cup	282	254	9	36	1	8	4.7	25
46	Hot cocoa, sugar free, w/aspartame, prepared w/water	1 cup	256	74	3	14	2	1	0.4	0
21	Hot cocoa, prepared from recipe, w/milk	1 cup	250	192	9	27	2	6	3.6	20
48	Hot cocoa, prepared from dry mix	1 cup	274.7	151	3	32	1	2	0.9	0
166	Hot cocoa, w/marshmallows, dry packet	1 ea	28	112	1	21	1	4	4.2	0
29	Malted milk, natural, w/o add nutrients, prepared from powder w/milk	1 cup	265	233	10	27	0	10	5.4	32
41	Drink, strawberry, prepared from dry mix w/whole milk	1 cup	266	234	8	33	0	8	5.1	32
	Fruit and Vegetable Beverages and Juices									
20965	Apple cider, flavored, low calorie, w/vitamin C, prepared from instant	8 fl-oz	240	2	0	1	0	0	0	0
71080	Apple juice, unsweetened	1 ea	262	121	0	30	1	0	0.1	0
3015	Apricot nectar, canned	1 cup	251	141	1	36	2	0	0	0
72092	Blackberry juice, canned	0.5 cup	120	46	0	9	0	1	0	0
5226	Carrot juice, canned	1 cup	236	94	2	22	2	0	0.1	0
20042	Clam and tomato juice, canned	1 ea	166.1	80	1	18	1	0		0
3042	Cranberry juice cocktail, bottled	1 cup	252.8	137	0	34	0	0		0
20115	Cranberry juice cocktail, from frozen concentrate	1 cup	249.6	117	0	29	0	0	0	0
3275	Cranberry-grape juice	1 cup	244.8	137	0	34	0	0	0.1	0
20024	Fruit punch, w/added nutrients, canned	1 cup	248	117	0	30	0	0	0	0
20035	Fruit punch, from frozen concentrate	1 cup	247.2	114	0	29	0	0	0	0
20101	Grape drink, canned	1 cup	250.4	153	0	39	0	0	0	0
3052	Grapefruit juice, unsweetened, canned	1 cup	247	94	1	22	0	0	0	0
3053	Grapefruit juice, unsweetened, from frozen concentrate	1 cup	247	101	1	24	0	0	0	0
3068	Lemon juice, fresh	1 Tbs	15.2	4	0	1	0	0	0	0

MDA Code	Food Name	Amt	Wt (g)	Ener (kcal)	Prot (g)	Carb (g)	Fiber (g)	Fat (g)	Sat (g)	Chol (mg)
20045	Lemonade, prepared from powder	1 cup	266	69	0	18	0	0	0	0
20047	Lemonade, low-calorie, w/aspartame, prepared from powder	1 cup	236.8	7	0	2	0	0	0	0
20117	Lemonade, pink, from frozen concentrate	1 cup	247.2	99	0	26	0	0	0	0
3072	Lime juice, fresh	1 Tbs	15.4	4	0	1	0	0	0	0
20002	Limeade, from frozen concentrate	1 cup	247.2	129	0	34	0	0	0	0
20070	Orange drink, w/added vitamin C, canned	1 cup	248	122	0	31	0	0	0	0
20004	Orange breakfast drink, from powder	1 cup	248	122	0	31	0	0	0	0
71108	Orange juice, unsweetened, box	1 ea	263	124	2	29	1	0	0	0
3090	Orange juice, fresh	1 cup	248	112	2	26	0	0	0.1	0
3091	Orange juice, unsweetened, from frozen concentrate	1 cup	249	112	2	27	0	0	0	0
3170	Orange-grapefruit juice, unsweetened, canned	1 cup	247	106	1	25	0	0	0	0
3101	Peach nectar, canned	1 cup	249	134	1	35	1	0	0	0
20059	Pineapple-grapefruit juice, canned	1 cup	250.4	118	1	29	0	0	0	0
20025	Pineapple-orange juice, canned	1 cup	250.4	125	3	30	0	0	0	0
3120	Pineapple juice, unsweetened, canned	1 cup	250	132	1	32	1	0	0	0
3128	Prune juice, canned	1 cup	256	182	2	45	3	0	0	0
3985	Punch, fruit	1 cup	247.2	128	0	31	0	0	0	0
20106	Punch, fruit, prepared from frozen concentrate, w/water	8 fl-oz	234.4	98	0	24	0	0	0	0
14594	Punch, tropical, w/artificial sweetener, from dry packet	1 indv pkt	8	30	0	7	0	0	0	0
3140	Tangerine juice, sweetened, canned	1 cup	249	124	1	30	0	0	0	0
5397	Tomato juice, unsalted, canned	1 cup	243	41	2	10	1	0	0	0
20849	Vegetable-fruit juice, mixed	4 oz	113.4	33	0	8	0	0		0
20080	Vegetable juice, mixed, canned	1 cup	242	46	2	11	2	0	0	0
	Soft Drinks									
20006	Club soda	1 cup	236.8	0	0	0	0	0	0	0
20685	Low-calorie caffeine-free cola, w/aspartame	12 fl-oz	355.2	4	0	1	0	0	0	0
20843	Cola, w/higher caffeine	12 fl-oz	370	152	0	39	0	0	0	0
20028	Cream soda	1 cup	247.2	126	0	33	0	0	0	0
20008	Ginger ale	1 cup	244	83	0	21	0	0	0	0
20031	Grape soda	1 cup	248	107	0	28	0	0	0	0
20032	Lemon-lime soft drink	1 cup	245.6	98	0	25	0	0		0
20027	Pepper-type soft drink	1 cup	245.6	101	0	26	0	0	0.2	0
20009	Root beer	1 cup	246.4	101	0	26	0	0	0	0
	Teas									
20436	Iced tea, lemon flavor	1 cup	240	86	0	22	0	0	0	
20040	Instant tea powdered mix, lemon flavor, w/saccharin	1 cup	236.8	5	0	1	0	0	0	0
20014	Tea, brewed	1 cup	236.8	2	0	1	0	0	0	0
444	Tea, decaffeinated, brewed	1 cup	236.8	2	0	1	0	0	0	0
20118	Tea, herbal, chamomile, brewed	1 cup	236.8	2	0	0	0	0	0	0
20036	Tea, herbal (not chamomile), brewed	1 cup	236.8	2	0	0	0	0	0	0
	Other Drinks									
22606	Beer, nonalcoholic	12 fl-oz	352.9	73	1	14	0	0	0	0
17	Eggnog	1 cup	254	343	10	34	0	19	11.3	150
8889	Rice milk, enriched, original	8 fl-oz	248	120	1	25	0	2	0	0
20033	Soy milk	1 cup	245	132	8	15	1	4	0.5	0

MDA Code	Food Name	Amt	Wt (g)	Ener (kcal)	Prot (g)	Carb (g)	Fiber (g)	Fat (g)	Sat (g)	Chol (mg)
21070	Soy milk, plain, "lite"	1 cup	245	90	4	15	2	2	0	0
21064	Soy milk, vanilla	1 cup	245	190	11	25	5	5	0.5	0
20041	Water, tap, (municipal)	1 cup	236.6	0	0	0	0	0	0	0
	BREAKFAST CEREALS									
61211	Bran, w/malted flour	0.33 cup	29	83	4	23	8	1	0.1	0
40095	All-Bran/Kelloggs	0.5 cup	30	78	4	22	9	1	0.2	0
40295	Apple Cinnamon Cheerios/General Mills	0.75 cup	30	120	2	25	1	2	0	0
40098	Apple Jacks/Kelloggs	1 cup	30	117	1	27	0	0	0.1	0
40394	Basic 4/General Mills	1 cup	55	210	4	44	3	3	0.5	0
40259	Bran Flakes/Post	0.75 cup	30	96	3	24	5	1	0.1	0
40032	Capn' Crunch/Quaker Oats	0.75 cup	27	109	1	23	1	2	1.1	0
40297	Cheerios/General Mills	1 cup	30	110	3	22	3	2	0.3	0
40414	Cinnamon Grahams/General Mills	0.75 cup	30	113	2	26	1	1	0.2	0
60924	Chex, multi-bran/General Mills	0.75 cup	47	154	3	40	6	1	0.2	0
40126	Cinnamon Toast Crunch/General Mills	0.75 cup	30	130	2	24	1	3	0.4	0
40102	Cocoa Krispies/Kelloggs	0.75 cup	31	118	2	27	1	1	0.6	0
40425	Cocoa Puffs/General Mills	1 cup	30	120	1	26	2	2	0	0
40325	Corn Chex/General Mills	1 cup	30	110	2	26	1	1	0.1	0
40195	Corn Flakes/Kelloggs	1 cup	28	101	2	24	1	0	0.1	0
40089	Corn Grits, instant, plain, prepared/Quaker Oats	1 ea	137	93	2	21	1	0	0	0
40206	Corn Pops/Kelloggs	1 cup	31	117	1	28	0	0	0.1	0
40205	Cracklin' Oat Bran/Kelloggs	0.75 cup	55	221	4	39	7	8	3.4	0
40179	Rice cereal, hot, prepared with salt	1 cup	244	127	2	28	0	0	0	0
40182	Farina, hot, instant, prepared with salt	1 cup	241	149	4	32	1	1	0.1	0
40104	Crispix/Kelloggs	1 cup	29	109	2	25	0	0	0.1	0
40130	Fiber One/General Mills	0.5 cup	30	60	2	25	14	1	0.1	0
40218	Froot Loops/Kelloggs	1 cup	30	118	1	26	1	1	0.6	0
40217	Frosted Flakes/ Kelloggs	0.75 cup	31	114	1	28	1	0	0	0
11916	Frosted Mini Wheats, bite-size/Kelloggs	1 cup	55	189	6	45	6	1	0.2	0
40197	Granola, lowfat w/raisins/Kelloggs	0.66 cup	55	211	4	45	4	3	0.8	0
40265	Grape Nuts Flakes	0.75 cup	29	106	3	24	3	1	0.2	0
61155	Honey Bunches Of Oats	0.75 cup	30	118	2	25	1	1	0.1	0
40378	Honey Nut Clusters	1 cup	57	218	4	48	3	3	0	0
40010	Kix/General Mills	1.33 cup	30	110	2	25	3	1	0.2	0
40011	Life, plain/Quaker Oats	0.75 cup	32	119	3	25	2	1	0.3	0
40300	Lucky Charms/General Mills	1 cup	30	122	2	25	1	1	0.2	0
40186	Wheat cereal, hot, prepared w/salt	1 cup	249	189	6	39	2	1	0.2	0
40434	Oat Bran/Quaker Oats	1.25 cup	57	212	7	43	6	3	0.5	0
61223	Oat, corn & wheat squares, maple flavor, w/add sugar	1 cup	30	129	2	24	1	3	0.4	0
40358	Oatmeal Squares, cinnamon	1 cup	60	227	6	48	5	3	0.5	0
40430	Oatmeal Squares/Quaker Oats	1 cup	56	212	6	44	4	2	0.5	0
40073	Oatmeal, hot, apple-cinnamon, instant Quaker Oats	1 ea	149	130	3	26	3	1	0.2	0
40343	Peanut Butter Puffs (Reeses)/General MIlls	0.75 cup	30	130	2	23	1	4	0.5	0
40018	Puffed Rice/Quaker Oats	1 cup	14	54	1	12	0	0	0	0
40242	Puffed Wheat, fortified	1 cup	12	44	2	10	1	0	0	0
40209	Raisin Bran/Kelloggs	1 cup	61	196	5	47	7	1	0.2	0
40117	Raisin Squares, mini wheats	0.75 cup	55	188	5	44	5	1	0.2	0

MDA Code	Food Name	Amt	Wt (g)	Ener (kcal)	Prot (g)	Carb (g)	Fiber (g)	Fat (g)	Sat (g)	Chol (mg)
40333	Rice Chex/General Mills	1.25 cup	31	118	2	26	0	0	0.1	0
40210	Rice Krispies/Kelloggs	1.25 cup	33	128	2	28	0	0	0.1	0
60887	Shredded Wheat, no added sugar or salt, round biscuits	2 ea	37.8	127	4	30	5	1	0.2	0
40288	Shredded Wheat 'N Bran	1 cup	237	792	30	189	32	3	0.5	0
60879	Smart Start/Kelloggs	1 cup	50	182	4	43	3	1	0.1	0
40211	Special K/Kelloggs	1 cup	31	117	7	22	1	0	0.1	0
40413	Toasty Os/Malt-O-Meal	1 cup	30	121	4	22	3	2	0.4	0
40382	Total Raisin Bran/General Mills	1 cup	55	170	3	42	5	1	0.2	0
40021	Total Wheat/General Mills	0.75 cup	30	100	2	23	3	1	0.1	0
40306	Trix/General Mills	1 cup	30	120	1	26	1	2	0.2	0
40202	Wheat Bran Flakes, complete	0.75 cup	29	92	3	23	5	1	0.1	0
40335	Wheat Chex/General Mills	1 cup	30	108	3	24	3	1	0.1	0
61208	Wheat & malt barley flakes	0.75 cup	29	106	3	24	3	1	0.2	0
40307	Wheaties/General Mills	1 cup	30	110	3	24	3	1	0.1	0
	DAIRY									
7	Buttermilk, lowfat, cultured	1 cup	245	98	8	12	0	2	1.3	10
500	Cream, half & half	2 Tbs	30	39	1	1	0	3	2.1	11
218	Milk, 2% w/added vitamins A & D	1 cup	245	130	8	13	0	5	3	20
21109	Milk, chocolate, reduced fat w/added calcium	1 cup	250	195	7	30	2	5	2.9	20
19	Milk, chocolate, reduced fat	1 cup	250	158	8	26	1	2	1.5	8
11	Milk, condensed, sweetened	2 Tbs	38.2	123	3	21	0	3	2.1	13
134	Milk, evaporated, whole, w/added vitamin A	2 Tbs	31.5	42	2	3	0	2	1.4	9
68	Milk, nonfat/skim, w/added vitamin D, dry	0.5 cup	60	217	22	31	0	0	0.3	12
6	Milk, nonfat/skim, w/added vitamin A	1 cup	245	83	8	12	0	0	0.1	5
1	Milk, whole, 3.25%	1 cup	244	146	8	11	0	8	4.6	24
20	Milk, whole, chocolate	1 cup	250	208	8	26	2	8	5.3	30
2834	Yogurt, blueberry, fruit on the bottom	1 ea	227	220	9	41	1	2	1	10
2315	Yogurt, blueberry, lowfat	1 ea	113	110	3	23	0	1	0.5	10
72636	Yogurt, blueberry, nonfat	1 ea	227	120	7	21	0	0	0	5
72639	Yogurt, creamy vanilla, nonfat	1 ea	227	120	7	21	0	0	0	5
2001	Yogurt, fruit, lowfat	1 cup	245	250	11	47	0	3	1.7	10
15408	Yogurt, fruit, nonfat	1 cup	245	233	11	47	0	0	0.3	5
2450	Yogurt, lemon, nonfat	1 cup	227	130	8	24	0	0	0	5
	Cheese									
1287	American, nonfat, slice/Kraft	1 pce	21.3	32	5	2	0	0	0.1	3
47855	Blue, 1" cube	1 ea	17.3	61	4	0	0	5	3.2	13
47859	Brie, 1" cube	1 ea	17	57	4	0	0	5	3	17
48333	Cheddar, 1" cube, processed, pasterized, fat-free	1 ea	16	24	4	2	0	0	0.1	2
1440	Cheese, fondue	2 Tbs	26.9	62	4	1	0	4	2.3	12
48313	Cheese spread, cream cheese base	1 Tbs	15	44	1	1	0	4	2.7	14
13349	Cheese sauce, pasturized, processed/Kraft	2 Tbs	33	91	4	3	0	7	4.3	25
1014	Cottage cheese, 2% fat	0.5 cup	113	97	13	4	0	3	1.1	11
47867	Cottage cheese, fat-free, small curd, dry	0.5 cup	113	81	12	8	0	0	0.2	8
1015	Cream cheese	2 Tbs	29	99	2	1	0	10	5.6	32
1452	Cream cheese, fat-free	2 Tbs	29	30	5	2	0	0	0.2	3
1016	Feta, crumbled	0.25 cup	37.5	99	5	2	0	8	5.6	33
1054	Gouda	1 oz	28.4	101	7	1	0	8	5	32

MDA Code	Food Name	Amt	Wt (g)	Ener (kcal)	Prot (g)	Carb (g)	Fiber (g)	Fat (g)	Sat (g)	Chol (mg)
1442	Mexican, queso anejo, crumbled	0.25 cup	33	123	7	2	0	10	6.3	35
47885	Monterey jack, slice	1 ea	28.4	106	7	0	0	9	5.4	25
47887	Mozzarella, whole milk, slice	1 ea	34	102	8	1	0	8	4.5	27
1075	Parmesan, grated	1 Tbs	5	22	2	0	0	1	0.9	4
47900	Provolone, slice	1 ea	28.4	100	7	1	0	8	4.9	20
1064	Ricotta, whole milk	0.25 cup	62	108	7	2	0	8	5.1	32
	EGGS AND EGG SUBSTITUTES									
19510	Egg, hard boiled, large	1 ea	50	78	6	1	0	5	1.6	212
19517	Egg, poached, large	1 ea	50	71	6	0	0	5	1.5	211
19525	Egg substitute, liquid	0.25 cup	62.8	53	8	0	0	2	0.4	1
19506	Egg whites, raw, large	1 ea	33.4	16	4	0	0	0		0
19509	Egg, whole, large, fried	1 ea	46	90	6	0	0	7	2	210
19516	Egg, scrambled	1 ea	61	102	7	1	0	7	2.2	215
19508	Egg yolk, raw, large	1 ea	16.6	53	3	1	0	4	1.6	205
	FRUIT									
71079	Apples, fresh, chopped w/peel	1 cup	125	65	0	17	3	0	0	0
3004	Apples, fresh, peeled, slices	1 cup	110	53	0	14	1	0	0	0
3001	Apple, fresh, w/peel, medium, 3"	1 ea	182	95	0	25	4	0	0.1	0
3330	Applesauce, unsweetened, w/vitamin C, canned	1 cup	244	102	0	27	3	0	0	0
72101	Apricots, w/heavy syrup, canned, drained	1 cup	182	151	1	39	5	0	0	0
3657	Apricots, raw, sliced	1 cup	165	79	2	18	3	1	0	0
3210	Avocado, California, raw	1 ea	173	289	3	15	12	27	3.7	0
3024	Blackberries, fresh	1 cup	144	62	2	14	7	1	0	0
3032	Boysenberries, w/heavy syrup, canned	0.5 cup	128	113	1	29	3	0	0	0
3026	Boysenberries, fresh	0.5 cup	72	31	1	7	4	0	0	0
71082	Banana, fresh, extra small, 6" or shorter	1 ea	81	72	1	19	2	0	0.1	0
3642	Cantaloupe, fresh, wedge, 1/8 of a medium melon	1 pce	69	23	1	6	1	0	0	0
72094	Cherries, maraschino, canned, drained	1 ea	4	7	0	2	0	0	0	0
3336	Cherries, sweetened, canned, w/juice	0.5 cup	125	68	1	17	2	0	0	0
3045	Fruit cocktail, canned, w/heavy syrup	0.5 cup	124	91	0	23	1	0	0	0
3164	Fruit cocktail, canned, w/juice	0.5 cup	118.5	55	1	14	1	0	0	0
3414	Fruit salad, canned, w/heavy syrup	0.5 cup	127.5	93	0	24	1	0	0	0
44023	Fuit salad, canned, w/juice	0.5 cup	124.5	62	1	16	1	0	0	0
72093	Cranberries, dried, sweetened	0.25 cup	30.3	93	0	25	2	0	0	0
3673	Cranberries, fresh, chopped	0.5 cup	55	25	0	7	3	0	0	0
3192	Currants, zante, dried	0.25 cup	36	102	1	27	2	0	0	0
72111	Dates, medjool, w/o pit	1 ea	40	111	1	30	3	0		
3677	Figs, fresh, small, 1-½"	1 ea	40	30	0	8	1	0	0	0
71976	Grapefruit, fresh, medium	0.5 ea	154	60	1	16	6	0	0	0
3634	Guava, fresh	0.5 cup	82.5	56	2	12	4	1	0.2	0
3055	Grapes, Thompson seedless, fresh	0.5 cup	80	55	1	14	1	0	0	0
3342	Grapefruit, canned, w/juice, sections	0.5 cup	124.5	46	1	11	0	0	0	0
3644	Honeydew, fresh, 6"–7"	1 ea	1280	461	7	116	10	2	0.5	0
71979	Lemon, fresh, medium	1 ea	58	15	0	5	1	0	0	0
3071	Lime, fresh, peeled, 2"	1 ea	67	20	0	7	2	0	0	0
71743	Lychee (Litchi), dried, shelled	1 ea	2.5	7	0	2	0	0	0	0

MDA Code	Food Name	Amt	Wt (g)	Ener (kcal)	Prot (g)	Carb (g)	Fiber (g)	Fat (g)	Sat (g)	Chol (mg)
71990	Mandarin orange, fresh, medium	1 ea	109	50	1	15	3	0	0	0
71927	Mango, dried	0.33 cup	40	140	0	34	1	0	0	0
3221	Mango, fresh, whole	1 ea	207	135	1	35	4	1	0.1	0
3644	Melon, honeydew, fresh, 6"–7"	1 ea	1280	461	7	116	10	2	0.5	0
3085	Orange, all types, fresh, large, 3-1/16"	1 ea	184	86	2	22	4	0	0	0
71990	Orange, mandarin, fresh, medium	1 ea	109	50	1	15	3	0	0	0
3228	Orange, navel, fresh, 2-7/8"	1 ea	140	69	1	18	3	0	0	12
3098	Peaches, canned, w/heavy syrup	1 cup	262	194	1	52	3	0	0	0
3194	Persimmon, native, fresh	1 ea	25	32	0	8	0	0		0
3168	Mixed fruit, prunes apricots & pears, dried	1 ea	293	712	7	188	23	1	0.1	0
3216	Nectarines, fresh, slices	0.5 cup	71.5	31	1	8	1	0	0	0
3721	Papaya, fresh, small, 4 1/2" × 2 3/4"	1 ea	152	59	1	15	3	0	0.1	0
3726	Peaches, fresh, small, w/o skin, 2.5"	1 cup	130	51	1	12	2	0	0	0
3106	Pear, fresh, large	1 ea	209	121	1	32	6	0	0	0
72113	Pineapple, fresh, slice	1 pce	84	38	0	10		0		
3748	Plantain, cooked, mashed	1 cup	200	232	2	62	5	0	0.1	0
3121	Plum, fresh	1 ea	66	30	0	8	1	0	0	0
3197	Pomegranate, fresh	1 ea	154	128	3	29	6	2	0.2	0
3766	Raisins, seedless	50 ea	26	78	1	21	1	0	0	0
9758	Raisins, golden, seedless	0.25 cup	40	130	1	31	2	0	0	0
71987	Raspberries, fresh	1 cup	125	50	1	17	8	0	0	0
3354	Strawberries, frozen, sweetened, thawed, whole	0.5 cup	127.5	99	1	27	2	0	0	0
3135	Strawberries, fresh, slices	1 cup	166	53	1	13	3	0	0	0
3717	Tangerine, fresh, large	1 ea	98	52	1	13	2	0	0	0
3143	Watermelon, fresh, 1/16 melon	1 pce	286	86	2	22	1	0	0	0
	GRAIN AND FLOUR PRODUCTS									
	Breads, Rolls, Bread Crumbs, and Croutons									
62740	Bagel, blueberry	1 ea	85	190	7	40	5	2	0	0
71170	Bagel, cinnamon raisin, mini, 2-1/2"	1 ea	26	71	3	14	1	0	0.1	0
71167	Bagel, egg, mini, 2-1/2"	1 ea	26	72	3	14	1	1	0.1	6
71152	Bagel, sesame, mini, enriched, w/calcium propionate, 2-1/2"	1 ea	26	67	3	13	1	0	0.1	0
42039	Banana bread, homemade w/margarine, slice	1 pce	60	196	3	33	1	6	1.3	26
42433	Biscuit	1 ea	82	273	5	28	1	16	3.9	1
47709	Biscuit, buttermilk, refrigerated dough/Pillsbury	1 ea	64	150	4	29	1	2	0.3	0
71192	Biscuit, plain, lowfat, refrigerated dough	1 ea	21	63	2	12	0	1	0.3	0
42004	Bread crumbs, dry	1 Tbs	6.8	27	1	5	0	0	0.1	0
49144	Bread, garlic, Italian, crusty	1 pce	50	186	4	21		10	2.4	6
42090	Bread, egg, slice	1 pce	40	113	4	19	1	2	0.6	20
42069	Bread, oat bran, slice	1 pce	30	71	3	12	1	1	0.2	0
42076	Bread, oat bran, reduced calorie, slice	1 pce	23	46	2	9	3	1	0.1	0
42136	Bread, wheat bran, slice	1 pce	36	89	3	17	1	1	0.3	0
42095	Bread, whole wheat, reduced calorie, slice	1 pce	23	46	2	10	3	1	0.1	0

MDA Code	Food Name	Amt	Wt (g)	Ener (kcal)	Prot (g)	Carb (g)	Fiber (g)	Fat (g)	Sat (g)	Chol (mg)
71247	Bread, white, soft, w/o crust, thin slice	1 pce	9	24	1	5	0	0	0.1	0
42084	Bread, white, reduced calorie, slice	1 pce	23	48	2	10	2	1	0.1	0
71259	Breadsticks, plain, small, 4-1/4" Long	1 ea	5	21	1	3	0	0	0.1	0
26561	Buns, hamburger/Wonder	1 ea	43	117	3	22	1	2	0.4	
42021	Buns, hot dog/frankfurter	1 ea	43	120	4	21	1	2	0.5	0
71364	Buns, whole wheat, hot dog/frankfurter	1 ea	43	114	4	22	3	2	0.4	0
42115	Cornbread, prepared from dry mix	1 pce	60	188	4	29	1	6	1.6	37
42016	Croutons, plain, dry	0.25 cup	7.5	31	1	6	0	0	0.1	0
71227	Pita bread, white, enriched, small, 4"	1 ea	28	77	3	16	1	0	0	0
71228	Pita bread, whole wheat, small, 4"	1 ea	28	74	3	15	2	1	0.1	0
42159	Roll, dinner, egg, 2-1/2"	1 ea	35	107	3	18	1	2	0.6	18
42161	Roll, dinner, french	1 ea	38	105	3	19	1	2	0.4	0
71056	Roll, Kaiser	1 ea	57	167	6	30	1	2	0.3	0
42297	Tortilla, corn, unsalted, medium, 6"	1 ea	26	58	1	12	1	1	0.1	0
90645	Taco shells, baked, medium, 6"	1 ea	10	46	0	6	0	2	0.4	0
	Crackers									
71277	Cheese crackers, bite size	1 cup	62	312	6	36	1	16	5.8	8
71451	Goldfish cheese crackers, low sodium	55 pce	33	166	3	19	1	8	3.2	4
43532	Rye crispbread crackers	1 ea	10	37	1	8	2	0	0	0
71284	Melba toast crackers, plain, peices	1 cup	30	117	4	23	2	1	0.1	0
43507	Oyster crackers	1 cup	45	189	4	33	1	4	0.9	0
70963	Butter crackers, original/Kraft	5 ea	16	79	1	10	0	4	0.9	
43587	Saltine crackers, original/Kraft	5 ea	14	56	1	10	0	1	0	0
43664	Saltine crackers, fat free, low sodium	6 ea	30	118	3	25	1	0	0.1	0
43659	Oyster crackers, low sodium	1 cup	45	189	4	33	1	4	0.9	0
43545	Crackers w/cheese filling	4 ea	28	134	3	17	1	6	1.7	1
43501	Crackers, cheese, w/peanut butter filling	4 ea	28	139	3	16	1	7	1.2	0
43546	Crackers w/peanut butter filling	4 ea	28	138	3	16	1	7	1.4	
43581	Crackers, wheat, original/Kraft	16 ea	29	140	3	20	1	6	0.9	0
12683	Crackers, Wheat Thins/Kraft	5 ea	16	80	1	10	0	4	1	0
43508	Crackers, whole wheat	4 ea	32	142	3	22	3	6	1.1	0
	Muffins									
42723	English muffin, plain/Thomas'	1 ea	57	132	5	26		1	0.2	
42153	English muffin, wheat	1 ea	57	127	5	26	3	1	0.2	0
62916	Muffin, blueberry, mini, 1-1/4"	1 ea	11	43	1	5	0	2	0.4	4
44521	Muffin, corn, 2-1/4" × 2-1/2"	1 ea	57	174	3	29	2	5	0.8	15
44514	Muffin, oat bran, 2-1/4" × 2-1/2"	1 ea	57	154	4	28	3	4	0.6	0
44518	Toaster muffin, blueberry	1 ea	33	103	2	18	1	3	0.5	2
44522	Toaster muffin, cornmeal	1 ea	33	114	2	19	1	4	0.6	4
	Noodles and Pasta									
66103	Angel hair pasta, semolina, dry	2 oz	56	201	7	41	2	1	0.3	0
91313	Bow tie pasta, enriched, dry	1.5 cup	56	204	8	42	2	1	0.2	0

MDA Code	Food Name	Amt	Wt (g)	Ener (kcal)	Prot (g)	Carb (g)	Fiber (g)	Fat (g)	Sat (g)	Chol (mg)
38048	Chow mein noodles, dry	1 cup	45	237	4	26	2	14	2	0
38047	Egg pasta, enriched, cooked	0.5 cup	80	110	4	20	1	2	0.3	23
91316	Elbow pasta, enriched, dry	0.5 cup	56	204	8	42	2	1	0.2	0
38356	Fettuccine pasta, frozen/Kraft	70 g	70	200	8	38	2	2	0	0
91293	Fettuccine pasta, spinach, enriched, dry	1.33 cup	56	202	8	40	2	1	0.3	1
38102	Macaroni pasta, enriched, cooked	1 cup	140	221	8	43	3	1	0.2	0
66121	Pasta shells, low protein, wheat free, dry, small	2 oz	56.7	194	0	48	0	0	0	0
92830	Penne pasta, dry	2 oz	57	210	7	41	1	1		0
38067	Ramen noodles, cooked	0.5 cup	113.5	77	2	10	1	3	0.8	0
38551	Rice pasta, cooked	0.5 cup	88	96	1	22	1	0	0	0
38094	Soba noodles, cooked	1 cup	114	113	6	24		0	0	0
38118	Spaghetti, enriched, cooked	0.5 cup	70	111	4	22	1	1	0.1	0
38066	Spaghetti, spinach, cooked	1 cup	140	182	6	37	5	1	0.1	0
38060	Spaghetti, whole wheat, cooked	1 cup	140	174	7	37	6	1	0.1	0
	Grains									
38003	Barley, pearled, cooked	0.5 cup	78.5	97	2	22	3	0	0.1	0
38028	Bulgur, wheat, cooked	1 cup	182	151	6	34	8	0	0.1	0
38279	Cornmeal, yellow, dry	0.25 cup	41.5	151	4	31	3	2	0.3	0
38076	Couscous, cooked	0.5 cup	78.5	88	3	18	1	0	0	0
5470	Hominy, yellow, canned	0.5 cup	80	58	1	11	2	1	0.1	0
38078	Oat bran, cooked	0.5 cup	109.5	44	4	13	3	1	0.2	0
38080	Oats, whole grain, unprocessed	0.25 cup	39	152	7	26	4	3	0.5	0
38010	Rice, brown, long grain, cooked	1 cup	195	216	5	45	4	2	0.4	0
38082	Rice, brown, medium grain, cooked	0.5 cup	97.5	109	2	23	2	1	0.2	0
38256	Rice, white, enriched, long grain, cooked w/salt	1 cup	158	205	4	45	1	0	0.1	0
38019	Rice, white, enriched, long grain, instant, cooked	1 cup	165	193	4	41	1	1	0	0
38097	Rice, white, medium grain, cooked	0.5 cup	93	121	2	27	0	0	0.1	0
38034	Tapioca, pearl, dry	0.25 cup	38	136	0	34	0	0	0	0
38025	Wheat, germ, crude, raw	0.25 cup	28.8	104	7	15	4	3	0.5	0
	Pancakes, French Toast, and Waffles									
42155	French toast, frozen	1 pce	59	126	4	19	1	4	0.9	48
42156	French toast, homemade w/2% milk	1 pce	65	149	5	16		7	1.8	75
45192	Pancakes, buttermilk, frozen/Eggo	1 ea	42.5	99	3	16	0	3	0.6	5
45118	Pancakes, blueberry, homemade, 6"	1 ea	77	171	5	22	1	7	1.5	43
45117	Pancakes, plain, homemade, 6"	1 ea	77	175	5	22	1	7	1.6	45
45193	Waffles, homestyle, low fat, frozen/Eggo	1 ea	35	83	2	15	0	1	0.3	9
45003	Waffles, homemade, 7"	1 ea	75	218	6	25	1	11	2.1	52
	MEAT AND MEAT SUBSTITUTES									
	Beef									
10093	Beef, average of all cuts, cooked, 1/4" trim	3 oz	85.1	260	22	0	0	18	7.3	75
10705	Beef, average of all cuts, lean, cooked, 1/4" trim	3 oz	85.1	184	25	0	0	8	3.2	73
10108	Beef, brisket, whole, braised, 1/4" trim	3 oz	85.1	328	20	0	0	27	10.5	80

MDA Code	Food Name	Amt	Wt (g)	Ener (kcal)	Prot (g)	Carb (g)	Fiber (g)	Fat (g)	Sat (g)	Chol (mg)
10035	Beef, breakfast strips, cured, cooked	3 ea	34	153	11	0	0	12	4.9	40
58099	Beef, chuck tender steak, broiled, 0" trim	3 oz	85.1	136	22	0	0	5	1.6	54
10264	Beef, cured, thin sliced	5 pce	21	37	6	1	0	1	0.3	9
10624	Beef, short ribs, braised, choice	3 oz	85.1	401	18	0	0	36	15.1	80
10133	Beef, whole rib, roasted, 1/4" trim	3 oz	85.1	305	19	0	0	25	10	71
10008	Corned beef, cured, slices, canned	3 oz	85.1	213	23	0	0	13	5.3	73
58129	Ground beef, hamburger, pan browned, 25% fat	3 oz	85.1	236	22	0	0	15	6	76
58114	Ground beef, hamburger, pan browned, 10% fat	3 oz	85.1	196	24	0	0	10	4	76
58109	Ground beef, hamburger, pan browned, 5% fat	3 oz	85.1	164	25	0	0	6	2.9	76
10791	Porterhouse steak, broiled, 1/4" trim	3 oz	85.1	280	19	0	0	22	8.7	61
58257	Rib eye steak, broiled, 0" trim	3 oz	85.1	210	23	0	0	13	4.9	94
58094	Skirt steak, broiled, 0" trim	3 oz	85.1	187	22	0	0	10	4	51
58328	Strip steak, top loin, lean, broiled, choice, 1/8" trim	3 oz	85.1	171	25	0	0	7	2.7	67
10805	T-bone steak, broiled, 1/4" trim	3 oz	85.1	260	20	0	0	19	7.6	55
58299	Top round steak, lean, broiled, select, 1/8" trim	3 oz	85.1	151	27	0	0	4	1.4	52
58098	Tri-tip steak, loin, broiled, 0" trim	3 oz	85.1	226	26	0	0	13	4.9	58
11531	Veal, average of all cuts, cooked	3 oz	85.1	197	26	0	0	10	3.6	97
	Chicken									
81185	Chicken, breast, mesquite flavor, fat free, sliced	2 pce	42	34	7	1	0	0	0.1	15
81186	Chicken, breast, oven roasted, fat free, sliced	2 pce	42	33	7	1	0	0	0.1	15
15013	Chicken breast, w/skin, batter fried	3 oz	85.1	221	21	8	0	11	3	72
15057	Chicken breast, w/o skin, fried	3 oz	85.1	159	28	0	0	4	1.1	77
15113	Chicken, dark meat, w/skin, batter fried	3 oz	85.1	254	19	8		16	4.2	76
15080	Chicken, dark meat, w/skin, roasted	3 oz	85.1	215	22	0	0	13	3.7	77
15030	Chicken drumstick, w/skin, batter fried	3 oz	85.1	228	19	7	0	13	3.5	73
15042	Chicken drumstick, w/o skin, fried	3 oz	85.1	166	24	0	0	7	1.8	80
15111	Chicken, light meat, w/skin, batter fried	3 oz	85.1	236	20	8	0	13	3.5	71
15077	Chicken, light meat, w/skin, roasted	3 oz	85.1	189	25	0	0	9	2.6	71
15072	Chicken, whole, w/skin, batter fried	3 oz	85.1	246	19	8	0	15	3.9	74
15000	Chicken, whole, w/o skin, roasted	3 oz	85.1	162	25	0	0	6	1.7	76
15036	Chicken thigh, w/skin, batter fried	3 oz	85.1	236	18	8	0	14	3.8	79
15011	Chicken thigh, w/o skin, fried	3 oz	85.1	186	24	1	0	9	2.4	87
15034	Chicken wing, w/skin, batter fried	3 oz	85.1	276	17	9	0	19	5	67
15048	Chicken wing, w/o skin, fried	3 oz	85.1	180	26	0	0	8	2.1	71
15059	Chicken wing, w/o skin, roasted	3 oz	85.1	173	26	0	0	7	1.9	72
	Turkey									
51151	Turkey bacon, cooked	1 oz	28.4	108	8	1	0	8	2.4	28
51098	Turkey, thick slice, breaded & batter fried, 3" × 2" × 3/8"	1 ea	42	119	6	7	0	8	2	32
16308	Turkey, roast, light & dark meat, from frozen	1 cup	135	209	29	4	0	8	2.6	72
16110	Turkey breast, w/skin, roasted	3 oz	85.1	130	25	0	0	3	0.7	77
16038	Turkey breast, w/o skin, roasted	3 oz	85.1	115	26	0	0	1	0.2	71
16101	Turkey, dark meat, w/skin, roasted	3 oz	85.1	155	24	0	0	6	1.8	100
16099	Turkey, light meat, w/skin, roasted	3 oz	85.1	140	24	0	0	4	1.1	81
16003	Turkey, ground patty, 13% fat, raw	1 ea	113.4	193	22	0	0	11	2.8	84
	Lamb									
13604	Lamb, average of all cuts, cooked, choice, 1/4" trim	3 oz	85.1	250	21	0	0	18	7.5	83
13616	Lamb, average of all cuts, cooked, choice, lean 1/4" trim	3 oz	85.1	175	24	0	0	8	2.9	78

MDA Code	Food Name	Amt	Wt (g)	Ener (kcal)	Prot (g)	Carb (g)	Fiber (g)	Fat (g)	Sat (g)	Chol (mg)
13522	Lamb, kabob meat, lean, broiled, 1/4" trim	3 oz	85.1	158	24	0	0	6	2.2	77
13524	Lamb, ground, broiled, 20% Fat	3 oz	85	241	21	0	0	17	6.9	82
	Pork									
12000	Bacon, medium slice, cooked	3 pce	19	103	7	0	0	8	2.6	21
28143	Bacon, Canadian/Hormel	1 ea	56	68	9	1		3	1	27
12212	Ham, extra lean, 5% fat, roasted	1 cup	140	203	29	2	0	8	2.5	74
12211	Ham, 11% fat, roasted	1 cup	140	249	32	0	0	13	4.4	83
12309	Pork, loin & spareribs, average of retail cuts, cooked	3 oz	85.1	232	23	0	0	15	5.3	77
12097	Pork, backribs, roasted	3 oz	85.1	315	21	0	0	25	9.4	100
12099	Pork, ground, cooked	3 oz	85.1	253	22	0	0	18	6.6	80
	Lunch Meats									
13103	Beef, chopped, smoked, cured, 1oz slice	1 pce	28.4	38	6	1	0	1	0.5	13
13335	Beef, smoked, sliced, package/Carl Buddig	1 pce	71	99	14	0	0	5	1.8	48
13000	Beef, thin slice	1 oz	28.4	33	5	1	0	1	0.3	14
58275	Bologna, beef & pork, lowfat, 1" cube	1 ea	14	32	2	0	0	3	1	5
58280	Bologna, beef, lowfat, medium slice	1 ea	28	57	3	1	0	4	1.5	12
58212	Bologna, beef, reduced sodium, thin slice	1 pce	14	44	2	0	0	4	1.6	8
13176	Bologna, beef, light	1 pce	28	56	3	2	0	4	1.6	12
13152	Chicken, oven roasted, breast (white) meat, serving	1 oz	28	36	5	1	0	2	0.4	17
13306	Corned beef, chopped, cooked, serving, packaged/Carl Buddig	1 ea	71	101	14	1	0	5	2	46
13263	Ham, 11% fat	1 oz	28	46	5	1	0	2	0.8	16
13264	Ham, slices, regular, 11% fat	1 cup	135	220	22	5	2	12	4	77
13049	Olive loaf, w/pork, 4" × 4" × 3/32" slice	1 pce	28.4	67	3	3	0	5	1.7	11
13337	Pastrami, beef, smoked, chopped, package/Carl Buddig	1 oz	28.4	40	6	0	0	2	0.9	18
13101	Pastrami, beef, cured, 1 oz slice	1 oz	28.4	41	6	0	0	2	0.8	19
13020	Pastrami, turkey, slices	2 pce	56.7	75	9	1	0	4	1	39
11913	Pork & ham, canned/Spam	2 oz	56.7	176	8	2	0	15	5.6	40
13123	Bologna, turkey/Louis Rich	1 oz	28.4	52	3	1	0	4	1.1	19
16160	Turkey, breast, 3-1/2" slice	1 pce	21	22	4	1	0	0	0.1	9
58279	Turkey ham, extra lean, package	1 cup	138	171	27	4	0	5	1.5	92
13014	Turkey ham, thigh, cured	1 oz	28	35	5	1	0	1	0.4	20
	Sausage & Wursts									
58009	Bacon & beef stick	2 oz	56.7	293	16	0	0	25	9.1	58
58230	Beef sausage, cooked from fresh	2 oz	56.7	188	10	0	0	16	6.2	46
58228	Beef sausage, precooked	2 oz	56.7	230	9	0	0	21	8.6	47
13035	Beerwurst, salami, pork & beef	2 oz	56.7	157	8	2	1	13	4.8	35
13077	Blood sausage, 5" × 4-5/8" × 1/16" slice	1 pce	25	95	4	0	0	9	3.3	30
13079	Bratwurst, pork, cooked	1 ea	85	283	12	2	0	25	8.5	63
58012	Bratwurst, pork, beef & turkey, light, smoked	3 oz	85.1	158	12	1	0	12		48
13070	Chorizo, pork & beef sausage, 4" link	1 ea	60	273	14	1	0	23	8.6	53
13190	Frankfurter, beef, bun length/Kraft	1 ea	57	185	6	2	0	17	7.1	34
13191	Hot dog, beef/Kraft	1 ea	45	147	5	1	0	14	5.6	25
13129	Frankfurter, turkey & chicken/Kraft	1 ea	45	85	5	2	0	6	1.7	41
57877	Frankfurter, beef, 5" × 3/4"	1 ea	45	148	5	2	0	13	5.3	24
57966	Frankfurter, beef, 97% fat free	1 ea	49	45	6	3	0	2	1	15
13260	Frankfurter, chicken	1 ea	45	100	7	1	0	7	1.7	43
13012	Frankfurter, turkey	1 ea	45	100	6	2	0	8	1.8	35

MDA Code	Food Name	Amt	Wt (g)	Ener (kcal)	Prot (g)	Carb (g)	Fiber (g)	Fat (g)	Sat (g)	Chol (mg)
57890	Pork sausage, Italian, link, cooked, 1/4 lb (before cooking)	1 ea	83	286	16	4	0	23	7.9	47
13043	Kielbasa beef & pork sausage, link	1 pce	26	80	3	1	0	7	2.4	17
58020	Kielbasa turkey & beef sausage, smoked	3 oz	85.1	192	11	3	0	15	5.3	60
13044	Knockwurst beef & pork sausage, link	1 ea	68	209	8	2	0	19	6.9	41
13019	Liverwurst pork sausage, 2.5" × 1/4" slice	1 pce	18	59	3	0	0	5	1.9	28
13021	Pepperoni, beef & pork, slice	1 pce	5.5	27	1	0	0	2	0.8	6
13022	Polish sausage, pork, 10" × 1.25"	1 ea	227	740	32	4	0	65	23.4	159
58227	Pork sausage, precooked	3 oz	85	321	12	0	0	30	9.9	63
13184	Smokie sausage links/Oscar Mayer	1 ea	43	130	5	1	0	12	4	27
13200	Summer sausage, slice/Kraft	2 ea	46	140	7	0	0	12	4.9	39
13066	Sausage, liver, braunschweiger, slice, 2-1/2" × 1/4"	1 pce	18	59	3	1	0	5	1.7	32
13025	Salami, turkey, cooked, serving	1 oz	28.4	48	5	0	0	3	0.8	22
13267	Sausage, pork, cooked	2 oz	56	190	11	0	0	16	5.1	47
17345	Salami, beef cotto	1 slc	23	47	3	0	0	4	1.6	19
58007	Turkey sausage, breakfast link, mild	2 ea	56	129	9	1	0	10	2.1	90
	Meat Substitutes									
27044	Bacon bits, meatless	1 Tbs	7	33	2	2	1	2	0.3	0
7509	Bacon strips, meatless	3 ea	15	46	2	1	0	4	0.7	0
7561	Beef substitute, patty	1 ea	56	110	12	4	3	5	0.8	0
62359	Breakfast sausage patty, meatless, frozen/Morningstar Farms	1 ea	38	80	10	3	2	3	0.4	1
91055	Burger, vegetarian, frozen, Grillers Vegan/Morningstar Farms	1 ea	85	112	14	8	4	3	0.4	0
91489	Burger, vegan, original	1 ea	71	70	13	6	4	1		0
7547	Chicken, vegetarian	1 cup	168	376	40	6	6	21	3.1	0
7722	Garden Veggie Patties, vegetarian, frozen/Morningstar Farms	1 ea	67	118	12	9	3	4	0.5	1
7674	Harvest Burger, vegetarian, original, frozen/Gardetto's	1 ea	90	138	18	7	6	4	1	0
90626	Sausage, vegetarian, slices	1 ea	28	72	5	3	1	5	0.8	0
7726	Spicy Black Bean Burger, vegetarian, frozen/Morningstar Farms	1 ea	78	133	13	15	5	4	0.6	1
7549	Vegetarian fish sticks	1 ea	28	81	6	3	2	5	0.8	0
	NUTS AND SEEDS									
63195	Cashews, raw	2 oz	56.7	314	10	17	2	25	4.4	0
4519	Cashews, whole dry roasted, salted	0.25 cup	34.2	196	5	11	1	16	3.1	0
4645	Chinese chestnuts, dried	1 oz	28.4	103	2	23		1	0.1	0
63081	Flaxseeds, whole	0.25 cup	42	224	8	12	11	18	1.5	0
4728	Macadamias, whole, dry roasted, unsalted	1 cup	134	962	10	18	11	102	16	0
4592	Mixed nuts, dry roasted, salted	0.25 cup	34.2	203	6	9	3	18	2.4	0
4626	Peanut butter, chunky	2 Tbs	32	188	8	7	3	16	2.6	0
4756	Peanuts, dry roasted, unsalted	30 ea	30	176	7	6	2	15	2.1	0
4696	Peanuts, raw	0.25 cup	36.5	207	9	6	3	18	2.5	0
4540	Pistachios, dry roasted, salted	0.25 cup	32	182	7	9	3	15	1.8	0
4523	Sesame seeds, whole, dried	0.25 cup	36	206	6	8	4	18	2.5	0
4551	Sunflower seeds, kernels dry roasted, unsalted	0.25 cup	32	186	6	8	4	16	1.7	0
	SEAFOOD									
19041	Abalone, fried, mixed species	3 oz	85.1	161	17	9	0	6	1.4	80
17029	Bass, freshwater, mixed species, fillet, baked/broiled	3 oz	85.1	124	21	0	0	4	0.9	74
17104	Bass, striped, fillet, baked/broiled	3 oz	85.1	106	19	0	0	3	0.6	88
17088	Catfish, channel, fillet, breaded, fried	3 oz	85.1	195	15	7	1	11	2.8	69
19002	Clams, mixed species, canned, drained	3 oz	85.1	126	22	4	0	2	0.2	57

MDA Code	Food Name	Amt	Wt (g)	Ener (kcal)	Prot (g)	Carb (g)	Fiber (g)	Fat (g)	Sat (g)	Chol (mg)
71140	Clams, mixed species, raw	4 oz	113.4	84	14	3	0	1	0.1	39
17037	Cod, Atlantic, fillet, baked/broiled	3 oz	85.1	89	19	0	0	1	0.1	47
19036	Crab, Alaska king, leg, steamed	3 oz	85.1	83	16	0	0	1	0.1	45
19037	Crab, Alaska king, imitation	3 oz	85.1	81	6	13	0	0	0.1	17
17289	Eel, mixed species, fillet, w/o bone, baked/broiled, 1" cube	3 oz	85.1	201	20	0	0	13	2.6	137
17291	Halibut, Atlantic/Pacific, fillet, baked/broiled	3 oz	85.1	119	23	0	0	3	0.4	35
17049	Mackerel, Atlantic, fillet, baked/broiled	3 oz	85.1	223	20	0	0	15	3.6	64
17115	Mackerel, king, fillet, baked/broiled	3 oz	85.1	114	22	0	0	2	0.4	58
19044	Mussels, blue, steamed	3 oz	85.1	146	20	6	0	4	0.7	48
17093	Perch, ocean, Atlantic, fillet, baked/broiled	3 oz	85.1	103	20	0	0	2	0.3	46
19048	Octopus, steamed	3 oz	85.1	140	25	4	0	2	0.4	82
19089	Oysters, eastern, farmed, medium, raw	4 oz	113.4	67	6	6	0	2	0.5	28
17095	Pike, northern, fillet, baked/broiled	3 oz	85.1	96	21	0	0	1	0.1	43
17074	Rockfish, Pacific, mixed species, fillet, baked/broiled	3 oz	85.1	103	20	0	0	2	0.4	37
17121	Orange Roughy, orange fillet, baked/broiled	3 oz	85.1	89	19	0	0	1	0	68
17181	Salmon, Atlantic, farmed, fillet, baked/broiled	3 oz	85.1	175	19	0	0	11	2.1	54
17123	Salmon, Atlantic, fillet, baked/broiled, wild	3 oz	85.1	155	22	0	0	7	1.1	60
17099	Salmon, sockeye, fillet, baked/broiled	3 oz	85.1	184	23	0	0	9	1.6	74
17086	Sea bass, mixed species, fillet, baked/broiled	3 oz	85.1	106	20	0	0	2	0.6	45
17023	Sea trout, mixed species, fillet, baked/broiled	3 oz	85.1	113	18	0	0	4	1.1	90
17076	Shark, mixed species, Batter Fried	3 oz	85.1	194	16	5	0	12	2.7	50
17022	Snapper, mixed species, fillet, baked/broiled	3 oz	85.1	109	22	0	0	1	0.3	40
71707	Calamari, mixed species, fried	3 oz	85.1	149	15	7	0	6	1.6	221
71139	Sturgeon, mixed species, baked/broiled	3 oz	85.1	115	18	0	0	4	1	66
17066	Swordfish, fillet, baked/broiled	3 oz	85.1	132	22	0	0	4	1.2	43
17185	Trout, rainbow, farmed, fillet, baked/broiled	3 oz	85.1	144	21	0	0	6	1.8	58
17082	Trout, rainbow, wild, fillet, baked/broiled	3 oz	85.1	128	20	0	0	5	1.4	59
56007	Tuna salad spread	2 Tbs	25.6	48	4	2	0	2	0.4	3
17101	Tuna, bluefin, fillet, baked/broiled	3 oz	85.1	157	25	0	0	5	1.4	42
17151	Tuna, white, w/water, drained, canned	3 oz	85.1	109	20	0	0	3	0.7	36
17083	Tuna, white, w/oil, canned, drained	3 oz	85.1	158	23	0	0	7	1.1	26
17162	Whitefish, mixed species, fillet, baked/broiled	3 oz	85.1	146	21	0	0	6	1	66
17164	Yellowtail, mixed species, fillet, baked/broiled	3 oz	85.1	159	25	0	0	6		60
	VEGETABLES AND LEGUMES									
	Beans									
7038	Baked beans, plain/vegetarian, canned	1 cup	254	239	12	54	10	1	0.2	0
56101	Baked beans, w/frankfurters, canned	0.5 cup	129.5	184	9	20	9	9	3	8
5197	Bean sprouts, mung, mature, canned, drained	1 cup	125	15	2	3	1	0	0	0
7012	Black beans, mature, cooked	1 cup	172	227	15	41	15	1	0.2	0
92152	Chili beans, ranch style, bbq, cooked	1 cup	253	245	13	43	11	3	0.4	0
9574	Black eyed peas, immature, cooked w/salt, drained	1 cup	165	155	5	33	8	1	0.2	0
90018	Cowpeas, mature, cooked w/salt	1 cup	171	198	13	35	11	1	0.2	0
7913	Fava beans, immature, in pod	1 cup	126	111	10	22		1	0.1	0
7081	Hummus (garbanzo or chickpea spread), homemade	1 Tbs	15.4	27	1	3	1	1	0.2	0
7087	Kidney beans, all types, mature, canned	1 cup	256	215	13	37	14	2	0.3	0
7006	Lentils, mature, cooked	1 cup	198	230	18	40	16	1	0.1	0
7011	Lima beans, large, mature, canned	1 cup	241	190	12	36	12	1	0.1	0

MDA Code	Food Name	Amt	Wt (g)	Ener (kcal)	Prot (g)	Carb (g)	Fiber (g)	Fat (g)	Sat (g)	Chol (mg)
7022	Navy beans, mature, cooked	1 cup	182	255	15	47	19	1	0.2	0
7122	Navy beans, mature, canned	1 cup	262	296	20	54	13	1	0.3	0
7051	Pinto beans, mature, canned	1 cup	240	206	12	37	11	2	0.4	0
5854	Pinto beans, immature, cooked from frozen w/salt, drained	3 oz	85.1	138	8	26	7	0	0	0
5856	Snap beans, green, cooked w/salt, drained	1 cup	125	44	2	10	4	0	0.1	0
6748	Snap beans, green, fresh, 4" Long	10 ea	55	17	1	4	2	0	0	0
90026	Green peas, mature, split, cooked w/salt	0.5 cup	98	114	8	20	8	0	0.1	0
7053	White beans, mature, cooked	1 cup	179	249	17	45	11	1	0.2	0
7054	White beans, mature, canned	1 cup	262	299	19	56	13	1	0.2	0
	Vegetables									
9577	Artichoke, French, fresh, cooked w/salt, drained	1 ea	20	11	1	2	2	0	0	0
5723	Artichoke, globe, frozen	3 oz	85.1	32	2	7	3	0	0.1	0
6033	Arugula greens, fresh, chopped	1 cup	20	5	1	1	0	0	0	0
5841	Asparagus, cooked w/salt, drained	0.5 cup	90	20	2	4	2	0	0	0
6755	Beet slices, canned, drained	1 cup	170	53	2	12	3	0	0	0
5573	Beet slices, fresh	0.5 cup	68	29	1	7	2	0	0	0
5558	Broccoli, stalks, fresh	1 ea	114	32	3	6	3	0	0.1	0
6091	Broccoli, chopped, cooked w/salt, drained	0.5 cup	78	27	2	6	3	0	0.1	0
5870	Brussels sprouts, cooked w/salt, drained	0.5 cup	78	28	2	6	2	0	0.1	0
5036	Cabbage, fresh, shredded	1 cup	70	18	1	4	2	0	0	0
5042	Cabbage, red, fresh, shredded	0.5 cup	35	11	1	3	1	0	0	0
90605	Carrots, fresh, baby, large	1 ea	15	5	0	1	0	0	0	0
5281	Carrots, w/peas, in liquid, canned	0.5 cup	127.5	48	3	11	3	0	0.1	0
5887	Carrot slices, cooked w/salt, drained	0.5 cup	78	27	1	6	2	0	0	0
5199	Carrot slices, canned, drained	0.5 cup	73	18	0	4	1	0	0	0
5045	Carrots, fresh, whole, 7-1/2" long	1 ea	72	30	1	7	2	0	0	0
5049	Cauliflower, fresh	0.5 cup	50	12	1	3	1	0	0	0
5891	Cauliflower, cooked w/salt, drained, 1" pieces	0.5 cup	62	14	1	3	1	0	0	0
90436	Celery stalk, fresh, small, 5" long	1 ea	17	3	0	1	0	0	0	0
6093	Greens, collard, chopped, cooked w/salt, drained	1 cup	190	49	4	9	5	1	0.1	0
6801	Corn, sweet, yellow, fresh, small ear, 5.5"–6.5" long	1 ea	73	63	2	14	2	1	0.1	0
7202	Corn, sweet, white, fresh, kernels from small ear	1 ea	73	63	2	14	2	1	0.1	0
5900	Corn, sweet, yellow, cooked w/salt, drained	0.5 cup	82	89	3	21	2	1	0.2	0
5908	Eggplant, cubes, cooked w/salt, drained	1 cup	99	33	1	8	2	0	0	0
5450	Fennel, bulb, fresh, slices	0.5 cup	43.5	13	1	3	1	0		0
9182	Jicama, fresh, slices	1 cup	120	46	1	11	6	0	0	0
5915	Kale, chopped, cooked w/salt, drained	0.5 cup	65	18	1	4	1	0	0	0
90445	Lettuce, butterhead, small leaf	1 pce	5	1	0	0	0	0	0	0
5089	Lettuce, romaine, fresh, inner leaf	2 pce	20	3	0	1	0	0	0	0
9545	Lettuce, red leaf, fresh, shredded	1 cup	28	4	0	1	0	0		
5926	Mushrooms, shiitake, cooked w/salt, pieces	1 cup	145	78	2	20	3	0	0.1	0
51069	Mushrooms, crimini, fresh	2 ea	28	8	1	1	0	0	0	0
90457	Mushrooms, canned, drained, caps	8 ea	47	12	1	2	1	0	0	0
51067	Mushrooms, portabella, fresh	1 oz	28	7	1	1	0	0	0	0
5927	Mustard greens, chopped, cooked w/salt, drained	0.5 cup	70	10	2	1	1	0	0	0
6971	Okra, pod, cooked w/salt, drained, sliced	0.5 cup	80	18	1	4	2	0	0	0
6074	Onion, cooked w/salt, drained	0.5 cup	105	44	1	10	1	0	0	0

MDA Code	Food Name	Amt	Wt (g)	Ener (kcal)	Prot (g)	Carb (g)	Fiber (g)	Fat (g)	Sat (g)	Chol (mg)
9548	Onion, sweet, fresh	1 oz	28	9	0	2	0	0		0
9547	Onion, green, fresh, stalk-top only	1 Tbs	6	2	0	0	0	0	0	0
7270	Palm hearts, canned	0.5 cup	73	20	2	3	2	0	0.1	0
5938	Peas, green, cooked w/salt, drained	0.5 cup	80	67	4	13	4	0	0	0
5116	Peas, green, fresh	1 cup	145	117	8	21	7	1	0.1	0
9611	Peppers, green chili, canned	0.5 cup	69.5	15	1	3	1	0	0	0
7932	Peppers, jalapeno, fresh, sliced	1 cup	90	27	1	5	2	1	0.1	0
9632	Peppers, serrano chili, fresh, chopped	1 cup	105	34	2	7	3	0	0.1	0
90493	Peppers, bell, green, sweet, fresh, strips	10 pce	27	5	0	1	0	0	0	0
9549	Peppers, bell, green, sweet, sauteed	1 oz	28	36	0	1	1	3	0.4	0
6990	Peppers, bell, red, sweet, fresh, ring, 3" × 1/4" thick	1 ea	10	3	0	1	0	0	0	0
9551	Peppers, bell, red, sweet, sauteed	1 oz	28	37	0	2	1	4	0.4	0
90589	Pickles, sweet, spears	1 ea	20	18	0	4	0	0	0	0
9251	Potatoes, red, baked, w/skin, small	1 ea	138	123	3	27	2	0	0	0
9245	Potatoes, russet, baked, w/skin, small	1 ea	138	134	4	30	3	0	0	0
90564	Potatoes, peeled, cooked w/salt, large, 3" to 4-1/4"	1 ea	299.6	258	5	60	6	0	0.1	0
5950	Potatoes, skin, baked w/salt	1 ea	58	115	2	27	5	0	0	0
5964	Pumpkin, canned, salted	0.5 cup	122.5	42	1	10	4	0	0.2	0
90505	Radishes, fresh, red, small	10 ea	20	3	0	1	0	0	0	0
90508	Sauerkraut, canned, drained	0.5 cup	71	13	1	3	2	0	0	0
5260	Seaweed, spirulina, dried	0.5 cup	59.5	173	34	14	2	5	1.6	0
5972	Spinach, cooked w/salt, drained	0.5 cup	90	21	3	3	2	0	0	0
5149	Spinach, canned, drained	0.5 cup	107	25	3	4	3	1	0.1	0
5146	Spinach, fresh, chopped	1 cup	30	7	1	1	1	0	0	0
5984	Squash, butternut, baked w/salt, cubes	0.5 cup	102.5	41	1	11	3	0	0	0
5975	Squash, summer, all types, cooked w/salt, drained	0.5 cup	90	18	1	4	1	0	0.1	0
5981	Squash, winter, all types, baked w/salt, cubes	0.5 cup	102.5	40	1	9	3	1	0.1	0
90525	Squash, zucchini, fresh, w/skin, small	1 ea	118	19	1	4	1	0	0	0
6921	Squash, zucchini, w/skin, cooked w/salt, drained, mashed	0.5 cup	120	19	1	5	2	0	0	0
5989	Succotash, cooked w/salt, drained	0.5 cup	96	107	5	23	5	1	0.1	0
6924	Sweet potato, dark orange, baked in skin, w/salt	0.5 cup	100	92	2	21	3	0	0.1	0
5555	Sweet potato, dark orange, w/syrup, canned, drained	1 cup	196	212	3	50	6	1	0.1	0
5445	Tomatillo, fresh, medium	1 ea	34	11	0	2	1	0	0	0
5476	Tomato puree, canned	0.5 cup	125	48	2	11	2	0	0	0
5180	Tomato sauce, canned	0.5 cup	122.5	29	2	7	2	0	0	0
6887	Tomatoes, red, whole, w/juice, 6.7 oz can	1 ea	190	32	1	8	2	0	0	0
90532	Tomatoes, red, fresh, year round average, small, thin slice	1 pce	15	3	0	1	0	0	0	0
5447	Tomatoes, sun dried	10 pce	20	52	3	11	2	1	0.1	0
6002	Turnips, cooked w/salt, drained, mashed	0.5 cup	115	25	1	6	2	0	0	0
7955	Wasabi root, fresh	1 ea	169	184	8	40	13	1		0
5388	Water chestnuts, Chinese, whole w/liquid, canned	4 ea	28	14	0	3	1	0	0	0
5223	Watercress greens, fresh, sprig	10 ea	25	3	1	0	0	0	0	0
6010	Yams, tropical, baked w/salt, drained, cubes	0.5 cup	68	78	1	18	3	0	0	0
	Soy Products									
7503	Miso	1 Tbs	17.2	34	2	5	1	1	0.2	0
7564	Tempeh	0.5 cup	83	160	15	8		9	1.8	0
7015	Soybeans, mature, cooked	1 cup	172	298	29	17	10	15	2.2	0

MDA Code	Food Name	Amt	Wt (g)	Ener (kcal)	Prot (g)	Carb (g)	Fiber (g)	Fat (g)	Sat (g)	Chol (mg)
4707	Soybeans, mature, roasted, salted	0.25 cup	43	203	15	14	8	11	1.6	0
71584	Soy yogurt, peach/Silk	1 ea	170.1	160	4	32	1	2	0	0
7542	Tofu, firm, silken, 1" slice/Mori-Nu	3 oz	85.1	53	6	2	0	2	0.3	0
7799	Tofu, firm, silken, light, 1" slice/Mori-Nu	3 oz	85.1	31	5	1	0	1	0.1	0
7541	Tofu, soft, silken, 1" slice/Mori-Nu	3 oz	85.1	47	4	2	0	2	0.3	0
7546	Tofu yogurt	1 cup	262	246	9	42	1	5	0.7	0
	MEALS AND DISHES									
	Homemade									
57482	Coleslaw, homemade	0.5 cup	60	47	1	7	1	2	0.2	5
56102	Falafel, patty, homemade, 2-1/4"	1 ea	17	57	2	5		3	0.4	0
53125	Mole poblana, sauce, homemade	2 Tbs	30.3	50	1	4		3		0
56005	Potato salad, homemade	0.5 cup	125	179	3	14	2	10	1.8	85
5786	Potatoes au gratin, w/butter, homemade	1 cup	245	323	12	28	4	19	11.6	56
92216	Tortellini pasta, cheese filled	1 cup	108	332	15	51	2	8	3.9	45
	Packaged or Canned Meals or Dishes									
56634	Chimichanga, beef	1 ea	174	425	20	43		20	8.5	9
57705	Egg noodles, w/creamy alfredo sauce, dry mix/Lipton	1 ea	124	518	19	77		15	5.7	139
1753	Enchilada & tamale meal, beef	1 ea	311.9	450	10	56	9	20	8	30
90098	Beef ravioli, w/meat sauce, canned, serving/Chef Boyardee	1 ea	244	224	8	33	1	7	2.8	7
25279	Beefaroni, w/tomato sauce, canned, serving/Chef Boyardee	1 ea	212.6	196	7	29	1	6	2.5	6
82002	Burrito, mild, beef & bean	1 ea	142	294	9	43	5	10	3.5	7
70442	Chicken, orange glazed, low fat	1 serving	241	300	12	54	2	4	1	20
92265	Chicken & dumplings, canned	1 cup	247	230	11	24	2	10	4.5	35
57658	Chili con carne, w/beans, canned	1 cup	222	269	16	25	9	12	3.9	29
56001	Chili w/beans, canned	1 cup	256	287	15	30	11	14	6	44
57700	Chili w/o beans, canned/Hormel	1 cup	236	194	17	18	3	7	2.2	35
57701	Chili, turkey, w/beans, canned/Hormel	1 cup	247	203	19	26	6	3	0.7	35
57703	Chili, vegetarian, w/beans, canned/Hormel	1 cup	247	205	12	38	10	1	0.1	0
50317	Chili w/beans, canned/Chef-Mate	1 cup	253	420	18	34	8	24	10.1	40
90738	Cheeseburger macaroni pasta/Hamburger Helper	1.5 oz	42.5	168	5	27		4	1.2	4
57068	Macaroni & cheese, original, dry mix/Kraft	1 ea	70	259	11	48	1	3	1.3	10
57470	Meatloaf, w/gravy & mashed potatoes	1 ea	396.9	540	23	42	5	30	12	95
1751	Pasta, chicken alfredo	1 cup	194.4	270	11	28	3	12	7	40
83107	Pasta, chicken cacciatore	1.25 cup	295	330	23	44	3	6		40
57484	Potatoes, scalloped, from dry mix, w/milk & butter	1 ea	822	764	17	105	9	35	21.6	90
90103	Ravioli, beef, w/sauce, mini, canned, serving/Chef Boyardee	1 ea	252	232	8	31	3	8	3.5	8
47708	Spaghetti, w/meatballs canned/Chef Boyardee	1 ea	240	240	10	29	3	9	3.8	17
70959	Spinach au gratin, frozen	1 ea	155	222	7	11	2	17	7.6	42
70470	Stir fry, rice & vegetables	1 serving	226	350	7	45	3	16	4	15
42147	Stuffing, cornbread, from dry mix	0.5 cup	100	179	3	22	3	9	1.8	0
	Frozen Meals or Dishes									
11112	Beef macaroni, serving	1 ea	226.8	200	13	32	4	2	0.6	14
70893	Beef pot pie	1 ea	198	436	14	44	2	23	8.2	42
83051	Beef pot roast, w/potatoes & gravy/Stouffers	1 ea	255	184	13	21	3	5	1.4	20
70950	Beef w/gravy & vegetables, sliced	1 ea	255	207	15	26	4	5	1.3	31
11047	Beef, oriental, w/vegetables & rice	1 serving	255	189	13	28	4	3	1.1	23
57474	Beef stroganoff, w/noodles & vegetables/Marie Callender's	1 ea	368	420	25	40	7	18	7.2	63

MDA Code	Food Name	Amt	Wt (g)	Ener (kcal)	Prot (g)	Carb (g)	Fiber (g)	Fat (g)	Sat (g)	Chol (mg)
56915	Broccoli, w/cheese sauce/Gardettos	0.5 cup	84	56	2	7		2	0.4	
56738	Cabbage, stuffed, w/whipped potatoes/Lean Cuisine	1 ea	269	196	11	24	4	6	1.7	13
4104	Chicken & noodles, escalloped	1 ea	227	330	14	28	2	18	4	35
16195	Chicken & vegetables w/vermicelli/Lean Cuisine	1 ea	297	232	20	26	4	5	1.9	30
16262	Chicken, mesquite BBQ	1 ea	298	277	17	42	7	4	1.2	33
16198	Chicken enchilada w/rice & cheese sauce/Stouffer's	1 ea	283	424	15	61	4	13	7.4	51
83028	Chicken fajita kit, serving/Tyson	1 ea	107	128	7	17	2	4	0.9	12
1746	Chicken, thigh, fried, w/mashed potatoes & corn/Banquet	1 ea	228	388	22	30	4	20	4.4	68
70899	Chicken pot pie	1 ea	217	464	13	50	3	24	7.8	52
16266	Chicken teriaki/Healthy Choice	1 ea	312	250	16	36	9	5	1.6	22
70582	Chicken nuggets, w/macaroni & cheese	1 ea	257	457	19	51	7	20	5.6	57
70895	Egg, scrambled, & sausage, w/hash browns	1 ea	177	361	13	17	1	27	7.3	283
70917	Hot Pockets beef & cheddar pocket sandwich	1 ea	142	403	16	39		20	8.8	53
70918	Hot Pockets chicken broccoli cheddar pocket sandwich	1 ea	128	301	11	39	1	11	3.4	37
18119	Hot Pockets, chicken parmesan	1 ea	127	340	9	41	3	15	6	10
4096	Lasagna, w/Italian sausage	1 ea	308.4	410	18	41	4	19	9	50
56757	Lasagna w/meat sauce	1 ea	215	249	17	27	2	8	4.1	28
11029	Macaroni & beef, w/tomato sauce, serving/Lean Cuisine	1 ea	283	258	17	37	5	4	1.7	17
90491	Onion rings, cooked from frozen	1 cup	48	195	3	18	1	13	4.1	0
83156	Pasta, chicken, garlic, w/vegetables	1.67 cup	178	240	11	21	3	8	2	30
56762	Peppers, stuffed, w/beef & tomato sauce/Stouffers	0.5 ea	219.5	160	8	19	3	6	2.2	18
5587	Potatoes, mashed, granules w/milk, prepared w/water & margarine	0.5 cup	105	122	2	17	1	5	1.3	2
15972	Pot Pie, chicken	1 ea	283	733	20	64	4	44	17.8	62
70898	Pizza, pepperoni serving	1 ea	146	432	16	42	3	22	7.1	22
11034	Salisbury steak, w/potatoes & corn	1 ea	269	339	15	27	4	19	9.4	30
81146	Sausage w/biscuit sandwich/Jimmy Dean	1 ea	48	192	5	12	1	14	4.3	16
56703	Spaghetti w/meat sauce, serving/Lean Cuisine	1 ea	326	284	14	49	5	4	1.1	13
56760	Spaghetti, w/meatballs,12.6 oz	1 serving	357.2	360	19	45	6	12	3.5	35
6246	Spinach, creamed, w/real cream sauce	0.5 cup	124	100	3	7	1	7	3	35
11099	Swedish meatballs & pasta, serving/Lean Cuisine	1 ea	258	273	22	31	3	7	2.8	49
4128	Turkey beast, w/potatoes & vegetables	1 serving	453.6	460	22	51	5	19	6	65
70892	Turkey pot pie	1 ea	397	699	26	70	4	35	11.4	64
16306	Turkey w/gravy, 5 oz pkg	1 ea	141.8	95	8	7	0	4	1.2	26
6999	Vegetables, cooked, from frozen, w/salt, drained, 10 oz pkg	1 ea	275	165	8	36	12	0	0.1	0
	SNACK FOODS AND GRANOLA BARS									
3307	Banana chips	1 oz	28.4	147	1	17	2	10	8.2	0
10051	Beef jerky, large piece	1 ea	19.8	81	7	2	0	5	2.1	10
10052	Beef meat stick, smoked	1 ea	19.8	109	4	1		10	4.1	26
63331	Breakfast bar w/oats, raisins & coconut	1 ea	43	200	4	29	1	8	5.5	0
53227	Cereal bar, mixed berry/Kelloggs	1 ea	37	137	2	27	1	3	0.6	0
61251	Cheese puffs & twists, corn based, low fat	1 oz	28.4	123	2	21	3	3	0.6	0
44032	Chex snack mix, original	1 cup	42.5	180	4	32	2	4	0.6	
44034	Corn Nuts, BBQ	1 oz	28.4	124	3	20	2	4	0.7	0
44031	Corn Nuts, original	1 oz	28.4	127	2	20	2	4	0.7	0
11594	Fruit leather, bar	2 ea	28	104	0	24		1	0.3	
23404	Fruit leather, roll, large	1 ea	21	78	0	18	0	1	0.1	0

MDA Code	Food Name	Amt	Wt (g)	Ener (kcal)	Prot (g)	Carb (g)	Fiber (g)	Fat (g)	Sat (g)	Chol (mg)
23103	Granola bar, peanut butter, hard	1 ea	23.6	114	2	15	1	6	0.8	0
23059	Granola bar, plain, hard	1 ea	24.5	115	2	16	1	5	0.6	0
23101	Granola bar, chocolate chip, hard	1 ea	23.6	103	2	17	1	4	2.7	0
23096	Granola bar, chocolate chip, chocolate coated, soft	1 ea	35.4	165	2	23	1	9	5	2
23107	Granola bar, nut & raisin, soft	1 oz	28.4	129	2	18	2	6	2.7	0
72602	Nachos, cheese, serving	1 serving	57	120	4	5	0	9	4	10
44036	Oriental mix, rice based	1 oz	28.4	144	5	15	4	7	1.1	0
44012	Popcorn, air popped	1 cup	8	31	1	6	1	0	0	0
44014	Popcorn, caramel coated, w/o peanuts	1 oz	28.4	122	1	22	1	4	1	1
44038	Popcorn, cheese flavored	1 cup	11	58	1	6	1	4	0.7	1
44066	Popcorn, low fat, low sodium, microwaved	1 cup	8	34	1	6	1	1	0.1	0
44013	Popcorn, oil popped, microwaved	1 cup	11	64	1	5	1	5	0.8	0
61252	Popcorn, fat free, sugar syrup/caramel	1 cup	37.3	142	1	34	1	1	0.1	0
12080	Pork skins, plain	1 oz	28	153	17	0	0	9	3.2	27
44043	Potato chips, reduced fat	1 oz	28.4	134	2	19	2	6	1.2	0
44076	Potato chips, plain, unsalted	1 oz	28.4	152	2	15	1	10	3.1	0
5437	Potato chips, sour cream & onion	1 oz	28.4	151	2	15	1	10	2.5	2
61257	Potato chips, reduced fat, unsalted	1 oz	28.4	138	2	19	2	6	1.2	0
44015	Pretzels, hard	5 pce	30	113	3	24	1	1	0.1	0
44079	Pretzels, enriched, plain, hard, unsalted	10 ea	60	229	5	48	2	2	0.4	0
61182	Pretzels, soft, medium	1 ea	115	389	9	80	2	4	0.8	3
44021	Rice cake, brown rice, plain	1 ea	9	35	1	7	0	0	0.1	0
44020	Taro chips	1 oz	28.4	141	1	19	2	7	1.8	0
44058	Trail mix, regular	0.25 cup	37.5	173	5	17		11	2.1	0
44059	Trail mix, w/chocolate chips, salted nuts & seeds	0.25 cup	36.2	175	5	16		12	2.2	1
	SOUPS									
92160	Bean & ham, reduced sodium, canned, prepared w/water	0.5 cup	128	95	5	17	5	1	0.3	3
17776	Beef & barley	1 cup	242	140	9	18	2	4	1.5	15
92192	Beef mushroom, chunky, low sodium, canned	1 cup	251	173	11	24	1	6	4.1	15
50198	Beef mushroom, canned, prepared w/water	1 cup	244	73	6	6	0	3	1.5	7
57659	Beef stew, canned, serving	1 ea	232	220	11	16	3	12	5.2	37
50052	Chicken, chunky, ready to serve	1 cup	245	174	12	17	1	6	1.9	29
50077	Chicken gumbo, canned, prepared w/water	1 cup	244	56	3	8	2	1	0.3	5
50080	Chicken mushroom, canned, prepared w/water	1 cup	244	132	4	9	0	9	2.4	10
50081	Chicken noodle, chunky, canned, ready to serve	1 cup	240	89	8	10	1	2	1	12
50085	Chicken rice, chunky, canned, ready to serve	1 cup	240	127	12	13	1	3	1	12
50088	Chicken vegetable, chunky, canned, ready to serve	1 cup	240	166	12	19		5	1.4	17
40675	Cream of broccoli, microwave	1 serving	305	143	3	17	7	7	2	6
50049	Cream of mushroom, canned, prepared w/water	1 cup	244	102	2	8	0	7	1.6	0
50197	Cream of potato, canned, prepared w/water	1 cup	244	73	2	11	0	2	1.2	5
50050	Green pea, canned, prepared w/water	1 cup	250	152	8	25	5	3	1.3	0
50021	Clam chowder, Manhattan, canned, prepared w/water	1 cup	244	73	2	12	1	2	0.4	2
50009	Minestrone, canned, prepared w/water	1 cup	241	82	4	11	1	3	0.6	2
92163	Ramen noodle soup, any flavor, from dry packet	0.5 cup	38	172	4	25	1	6	2.9	0
28172	Ramen noodle soup, chicken flavor, from dry packet	1 serving	43	188	5	27	1	7	3.1	0
50025	Split pea & ham, canned, prepared w/water	1 cup	253	190	10	28	2	4	1.8	8
50028	Tomato, canned, prepared w/water	1 cup	244	85	2	16	1	1	0.2	0

MDA Code	Food Name	Amt	Wt (g)	Ener (kcal)	Prot (g)	Carb (g)	Fiber (g)	Fat (g)	Sat (g)	Chol (mg)
15774	Tomato & vegetable, from dry, prepared w/water	1 cup	245	54	2	10	1	1	0.4	0
50014	Vegetable beef, canned, prepared w/water	1 cup	244	76	5	10	2	2	0.8	5
92189	Vegetable chicken, low sodium	1 cup	241	166	12	21	1	5	1.4	17
7559	Vegetarian stew	1 cup	247	304	42	17	3	7	1.2	0
	DESSERTS, CANDIES, AND PASTRIES									
	Brownies and Fudge									
62904	Brownie, square, large, 2-3/4" × 7/8"	1 ea	56	227	3	36	1	9	2.4	10
47019	Brownie, homemade, 2" square	1 ea	24	112	1	12		7	1.8	18
23127	Fudge, chocolate marshmallow, w/nuts, homemade	1 pce	22	104	1	15	0	5	2.3	5
23025	Fudge, chocolate, homemade	1 pce	17	70	0	13	0	2	1.1	2
	Cakes, Pies, and Donuts									
46062	Cake, chocolate, homemade, w/o frosting, 9"	1 pce	95	352	5	51	2	14	5.2	55
12722	Cake, chocolate, w/cream, snack size	3 ea	85	280	3	54	0	6	2	75
46000	Cake, gingerbread, homemade, 8"	1 pce	74	263	3	36		12	3.1	24
46092	Coffee cake, w/cheese, 16 oz	1 pce	76	258	5	34	1	12	4.1	65
46003	Cake, white, w/coconut frosting, homemade, 9"	1 pce	112	399	5	71	1	12	4.4	1
46085	Cake, white, homemade, w/o frosting, 9"	1 pce	74	264	4	42	1	9	2.4	1
46091	Cake, yellow, homemade, w/o icing, 8"	1 pce	68	245	4	36	0	10	2.7	37
49001	Cheesecake, from dry mix, 9"	1 pce	99	271	5	35	2	13	6.6	29
46426	Cupcake, low fat, chocolate, w/frosting	1 ea	43	131	2	29	2	2	0.5	0
46011	Cupcake, snack, chocolate, w/frosting & cream filling	1 ea	50	200	2	30	2	8	2.4	0
71338	Doughnut, cake, chocolate, glazed, 3-3/4"	1 ea	60	250	3	34	1	12	3.1	34
71337	Doughnut, cake, w/chocolate icing, large, 3-1/2"	1 ea	57	258	3	29	1	14	7.7	11
45525	Doughnut, cake, glazed/sugared, medium, 3"	1 ea	45	192	2	23	1	10	2.7	14
71335	Doughnut holes	1 ea	14	59	1	6	0	3	1	1
45527	Doughnut, French cruller, glazed, 3"	1 ea	41	169	1	24	0	8	1.9	5
45563	Doughnut, creme filled, 3-1/2"oval	1 ea	85	307	5	26	1	21	4.6	20
48044	Pie filling, pumpkin, canned	0.5 cup	135	140	1	36	11	0	0.1	0
46001	Sponge cake, 1/12 of 16 oz	1 pce	38	110	2	23	0	1	0.3	39
	Candy									
51150	Candied fruit	1 oz	28.4	91	0	23	0	0	0	0
4148	Candy, Bit O Honey/Nestle	6 pce	40	150	1	32	0	3	2.2	0
23115	Candy, butterscotch	5 pce	30	117	0	27	0	1	0.6	3
23015	Candy, caramel	1 pce	10.1	39	0	8	0	1	0.3	1
92202	Candy, caramel, w/nuts, chocolate covered	1 ea	14	66	1	8	1	3	0.7	0
90671	Candy, jellybeans, large	10 ea	28.4	106	0	27	0	0		0
23480	Candy, milk chocolate, package, 1.69 oz	1 pkg	48	236	2	34	1	10	6.3	7
92212	Candy, milk chocolate covered coffee beans	1 oz	28.4	156	2	16	2	9	5.2	6
23022	Candy, milk chocolate covered raisins	1.5 oz	42.5	166	2	29	1	6	4.4	1
23047	Candy, milk chocolate w/peanuts	0.25 cup	42.5	219	4	26	2	11	4.3	3
23021	Candy, milk chocolate w/coated peanuts	10 ea	40	208	5	20	2	13	5.8	4
92201	Candy, nougat w/almonds	1 ea	14	56	0	13	0	0	0.2	0
23081	Candy, peanut brittle, homemade	1.5 oz	42.5	207	3	30	1	8	1.8	5
23152	Candy, Peppermint Patty/York 1-1/2 oz	1 ea	43	165	1	35	1	3	1.9	0
90698	Candy, Rolo, caramels in milk chocolate, 1.74 oz roll	1 ea	49.3	234	3	33	0	10	7.2	6
23142	Candy, sesame crunch	20 pce	35	181	4	18	3	12	1.6	0
23144	Candy, Starburst, original	8 ea	40	163	0	33	0	3	3.1	0
92198	Candy, strawberry, pkg, 8 oz	4 pce	45	158	1	36	0	1	0	0

MDA Code	Food Name	Amt	Wt (g)	Ener (kcal)	Prot (g)	Carb (g)	Fiber (g)	Fat (g)	Sat (g)	Chol (mg)
90682	Candy bar, milk chocolate w/almonds 1.55 oz	1 ea	43.9	231	4	23	3	15	7.8	8
91509	Candy, milk chocolate, w/almonds, bites/Hershey's Bites	17 pce	39	214	4	20	1	14	6.8	7
90681	Candy bar, milk chocolate, mini	1 ea	7	37	1	4	0	2	1.3	2
90685	Candy bar, milk chocolate, w/crisped rice, mini	1 ea	10	51	1	6	0	3	1.6	2
23145	Candy bar, sweet chocolate, 1.45 oz	1 ea	41.1	208	2	24	2	14	8.3	0
23405	Candy bar, Almond Joy, fun size, 7 oz	1 ea	19.8	95	1	12	1	5	3.5	1
23110	Candy bar, Baby Ruth, 2.1 oz	1 ea	60	275	3	39	1	13	7.3	0
23066	Candy bar, Butterfinger, 2.16 oz	1 ea	60	275	3	44	1	11	5.7	0
23116	Candy bar, Caramello, 1.6 oz	1 ea	45.4	210	3	29	1	10	5.8	12
23060	Candy bar, Kit Kat, 1.5 oz	1 ea	42.5	220	3	27	0	11	7.6	5
23061	Candy bar, Krackle, 1.45 oz	1 ea	42.5	218	3	27	1	11	6.8	5
23037	Candy bar, Mars, almonds, 1.76 oz	1 ea	50	234	4	31	1	12	3.6	8
90688	Candy bar, Milky Way, 2.05 oz	1 ea	58	262	2	41	1	10	7	5
23062	Candy bar, Mr. Goodbar, 1.75 oz	1 ea	49.6	267	5	27	2	16	7	5
23135	Candy bar, Oh Henry!, 2 oz	1 ea	56.7	262	4	37	1	13	5.4	4
23036	Candy bar, Skor, toffee, 1.4 oz	1 ea	39.7	212	1	25	1	13	7.5	21
23057	Candy bar, Special Dark, sweet chocolate, 1.45 oz	1 ea	41.1	229	2	25	3	13		2
23076	Candy bar, 3 Musketeers, fun size	2 ea	28	120	1	22	0	4	2.4	1
23149	Candy bar, Twix, caramel cookie, 2.06 oz pkg	1 ea	56.7	285	3	37	1	14	10.8	4
90712	Chewing gum, Chiclets	10 pce	16	40	0	11	0	0	0	0
	Cookies									
47026	Animal crackers	10 ea	12.5	56	1	9	0	2	0.4	0
90636	Chocolate chip cookie, enriched, higher fat, large, 3.5" to 4"	1 ea	40	190	2	26	1	9	4	0
47037	Chocolate chip cookie, homemade w/butter, 2-1/4"	2 ea	32	156	2	19		9	4.5	22
47032	Chocolate chip cookie, lower fat	3 ea	30	136	2	22	1	5	1.1	0
47001	Chocolate chip cookie, soft	2 ea	30	136	1	20	1	6	3	
45787	Chocolate peanut butter wafer, Nutty Bar	1 ea	57	312	5	31		19	3.6	
47006	Chocolate sandwich cookie, crème filled	3 ea	30	141	2	21	1	6	1.9	0
71272	Graham crackers, cinnamon, small rectangular peices	4 ea	14	59	1	11	0	1	0.2	0
47380	Graham crackers, chocolate, individual package	1 ea	31	144	2	22		5	1	
47526	Coconut macaroon cookie, home style	1 ea	22	101	1	13	1	5	4.4	0
62905	Fig bar, 2 oz pkg	1 ea	56.7	197	2	40	3	4	0.6	0
47043	Fortune cookie	3 ea	24	91	1	20	0	1	0.2	0
90638	Gingersnap, large, 3-1/2" to 4"	1 ea	32	133	2	25	1	3	0.8	0
90639	Molasses, cookie, large, 3-1/2" to 4"	1 ea	32	138	2	24	0	4	1	0
90640	Oatmeal cookie, big, 3-1/2" to 4"	1 ea	25	112	2	17	1	5	1.1	0
47003	Oatmeal raisin cookie, homemade, 2-5/8"	1 ea	15	65	1	10		2	0.5	5
47010	Peanut butter cookie, homemade, 3"	1 ea	20	95	2	12		5	0.9	6
47056	Peanut butter cookie, soft type	1 ea	15	69	1	9	0	4	0.9	0
47059	Peanut butter sandwich cookie	2 ea	28	134	2	18	1	6	1.4	0
47007	Shortbread cookie, plain, 1-5/8" square	4 ea	32	161	2	21	1	8	2	6
47559	Sugar cookie, home style/Archway	1 ea	24	99	1	17	0	3	0.7	4
62907	Sugar cookie, from refrigerated dough, pre-sliced	1 ea	23	111	1	15	0	5	1.4	7
90642	Sugar wafer cookie, crème filled, small	1 ea	3.5	18	0	2	0	1	0.1	0
90643	Vanilla sandwich cookie, crème filled, oval	2 ea	30	145	1	22	0	6	0.9	0
49065	Vanilla wafer cookie, golden, artificial flavor	1 ea	31	147	2	22		6	1.1	

MDA Code	Food Name	Amt	Wt (g)	Ener (kcal)	Prot (g)	Carb (g)	Fiber (g)	Fat (g)	Sat (g)	Chol (mg)
Custards, Gelatin, and Puddings										
2622	Custard, egg, from dry mix, w/2% milk	0.5 cup	133	148	5	23	0	4	1.8	64
57896	Custard, flan, dry mix, serving	1 ea	21	73	0	19	0	0	0	0
14734	Gelatin, strawberry, sugar free, from dry, serving	1 ea	2.9	10	2	1		0	0	
57894	Pudding, chocolate, ready to eat, 4 oz can	1 ea	113.4	161	2	26	0	5	1.4	1
2612	Pudding, vanilla, ready to eat, 4 oz can	1 ea	113.4	147	2	26	0	4	1.2	1
2651	Pudding, rice, ready to eat, 4 oz can	1 ea	141.8	167	5	28	1	4	2.5	26
57902	Pudding, tapioca, ready to eat, 3.5 oz can	1 ea	113.4	147	2	25	0	4	1.1	1
57989	Pudding, banana, snack cup	1 serving	98.9	130	1	21	0	5	2	0
57995	Pudding, vanilla, fat free, snack cup	1 ea	113.4	80	1	18	0	0	0	0
Ice Cream and Frozen Desserts										
71819	Frozen yogurt, chocolate, nonfat, w/artificial sweetener	1 cup	186	199	8	37	2	1	0.9	7
72124	Frozen yogurt, all flavors not chocolate	1 cup	174	221	5	38	0	6	4	23
70640	Ice cream bar, vanilla & dark chocolate	1 ea	85	300	4	23	1	21	13	70
49111	Ice cream cone, wafer/cake type, large	1 ea	29	121	2	23	1	2	0.4	0
49014	Ice cream cone, sugar, rolled type	1 ea	10	40	1	8	0	0	0.1	0
2010	Ice cream, vanilla, light, soft serve	0.5 cup	88	111	4	19	0	2	1.4	11
90723	Popsicle, 2 fl-oz bar	1 ea	59	47	0	11	0	0	0	0
Pastries										
45788	Apple turnover, frozen/Pepperidge Farm	1 ea	89	284	4	31	2	16	4	
42264	Cinnamon rolls, w/icing, refrigerated dough/Pillsbury	1 ea	44	145	2	23	0	5	1.5	0
45675	Éclair shell, homemade, 5"×; 2" × 1-3/4"	1 ea	48	174	4	11	0	12	2.7	94
71299	Croissant, butter, large	1 ea	67	272	5	31	2	14	7.8	45
71301	Croissant, cheese, large	1 ea	67	277	6	31	2	14	7.1	38
45572	Danish, cheese	1 ea	71	266	6	26	1	16	4.8	11
71330	Danish, cinnamon nut, 15 oz ring	1 pce	53.2	229	4	24	1	13	3.1	24
70913	Pie crust, Nilla, ready to use/Nabisco	1 ea	28	144	1	18	0	8	1.4	3
49015	Strudel, apple	1 pce	71	195	2	29	2	8	1.5	4
42164	Sweet roll, cheese	1 ea	66	238	5	29	1	12	4	50
71348	Sweet roll, honey bun, enriched, 5" × 13-1/2"	1 ea	85	339	5	43	2	16	4.6	26
42166	Sweet roll, cinnamon, frosted, from refrigerated dough	1 ea	30	109	2	17		4	1	0
71367	Sweet roll, cinnamon raisin, large	1 ea	83	309	5	42	2	14	2.6	55
45683	Toaster pastry, brown sugar & cinnamon	1 ea	50	206	3	34	0	7	1.8	0
45593	Toaster pastry, Pop Tarts, apple cinnamon	1 ea	52	205	2	37	1	5	0.9	0
45768	Toaster pastry, Pop Tarts, chocolate fudge, frosted, lowfat	1 ea	52	190	3	40	1	3	0.5	0
45601	Toaster pastry, Pop Tarts, chocolate fudge, frosted	1 ea	52	201	3	37	1	5	1	0
Toppings and Frostings										
23000	Apple butter	1 Tbs	18	31	0	8	0	0	0	0
23070	Caramel topping	2 Tbs	41	103	1	27	0	0	0	0
23014	Chocolate fudge topping, hot	2 Tbs	38	133	2	24	1	3	1.5	0
46039	Cream cheese frosting, creamy	1 oz	28.4	118	0	19	0	5	1.3	0
54334	Hazelnut spread, chocolate flavored	1 oz	28	151	2	17	2	8	8	0
23164	Strawberry topping	2 Tbs	42.5	108	0	28	0	0	0	0
510	Whipped cream topping, pressurized	2 Tbs	7.5	19	0	1	0	2	1	6
514	Dessert topping, pressurized	2 Tbs	8.8	23	0	1	0	2	1.7	0
508	Dessert topping, semi-solid, frozen	2 Tbs	9.4	30	0	2	0	2	2	0
54387	Whipped topping, low fat, frozen	2 Tbs	9.4	21	0	2	0	1	1.1	0

MDA Code	Food Name	Amt	Wt (g)	Ener (kcal)	Prot (g)	Carb (g)	Fiber (g)	Fat (g)	Sat (g)	Chol (mg)
	FATS AND OILS									
44469	Butter, light, salted	1 Tbs	13	66	0	0	0	7	4.5	14
44470	Butter, light, unsalted	1 Tbs	13	65	0	0	0	7	4.5	14
44952	Butter, organic, salted	1 Tbs	14	100	0	0	0	11	7	30
90210	Butter, unsalted, stick	1 Tbs	14	100	0	0	0	11	7.2	30
90209	Butter, salted, whipped, stick	1 Tbs	9.4	67	0	0	0	8	4.7	21
8003	Fat, bacon grease	1 tsp	4.3	39	0	0	0	4	1.7	4
8005	Fat, chicken	1 Tbs	12.8	115	0	0	0	13	3.8	11
8107	Fat, Lard	1 Tbs	12.8	115	0	0	0	13	5	12
8135	Margarine & butter, blend, w/soybean oil	1 Tbs	14.2	101	0	0	0	11	2	2
44476	Margarine, 80% fat, tub	1 Tbs	14.2	101	0	0	0	11	2	0
8067	Oil, fish, cod liver	1 Tbs	13.6	123	0	0	0	14	3.1	78
8084	Oil, canola	1 Tbs	14	124	0	0	0	14	1	0
8008	Oil, olive, salad/cooking	1 Tbs	13.5	119	0	0	0	14	1.9	0
8111	Oil, safflower, salad/cooking, more than 70% Oleic	1 Tbs	13.6	120	0	0	0	14	0.8	0
8027	Oil, sesame, salad/cooking	1 Tbs	13.6	120	0	0	0	14	1.9	0
44483	Shortening, vegetable, household	1 Tbs	12.8	113	0	0	0	13	3.2	0
8007	Shortening, household, hydrogenated soybean & cottonseed oil	1 Tbs	12.8	113	0	0	0	13	3.2	0
	CONDIMENTS, SAUCES, AND SYRUPS									
9713	Barbecue sauce, hickory smoked flavor	2 Tbs								
4936	Barbecue sauce, original flavor	2 Tbs	40	50	1	11	0	0	0	0
27001	Catsup, packet	1 ea	6	6	0	2	0	0	0	0
53523	Cheese sauce, ready to serve	0.25 cup	63	110	4	4	0	8	3.8	18
13095	Chicken spread, canned	1 oz	28.4	45	5	1	0	5	0.9	16
27019	Cranberry orange relish, canned	0.25 cup	68.8	122	0	32	0	0	0	0
54388	Cream substitute, light, powder	1 Tbs	5.9	25	0	4	0	1	0.2	0
9054	Enchilada sauce	0.25 cup	61	20	0	3	0	1	0	0
53474	Fish sauce	2 Tbs	36	13	2	1	0	0	0	0
53036	Gravy, brown, from dry mix	1 Tbs	6	22	1	4	0	1	0.2	0
53472	Hoisin sauce	2 Tbs	32	70	1	14	1	1	0.2	1
9533	Hollandaise sauce, w/butter fat, from dehydrated w/water, packet	1 ea	204	188	4	11	1	16	9.1	41
27004	Horseradish	1 tsp	5	2	0	1	0	0	0	0
92174	Hot sauce, chili, from immature green peppers	1 Tbs	15	3	0	1	0	0	0	0
92173	Hot sauce, chili, from mature red peppers	1 Tbs	15	3	0	1	0	0	0	0
23003	Jelly	1 Tbs	19	51	0	13	0	0	0	0
25002	Maple syrup	1 Tbs	20	52	0	13	0	0	0	0
23005	Marmalade, orange	1 Tbs	20	49	0	13	0	0	0	0
44697	Mayonnaise, light	1 Tbs	15	49	0	1	0	5	0.8	5
8145	Mayonnaise, w/safflower & soy oil	1 Tbs	13.8	99	0	0	0	11	1.2	8
8502	Miracle Whip, light/Kraft	1 Tbs	16	37	0	2	0	3	0.5	4
435	Mustard, yellow	1 tsp	5	3	0	0	0	0	0	0
27011	Olives, black, small, canned	1 ea	3.2	4	0	0	0	0	0	0
53473	Oyster sauce	2 Tbs	8	4	0	1	0	0	0	0
23042	Pancake syrup	1 Tbs	20	47	0	12	0	0	0	0
23172	Pancake syrup, reduced calorie	1 Tbs	15	25	0	7	0	0	0	0
53524	Pasta sauce, spaghetti/marinara, ready to serve	0.5 cup	125	109	2	17	3	3	0.9	2
53344	Pasta sauce, traditional	0.5 cup	130	81	2	13	3	3	1	0

MDA Code	Food Name	Amt	Wt (g)	Ener (kcal)	Prot (g)	Carb (g)	Fiber (g)	Fat (g)	Sat (g)	Chol (mg)
53470	Pepper/hot sauce	1 tsp	4.7	1	0	0	0	0	0	0
93303	Pickles, bread & butter, slices	1 ea	7.5	7	0	2	0	0	0	0
53461	Plum sauce	2 Tbs	38.1	70	0	16	0	0	0.1	0
92229	Preserves	1 Tbs	20	56	0	14	0	0	0	0
27019	Relish, cranberry orange, canned	0.25 cup	68.8	122	0	32	0	0	0	0
90594	Relish, sweet pickle, packet	1 ea	10	13	0	4	0	0	0	0
90280	Salsa, ready to serve, packet	1 ea	8.9	2	0	1	0	0	0	0
92614	Salsa, chipotle, chunky	2 Tbs	32	8	0	2	1	0	0	0
91457	Salsa, green chili & tomato, chunky	2 Tbs	31	7	0	3	0	0	0	0
91458	Salsa, picante, chunky	2 Tbs	31	7	0	1	0	0	0	0
26014	Salt, table	0.25 tsp	1.5	0	0	0	0	0	0	0
504	Sour cream, cultured	2 Tbs	28.8	56	1	1	0	6	3.3	15
54383	Sour cream, fat free	1 oz	28	21	1	4	0	0	0	3
54381	Sour cream, light	1 oz	28	38	1	2	0	3	1.8	10
515	Sour cream, cultured, reduced fat	2 Tbs	30	40	1	1	0	4	2.2	12
516	Sour dressing, non butterfat, cultured, filled cream type	1 Tbs	14.7	26	0	1	0	2	2	1
53063	Soy sauce, tamari	1 Tbs	18	11	2	1	0	0	0	0
90035	Soy sauce, low sodium, from wheat & soy	1 Tbs	18	10	1	2	0	0	0	0
53264	Sweet & sour sauce	1 Tbs	33	56	0	14	0	0	0	0
14867	Taco sauce, green	2 Tbs	16	4	0	1	0	0	0	0
14869	Taco sauce, red	1 Tbs	16	8	0	2	0	0	0	0
4655	Tahini sauce, from roasted & toasted kernels	1 Tbs	15	89	3	3	1	8	1.1	0
53004	Teriyaki sauce	1 Tbs	18	16	1	3	0	0		0
53468	White sauce, medium, homemade	1 cup	250	368	10	23	1	27	7.1	18
53099	Worcestershire sauce	1 Tbs	17	13	0	3	0	0	0	0
	Salad Dressing									
44497	Thousand island, fat free	1 Tbs	16	21	0	5	1	0	0	1
8024	Thousand island	1 Tbs	15.6	58	0	2	0	5	0.8	4
8013	Blue cheese	2 Tbs	30.6	146	0	1	0	16	2.5	9
92511	Caesar	2 Tbs	30	150	1	1	0	16	3	5
44467	French, fat free	1 Tbs	16	21	0	5	0	0	0	0
8255	French, reduced fat, unsalted	1 Tbs	16.3	38	0	5	0	2	0.2	0
90232	French, packet	1 ea	12.3	56	0	2	0	6	0.7	0
92510	Italian	2 Tbs	30	140	0	2	0	15	2.5	0
44498	Italian, fat free	1 Tbs	14	7	0	1	0	0	0	0
44720	Italian, reduced calorie	1 Tbs	14	28	0	1	0	3	0.4	0
44499	Ranch, fat free	1 oz	28.4	34	0	8	0	1		2
44696	Ranch, reduced fat	1 Tbs	15	29	0	3	0	2	0.2	2
8022	Russian	1 Tbs	15.3	54	0	5	0	4	0.4	0
8144	Sesame seed	2 Tbs	30.6	136	1	3	0	14	1.9	0
8035	Vinegar & oil, homemade	2 Tbs	31.2	140	0	1	0	16	2.8	0
	FAST FOOD									
	Generic Fast Food									
6178	Baked potato w/cheese sauce & bacon	1 ea	299	451	18	44		26	10.1	30
6177	Baked potato w/cheese sauce	1 ea	296	474	15	47		29	10.6	18
6181	Baked potato w/sour cream & chives	1 ea	302	393	7	50		22	10	24
66025	Burrito, bean	1 ea	108.5	224	7	36		7	3.4	2

MDA Code	Food Name	Amt	Wt (g)	Ener (kcal)	Prot (g)	Carb (g)	Fiber (g)	Fat (g)	Sat (g)	Chol (mg)
56629	Burrito, bean & cheese	1 ea	93	189	8	27		6	3.4	14
66023	Burrito, beef, bean & cheese	1 ea	101.5	165	7	20		7	3.6	62
66024	Burrito, beef	1 ea	110	262	13	29		10	5.2	32
56600	Breakfast biscuit w/egg sandwich	1 ea	136	373	12	32	1	22	4.7	245
56601	Breakfast biscuit w/egg & bacon sandwich	1 ea	150	458	17	29	1	31	8	352
56602	Breakfast biscuit w/egg & ham sandwich	1 ea	192	442	20	31	1	27	5.9	300
66028	Breakfast biscuit w/egg & sausage sandwich	1 ea	180	562	20	38	0	37	11.6	290
66029	Breakfast biscuit w/egg, cheese & bacon sandwich	1 ea	144	433	17	35	0	25	8.1	239
56604	Biscuit w/ham sandwich	1 ea	113	386	13	44	1	18	11.4	25
66030	Biscuit w/sausage sandwich	1 ea	124	460	12	37	0	30	9.2	35
66013	Cheeseburger, double patty, w/condiments & vegetables	1 ea	166	417	21	35		21	8.7	60
66016	Cheeseburger, double patty, plain	1 ea	155	477	27	32	1	27	11	85
56651	Cheeseburger, w/bacon & condiments, large	1 ea	195	550	31	37	3	31	11.9	98
56649	Cheeseburger, w/condiments & vegetables, large	1 ea	219	451	25	37	3	23	8.5	74
15063	Chicken drumstick & thigh, dark meat, breaded & fried	3 oz	85.1	248	17	9		15	4.1	95
15064	Chicken breast & wing, white meat, breaded & fried	3 oz	85.1	258	19	10		15	4.1	77
56656	Chicken fillet sandwich w/cheese	1 ea	228	632	29	42		39	12.4	78
56000	Chicken fillet sandwich, plain	1 ea	182	515	24	39		29	8.5	60
50312	Chili con carne	1 cup	253	256	25	22		8	3.4	134
56635	Chimichanga, beef & cheese	1 ea	183	443	20	39		23	11.2	51
19110	Clams, breaded & fried	3 oz	85.1	334	9	29		20	4.9	65
5461	Coleslaw	0.75 cup	99	147	1	13		11	1.6	5
6175	Corn cob w/butter	1 ea	146	155	4	32		3	1.6	6
56668	Corn dog	1 ea	175	460	17	56		19	5.2	79
56606	Croissant sandwich w/egg & cheese	1 ea	127	368	13	24		25	14.1	216
56607	Croissant sandwich w/egg, cheese & bacon	1 ea	129	413	16	24		28	15.4	215
56608	Croissant sandwich w/egg, cheese & ham	1 ea	152	474	19	24		34	17.5	213
45588	Cheese Danish, cheese	1 ea	91	353	6	29		25	5.1	20
45513	Danish, fruit	1 ea	94	335	5	45		16	3.3	19
66021	Enchilada, cheese	1 ea	163	319	10	29		19	10.6	44
66022	Enchilada, beef & cheese	1 ea	192	323	12	30		18	9	40
66020	Enchirito, beef, bean & cheese	1 ea	193	344	18	34		16	7.9	50
42064	English muffin w/butter	1 ea	63	189	5	30	2	6	2.4	13
66031	English muffin sandwich w/cheese & sausage	1 ea	115	389	15	29	1	24	9.4	49
66032	English muffin sandwich w/egg, cheese & Canadian bacon	1 ea	146	323	20	31	1	13	5.4	245
66010	Fish sandwich, w/tartar sauce	1 ea	158	431	17	41		23	5.2	55
66011	Fish sandwich w/tartar sauce & cheese	1 ea	183	523	21	48		29	8.1	68
90736	French fries, fried in vegetable oil, medium size	1 ea	134	427	5	50	5	23	5.3	0
90498	French fries, w/salt, from frozen, 9 oz pkg	1 pkg	198	265	5	55	6	10	2	0
42354	French toast sticks	5 pce	141	479	8	58	2	25	5.6	0
42353	French toast w/butter	2 pce	135	356	10	36		19	7.7	116
56638	Frijoles (refried beans) w/cheese	0.5 cup	83.5	113	6	14		4	2	18
42368	Garlic bread, from frozen, 2"	1 pce	50	170	5	21	1	8	2	6
56664	Ham & cheese sandwich	1 ea	146	352	21	33		15	6.4	58
56665	Ham, egg & cheese sandwich	1 ea	143	347	19	31		16	7.4	246
69150	Hamburger w/condiments, large	1 ea	171.5	439	27	38	2	20	8.2	69
56662	Hamburger, double patty, w/condiments & vegetables, large	1 ea	226	540	34	40		27	10.5	122

MDA Code	Food Name	Amt	Wt (g)	Ener (kcal)	Prot (g)	Carb (g)	Fiber (g)	Fat (g)	Sat (g)	Chol (mg)
56661	Hamburger w/condiments & vegetables, large	1 ea	218	512	26	40		27	10.4	87
56659	Hamburger w/condiments & vegetables, medium	1 ea	110	279	13	27		13	4.1	26
66007	Hamburger, plain	1 ea	90	266	13	30	1	10	3.2	30
5463	Hash browns	0.5 cup	72	235	2	23	2	16	3.6	0
56667	Hot dog w/chili & bun	1 ea	114	296	14	31		13	4.9	51
66004	Hot dog, plain,w/bun	1 ea	98	242	10	18		15	5.1	44
2032	Hot fudge sundae	1 ea	158	284	6	48	0	9	5	21
56666	Hush puppies	5 pce	78	257	5	35		12	2.7	135
6185	Mashed potatoes	0.5 cup	121	100	3	20		1	0.6	2
90214	Mayonnaise, w/soybean oil, packet	1 ea	10	72	0	0	0	8	1.2	4
71129	Milk shake, chocolate, small, 12 fl-oz	1 ea	249.6	317	8	51	5	9	5.8	32
71132	Milk shake, vanilla, small, 12 fl-oz	1 ea	249.6	369	8	49	2	16	9.9	57
56639	Nachos, w/cheese	7 pce	113	346	9	36		19	7.8	18
56641	Nachos w/cheese, beans, beef & peppers	7 pce	225	502	17	49		27	11	18
6176	Onion rings, serving	8 pce	78.1	259	3	29		15	6.5	13
19109	Oysters, breaded & battered, fried	3 oz	85.1	226	8	24		11	2.8	66
45122	Pancakes, w/butter & syrup	1 ea	116	260	4	45		7	2.9	29
6173	Potato salad	0.333 cup	95	108	1	13		6	1	57
56669	Roast beef sandwich, w/cheese	1 ea	176	473	32	45		18	9	77
66003	Roast beef sandwich, plain	1 ea	139	346	22	33		14	3.6	51
56643	Taco salad	1.5 cup	198	279	13	24		15	6.8	44
56644	Taco salad, w/chili con carne	1.5 cup	261	290	17	27		13	6	5
19115	Shrimp, breaded & fried	4 ea	93.7	260	11	23		14	3.1	114
56670	Steak sandwich	1 ea	204	459	30	52		14	3.8	73
56671	Submarine sandwich, w/cold cuts	1 ea	228	456	22	51		19	6.8	36
56673	Submarine sandwich, w/tuna salad	1 ea	256	584	30	55		28	5.3	49
57531	Taco, small	1 ea	171	371	21	27		21	11.4	56
66017	Tostada, bean & cheese	1 ea	144	223	10	27		10	5.4	30
56645	Tostada, beef & cheese	1 ea	163	315	19	23		16	10.4	41
	Arby's									
6429	Baked potato w/broccoli & cheese	1 ea	384	517	12	69	8	21	10.9	46
9011	Chicken tenders, 5 piece serving	1 ea	192	555	37	41	3	27	4.8	61
8987	French fries, curly, large	1 ea	198	631	8	73	7	37	6.8	0
9006	French fries, large	1 ea	212.6	565	6	82	6	37	6.7	0
9008	Cheese sticks, mozzarella, fried	1 ea	137	426	18	38	2	28	12.9	45
69055	Submarine sandwich, beef & swiss cheese	1 ea	311	678	35	47	4	36	10.9	91
9014	Breakfast biscuit, bacon, egg & cheese	1 ea	144	420	15	27	1	25	7.3	153
69043	Submarine sandwich, french dip, w/au jus	1 ea	285	453	29	49	3	18	7.2	59
8991	Submarine sandwich, hot, ham & swiss	1 ea	278	501	28	46	2	18	4.2	55
56336	Sandwich, roast beef	1 ea	157	326	20	35	1	14	5.5	45
81506	Sandwich, roast beef sourdough melt	1 ea	166	356	17	40	2	14	4.7	30
53256	Sauce, Arby's, packet	1 ea	14	15	0	4	0	0	0	0
9018	Sauce, barbecue, dipping, packet	1 serving	28.4	45	0	11	0	0	0	0
	Source: Arby's									
	Burger King									
56352	Cheeseburger	1 ea	133	380	19	32	4	20	9.1	60

MDA Code	Food Name	Amt	Wt (g)	Ener (kcal)	Prot (g)	Carb (g)	Fiber (g)	Fat (g)	Sat (g)	Chol (mg)
56355	Cheeseburger, Whopper	1 ea	316	790	35	53	3	48	18.3	114
56357	Cheeseburger, Whopper, double	1 ea	399	1061	58	54	6	68	27.9	188
9087	Chicken tenders, 4 piece serving	1 ea	62	179	11	11	1	10	2.6	32
9065	French fries, large	1 ea	160	530	6	64	5	28	7	
56351	Hamburger	1 ea	121	333	17	33	2	15	6.1	42
56354	Hamburger, Whopper	1 ea	291	678	31	54	5	37	12.4	87
9071	Hash browns, round, medium	1 ea	128	472	4	44	4	31	7.6	0
2127	Milk shake, chocolate, medium 16 fl-oz	1 ea	397	440	13	80	4	8	5	35
2129	Milk shake, vanilla, medium, 16 fl-oz	1 ea	397	667	13	76	0	35	21.2	123
9041	Onion rings, large	1 ea	137	480	7	60	5	23	6	0
69071	Breakfast biscuit, bacon, egg & cheese	1 ea	189	692	27	51	1	61	18.6	253
56360	Sandwich, chicken	1 ea	224	660	25	53	3	39	8	70
57002	Sandwich, Chicken Broiler	1 ea	258	550	30	52	3	25	5	105
9084	Sandwich, croissant w/sausage & cheese	1 ea	107	402	15	25	1	27	9.2	46
	Source: Burger King Corporation									
	Chik-Fil-A									
69185	Chargrilled Chicken breast fillet, chargrilled	1 ea	79	100	20	1	0	2	0	60
15263	Chicken nuggets, 8 piece serving	1 ea	113	260	26	12	1	12	2.5	70
15262	Chicken strips, 4 piece serving	1 ea	108	250	25	12	0	11	2.5	70
52138	Cole slaw, small	1 ea	105	210	1	14	2	17	2.5	20
48214	Lemon pie, slice	1 pce	113	320	7	51	3	10	3.5	110
52134	Salad, garden, chargrilled chicken	1 ea	278	180	23	8	3	6	3	70
52137	Salad, side	1 ea	164	80	5	6	2	5	2.5	15
69155	Sandwich, chicken salad, whole wheat	1 ea	153	350	20	32	5	15	3	65
69189	Sandwich, chicken, deluxe	1 ea	208	420	28	39	2	16	3.5	60
69176	Sauce, honey mustard, dipping, packet	1 ea	28	45	0	10	0	0	0	0
69182	Wrap, spicy chicken	1 ea	225	390	31	51	3	7	3.5	70
	Source: Chik-Fil-A									
	Dairy Queen									
56372	Cheeseburger, double, homestyle	1 ea	219	540	35	30	2	31	16	115
72142	Frozen dessert, banana split, large	1 ea	527	810	17	134	2	23	15	70
71693	Frozen dessert, Brownie Earthquake	1 ea	304	740	10	112	0	27	16	50
72139	Frozen dessert, chocolate cookie dough, large	1 ea	560	1320	21	193	0	52	26	90
72134	Frozen dessert, chocolate sundae, large	1 ea	333	580	11	100	1	15	10	45
72138	Frozen dessert, Oreo, large	1 ea	500	1010	19	148	2	37	18	70
72135	Frozen dessert, strawberry sundae, large	1 ea	333	500	10	83	1	15	9	45
72137	Frozen dessert, Triple Chocolate Utopia	1 ea	284	770	12	96	5	39	17	55
2222	Ice cream cone, chocolate, medium	1 ea	198	340	8	53	0	11	7	30
2136	Ice cream cone, dipped, medium	1 ea	220	490	8	59	1	24	13	30
2143	Ice cream cone, vanilla, medium	1 ea	213	355	9	57	0	10	6.5	32
2134	Ice cream sandwich	1 ea	85	200	4	31	1	6	3	10
72129	Milk shake, chocolate malt, large	1 ea	836	1320	29	222	2	35	22	110
	Source: International Dairy Queen, Inc.									
	Domino's Pizza									
91365	Breadsticks	1 ea	37.2	116	3	18	1	4	0.8	0
91369	Chicken, buffalo wings	1 ea	24.9	50	6	2	0	2	0.6	26
56386	Pizza, cheese, hand tossed, 12"	2 pce	159	375	15	55	3	11	4.8	23

MDA Code	Food Name	Amt	Wt (g)	Ener (kcal)	Prot (g)	Carb (g)	Fiber (g)	Fat (g)	Sat (g)	Chol (mg)
91356	Pizza, Deluxe Feast, hand tossed, 12"	2 pce	200.8	465	19	57	3	18	7.7	40
91358	Pizza, MeatZZa Feast, hand tossed, 12"	2 pce	216.2	560	26	57	3	26	11.4	64
91361	Pizza, Pepperoni Feast, hand tossed, 12"	2 pce	196.1	534	24	56	3	25	10.9	57
91357	Pizza, Veggie Feast, hand tossed, 12"	2 pce	203.2	439	19	57	4	16	7.1	34
	Source: Domino's Pizza Incorporated									
	Hardee's									
9295	Apple turnover	1 ea	91	270	4	38		12	4	0
42330	Biscuit, cinnamon raisin	1 ea	75	250	2	42		8	2	0
15201	Chicken wing, serving	1 ea	66	200	10	23	0	8	2	30
9278	Hot dog sandwich w/chili	1 ea	160	451	15	24	2	32	12	55
9284	Chicken strips, 5 piece serving	1 ea	92	201	18	13	0	8	1.7	25
9277	Hamburger, Monster	1 ea	278	949	53	35	2	67	25	185
9275	Hamburger, Six Dollar	1 ea	353	911	41	50	2	61	27	137
2247	Ice cream cone, twist	1 ea	118	180	4	34		2	1	10
6147	French fries, large	1 ea	150	440	5	59	0	21	3	0
9281	Chicken sandwich, barbecue, grilled	1 ea	171	268	24	34	2	3	1	60
56423	Sandwich, fish, Fisherman's Fillet	1 ea	221	530	25	45		28	7	75
	Source: Hardee's Food Systems, Inc.									
	Jack in the Box									
56437	Cheeseburger, Jumbo Jack	1 ea	296	714	26	56	3	43	16.6	72
62547	Cheeseburger, Bacon Ultimate	1 ea	302	974	41	47	2	69	26.8	125
56445	Egg roll, 3 piece serving	1 ea	170	400	14	44	6	19	6	15
62558	French toast sticks, original, serving	1 ea	120	466	7	58	4	23	5	25
56433	Hamburger	1 ea	104	273	14	26	1	12	5.3	35
2964	Milk shake, Oreo cookie, medium	1 ea	419	941	15	112	1	46	25.8	157
2165	Milk shake, vanilla, medium	1 ea	332	664	13	75	1	34	21	134
56446	Onion rings, serving	1 ea	120	504	6	51	3	30	6.1	0
6425	French fries, curly, medium	1 ea	125	404	6	44	4	23	4.4	0
6150	French fries, natural cut, small	1 ea	113	306	5	40	3	14	3.5	0
62551	Potato wedges, bacon & cheddar, serving	1 ea	268	692	21	53	6	44	14.8	49
56441	Sandwich, chicken fajita pita	1 ea	230	317	24	33	3	11	4.7	69
56431	Sandwich, breakfast, sausage croissant	1 ea	181	603	22	38	2	41	13.5	265
56377	Taco, beef, regular	1 ea	90	189	6	18	2	9	3.6	18
	Source: Jack in the Box									
	KFC									
42331	Biscuit, buttermilk	1 ea	57	203	4	24	1	10	2.4	1
15169	Chicken breast, extra crispy	1 ea	162	447	37	13	1	28	5.9	123
15185	Chicken breast, hot & spicy	1 ea	179	460	33	20	0	27	8	130
15163	Chicken breast, original recipe	1 ea	161	377	39	9	1	21	4.8	132
81292	Chicken breast, original recipe, w/o skin, breaded	1 ea	108	185	32	0	0	6	1.4	94
81293	Chicken, drumstick, original recipe	1 ea	59	145	13	3	0	9	2.1	69
15166	Chicken, thigh, original recipe	1 ea	126	335	24	9	1	23	5.4	125
416	Chicken, wing, honey barbecue, peices	6 ea	157	540	25	36	1	33	7	150
56451	Cole slaw, serving	1 ea	130	187	1	20	3	11	1.7	3
9535	Corn cob, small	1 ea	82	76	3	13	4	2	0.5	0
2897	Dessert, strawberry shortcake, LilBucket	1 ea	99	200	2	34	0	6	4	20
56681	Macaroni & cheese	1 ea	287	130	5	15	1	6	2	5

MDA Code	Food Name	Amt	Wt (g)	Ener (kcal)	Prot (g)	Carb (g)	Fiber (g)	Fat (g)	Sat (g)	Chol (mg)
56453	Potatoes, mashed w/gravy, serving	1 ea	136	130	2	18	1	4	1	0
45166	Pie, pecan, slice	1 pce	95	370	4	55	2	15	2.5	40
81090	Pot pie, chicken, chunky	1 ea	423	770	29	70	5	40	15	115
56454	Potato salad, serving	1 ea	128	180	2	22	1	9	1.5	5
49148	Sandwich, chicken, honey bbq flavor, w/sauce	1 ea	147	300	21	41	4	6	1.5	50
81301	Sandwich, chicken, tender roasted, w/o sauce	1 ea	177	260	31	23	1	5	1.5	65
81093	Sandwich, chicken roasted, w/sauce	1 ea	196	390	31	24	1	19	4	70
81302	Sandwich, chicken, Twister	1 ea	252	670	27	55	3	38	7	60
	Source: Yum! Brands, Inc.									
	Long John Silver's									
91388	Cheese sticks, fried	3 ea	45	140	4	12	1	8	2	10
91390	Clam chowder, serving	1 ea	227	220	9	23	1	10	4	25
56477	Hush puppies, serving	1 ea	23	60	1	9	1	2	0.5	0
56461	Fish, batter dipped, regular	1 pce	92	230	11	16	0	13	4	30
92415	Cod, baked, serving	1 ea	100.7	120	21	0	0	5	1	90
91392	Sandwich, fish, batter dipped, Ultimate	1 ea	199	500	20	48	3	25	8	50
92290	Battered Shrimp, battered, 4 piece serving	1 ea	65.8	197	7	14	0	13	4.1	64
92292	Shrimp, breaded, fried, basket	1 ea	114	340	12	32	2	19	5	105
	Source: Yum! Brands, Inc.									
	McDonald's									
81465	Breakfast, big, w/eggs, sausage, hash browns & biscuit	1 ea	266	758	27	47	3	52	17	460
56675	Burrito, sausage, breakfast	1 ea	113	296	13	24	1	17	6.1	173
69010	Cheeseburger, Big Mac	1 ea	219	563	26	44	4	33	8.3	79
81458	Cheeseburger, double	1 ea	173	458	26	34	1	26	10.5	83
69012	Cheeseburger, Quarter Pounder	1 ea	199	513	29	40	3	28	11.2	94
49152	Chicken McNuggets, 6 piece serving	6 pce	100	291	15	17	1	18	3.1	44
42334	Croutons, serving	1 ea	12	50	1	9	1	1	0	0
42335	Danish, apple	1 ea	105	340	5	47	2	15	3	20
72902	Dessert, apple dipper, w/low fat caramel sauce	1 ea	89	99	0	23		1	0.4	3
81440	French fries, large	1 ea	171	540	7	67	7	28	3.6	0
1747	Frozen dessert, Butterfinger	1 ea	348	620	16	90	1	22	14	70
2171	Frozen Dessert, hot fudge sundae	1 ea	179	333	7	54	1	11	6.4	23
69008	Hamburger	1 ea	105	265	13	32	1	10	3.1	28
69011	Hamburger, Quarter Pounder	1 ea	171	417	24	38	3	20	6.9	67
6155	Hash browns	1 ea	53	139	1	14	1	9	1.2	0
72913	Milk shake, chocolate, triple thick, large	1 ea	713	1162	26	199	1	32	16.4	100
81453	Pancakes, hotcake, w/2 pats margarine & syrup	1 ea	221	601	9	102	2	18	1.8	20
81154	Parfait, fruit n' yogurt, w/o granola	1 ea	142	128	4	25	1	2	0	7
48136	Pie, apple, snack	1 ea	77	249	2	34	2	12	3.1	
69218	Salad, bacon ranch, w/crispy chicken	1 ea	316	348	28	19	3	20	5.1	70
608	Salad, caesar, w/chicken, shaker	1 ea	163	100	17	3	2	2	1.5	40
61674	Salad, California cobb, w/grilled chicken	1 ea	325	273	34	11	3	11	4.8	143
57764	Salad, chef, Shaker	1 ea	206	150	17	5	2	8	3.5	95
61667	Salad, fruit & walnut	1 ea	264	312	5	44		13	1.8	5
81466	Sandwich, breakfast, McGriddle w/bacon, egg & cheese	1 ea	168	457	20	44	1	22	7.1	247
81532	Sandwich, chicken, grilled, classic	1 ea	229	419	32	51	3	10	2	78
69013	Sandwich, Filet O Fish, w/tartar sauce	1 ea	141	388	15	39	1	19	3.7	39

MDA Code	Food Name	Amt	Wt (g)	Ener (kcal)	Prot (g)	Carb (g)	Fiber (g)	Fat (g)	Sat (g)	Chol (mg)
81456	Sandwich, Filet O Fish w/o tartar sauce	1 ea	123	299	15	38	1	9	2.2	31
53176	Sauce, barbecue, packet	1 ea	28	46	0	10	0	0	0	
53177	Sauce, sweet & sour, packet	1 ea	28	48	0	11	0	0	0	
12230	Sausage, pork, serving	1 ea	43	170	6	0	0	16	5	35
42747	Sweet roll, cinnamon	1 ea	105	418	8	56	2	19	4.7	61
	Source: McDonald's Nutrition Information Center									
	Pizza Hut									
92497	Breadsticks, cheese	1 ea	67	200	7	21	1	10	3.5	15
92526	Dessert pizza, cherry, slice	1 pce	102	240	4	47	1	4	0.5	0
92519	Pasta Bakes, primavera w/chicken, serving	1 ea	540	1050	52	97	6	50	12	75
57394	Pizza, beef, medium, 12", slice	1 pce	91	230	11	21	2	11	5	25
56489	Pizza, cheese, medium, 12", slice	1 pce	96	260	11	30	2	10	4.8	23
56481	Pizza, cheese, pan, medium, 12", slice	1 pce	100	280	12	30	2	13	5.2	21
57781	Pizza, chicken supreme, 12", medium, slice	1 pce	120	230	14	30	2	6	3	25
830	Pizza, super supreme, medium, 12"	1 pce	127	309	14	33	3	14	5.8	25
92483	Pizza, green pepper, onion & tomato, 12", medium, slice	1 pce	104	150	6	24	2	4	1.5	10
92482	Pizza, ham, pineapple & tomato, 12" medium, slice	1 pce	99	160	8	24	2	4	2	15
57810	Pizza, Meat Lovers, 12", medium, slice	1 pce	169	450	21	43	3	21	10	55
56486	Pizza, pepperoni, 12" medium, slice	1 pce	77	210	10	21	1	10	4.5	25
57811	Pizza, Veggie Lovers, 12", medium, slice	1 pce	172	360	16	45	3	14	7	35
	Source: Yum! Brands, Inc.									
	Subway									
47658	Cookie, chocolate chip, M & M's	1 ea	45	220	2	30	1	10	4	15
52119	Salad, chicken breast, roasted	1 ea	303	140	16	12	3	3	1	45
52115	Salad, club	1 ea	322	150	17	12	3	4	1.5	35
52118	Salad, tuna, w/light mayonnaise	1 ea	314	240	13	10	3	16	4	40
52113	Salad, veggie delite	1 ea	233	50	2	9	3	1	0	0
91761	Sandwich, chicken teriyaki, w/sweet onion, white bread, 6"	1 ea	269	380	26	59	4	5	1.5	50
69117	Sandwich, club, white bread, 6"	1 ea	255	320	24	46	4	6	2	35
69113	Sandwich, cold cut trio, white bread, 6"	1 ea	257	440	21	47	4	21	7	55
91763	Sandwich, ham, w/honey mustard, white bread, 6"	1 ea	232	310	18	52	4	5	1.5	25
69139	Sandwich, Italian BMT, white bread, 6"	1 ea	248	480	23	46	4	24	9	55
69129	Sandwich, meatball, white bread, 6"	1 ea	287	530	24	53	6	26	10	55
69103	Sandwich, roast beef, deli style	1 ea	151	220	13	35	3	4	2	15
69143	Tuna Sandwich, tuna, w/Llight mayonnaise, white bread, 6"	1 ea	255	450	20	46	4	22	6	40
69101	Sandwich, turkey, deli style	1 ea	151	220	13	36	3	4	1.5	15
69109	Sandwich, veggie delight, white bread, 6"	1 ea	166	230	9	44	4	3	1	0
91778	Soup, roasted chicken noodle	1 cup	240	90	7	7	1	4	1	20
91791	Soup, cream of broccoli	1 cup	240	130	5	15	2	6	0	10
91783	Soup, minestrone	1 cup	240	70	3	11	2	1	0	10
91788	Soup, chicken w/ brown & wild rice	1 cup	240	190	6	17	2	11	4.5	20
	Source: Subway International									
	Taco Bell									
92107	Border Bowl, chicken, zesty, w/sauce	1 ea	417	730	23	65	12	42	9	45
56519	Burrito, bean	1 ea	198	404	16	55	8	14	4.8	18
56522	Burrito, beef, supreme	1 ea	248	469	20	52	8	20	7.6	40
57668	Burrito, chicken, fiesta	1 ea	184	370	18	48	3	12	3.5	30

MDA Code	Food Name	Amt	Wt (g)	Ener (kcal)	Prot (g)	Carb (g)	Fiber (g)	Fat (g)	Sat (g)	Chol (mg)
56691	Burrito, seven layer	1 ea	283	530	18	67	10	22	8	25
92113	Burrito, steak, grilled, Stuft	1 ea	325	680	31	76	8	28	8	55
92118	Chalupa, beef, nacho cheese	1 ea	153	380	12	33	3	22	7	20
92120	Chalupa, chicken, Baja	1 ea	153	400	17	30	2	24	6	40
92122	Chalupa, steak, supreme	1 ea	153	370	15	29	2	22	8	35
45585	Cinnamon twists, serving	1 ea	35	160	1	28	0	5	1	0
57666	Gordita, beef, Baja	1 ea	153	350	14	31	4	19	5	30
57669	Gordita, chicken, Baja	1 ea	153	320	17	29	2	15	3.5	40
57662	Gordita, steak, Baja	1 ea	153	320	15	29	2	16	4	30
56530	Guacamole, serving	1 ea	21	35	0	2	1	3	0	0
38561	Mexican rice, serving	1 ea	131	210	6	23	3	10	4	15
56534	Nachos, Bell Grande, serving	1 ea	308	780	20	80	12	43	13	35
56536	Pintos & cheese, serving	1 ea	128	180	10	20	6	7	3.5	15
56531	Pizza, Mexican	1 ea	216	550	21	46	7	31	11	45
57689	Quesadilla, chicken	1 ea	184	540	28	40	3	30	13	80
92098	Salsa, fiesta	1 ea	21	5	0	1		0	0	0
53186	Sauce, hot, Border, packet	1 ea	11	4	0	0	0	0	0	0
92105	Steak bowl, southwest	1 ea	443	700	30	73	13	32	8	55
56524	Taco	1 ea	78	184	8	14	3	11	3.6	24
57671	Taco, double decker, supreme	1 ea	191	380	15	40	6	18	8	40
56693	Taco, soft shell	1 ea	127	286	15	22	2	15	4.3	39
56537	Taco salad, w/salsa & shell	1 ea	533	906	36	80	16	49	15.9	101
56528	Tostada	1 ea	170	250	11	29	7	10	4	15
	Source: Taco Bell/Yum! Brands, Inc.									
	Wendy's									
56579	Baked potato w/bacon & cheese	1 ea	380	580	18	79	7	22	6	40
56582	Baked potato, w/sour cream & chives	1 ea	312	370	7	73	7	6	4	15
81445	Cheeseburger, single, classic	1 ea	236	522	35	34	3	27	12.3	90
56571	Cheeseburger, bacon, junior	1 ea	165	380	20	34	2	19	7	55
15176	Chicken nuggets, 5 piece serving	1 ea	75	250	12	12	1	17	3.7	38
50311	Chili, small	1 ea	227	200	17	21	5	6	2.5	35
6169	French fries, large	1 ea	159	507	6	63	6	26	5.1	
2177	Frozen dessert, dairy, medium	1 ea	298	393	10	70	10	8	4.9	48
56574	Hamburger, bacon big, classic	1 ea	282	570	34	46	3	29	12	100
56566	Hamburger, single, classic	1 ea	218	464	28	37	3	23	8	76
8457	Dressing, blue cheese, packet	1 ea	71	290	2	3	0	30	6	45
8461	Dressing, french, packet	1 ea	71	90	0	21	1	0	0	0
71595	Dressing, sesame, oriental, packet	1 ea	71	280	2	21	0	21	3	0
81444	Sandwich, Homestyle Chicken Fillet	1 ea	230	492	32	50	3	19	3.7	71
81443	Sandwich, Ultimate Grill Chicken	1 ea	225	403	33	42	2	11	2.3	90
52080	Salad, side, caesar, w/o dressing	1 ea	99	70	7	2	1	4	2	15
71592	Salad, chicken, mandarin, w/o dressing	1 ea	348	150	20	17	3	2	0	10
52083	Salad, side, garden, w/o dressing	1 ea	167	35	2	7	3	0	0	0
	Source: Wendy's Foods International									

Suggested Reading

Chapter 1

Blair, S., and M. Moore. Surgeon General's report on physical fitness: The inside story. *ACSM's Health and Physical Journal* 1:14–18, 1997.

Brooks, G. A., N. Butte, W. Rand, J. Flatt, and B. Caballero. Chronicle of the Institute of Medicine physical activity recommendation: How a physical activity recommendation came to be among dietary recommendations. *American Journal of Clinical Nutrition* 79:921S–930S, 2004.

Brown, D., D. Brown, G. Heath, L. Balluz, W. Giles, E. Ward, and A. Mokdad. Associations between physical activity dose and health-related quality of life. *Medicine and Science in Sports and Exercise* 36:890–896, 2004.

Bushman, B. (Ed.). *ACSM's Complete Guide to Health and Fitness.* Champaign, IL: Human Kinetics, 2011.

Franklin, B. Improved fitness = Increased longevity. *ACSM's Health and Fitness Journal* 5:32–33, 2001.

Haskell, W. L., et al. Physical activity and public health: Updated recommendation for adults from the American College of Sports Medicine and the American Heart Association. *Medicine and Science in Sports and Exercise* 39:1423–1434, 2007.

Howley, E., and D. Thompson. *Fitness Professional's Handbook*, 6th ed. Champaign, IL: Human Kinetics, 2012.

Powers, S., and E. Howley. *Exercise Physiology: Theory and Application to Fitness and Performance*, 8th ed. New York: McGraw-Hill, 2012.

Powers, S., S. Lennon, J. Quindry, and J. Mehta. Exercise and cardioprotection. *Current Opinion in Cardiology* 17:495–502, 2002.

Rahl, R. L. *Physical Activity and Health Guidelines.* Champaign, IL: Human Kinetics, 2010.

Chapter 2

Bushman, B. (Ed). *ACSM's Complete Guide to Fitness and Health.* Champaign, IL: Human Kinetics, 2011.

Blair, S. N. Physical inactivity: The biggest public health problem of the 21st century. *British Journal of Sports Medicine* 43:1–2, 2009.

Howley, E., and D. Thompson. *Fitness Professional's Handbook.* Champaign, IL: Human Kinetics, 2012.

Humphrey, R. Activity and fitness in health risk. *ACSM's Health and Fitness Journal* 11:36–37, 2007.

Murphy, M. H., S. N. Blair, and E. M. Murtagh. Accumulated versus continuous exercise for health benefit: A review of empirical studies. *Sports Medicine* 39:29–43, 2009.

Powell, K. A. Paluch, and S. Blair. Physical activity for health: What kind? How much? How intense? On top of what? *Annual Review of Public Health.* 32:349–395, 2011.

Powers, S., and E. Howley. *Exercise Physiology: Theory and Application to Fitness and Performance*, 8th ed. New York: McGraw Hill, 2012.

Chapter 3

Blair, S. N., M. J. LaMonte, and M. Z. Nichaman. The evolution of physical activity recommendations: How much is enough? *American Journal of Clinical Nutrition* 79(5):913S–920S, 2004.

Brisswalter J., M. Collardeau, and A. Rene. Effects of acute physical exercise characteristics on cognitive performance. *Sports Medicine* 32(9):555–566, 2002.

Chobanian, A. V., G. L. Bakris, H. R. Black, W. C. Cushman, L. A. Green, J. L. Izzo Jr., D. W. Jones, B. J. Materson, S. Oparil, J. T. Wright Jr., and E. J. Roccella. National Heart, Lung, and Blood Institute Joint National Committee on Prevention, Detection, Evaluation, and Treatment of High Blood Pressure; National High Blood Pressure Education Program Coordinating Committee. The seventh report of the Joint National Committee on Prevention, Detection, Evaluation, and Treatment of High Blood Pressure: The JNC 7 report. *Journal of the American Medical Association* 289(19):2560–2572, 2003.

Haskell, W. L., et al. Physical activity and public health: Updated recommendation for adults from the American College of Sports Medicine and the American Heart Association. *Medicine and Science in Sports and Exercise* 39:1423–1434, 2007.

Pollock, M. L., and J. H. Wilmore. *Exercise in Health and Disease*, 3rd ed. Philadelphia: W. B. Saunders, 1998.

Powers, S., and E. Howley. *Exercise Physiology: Theory and Application to Fitness and Performance*, 8th ed. New York: McGraw-Hill, 2012.

Rahl, R. L. *Physical Activity and Health Guidelines.* Champaign, IL: Human Kinetics, 2010.

Robertson, R. *Perceived Exertion for Practitioners: Rating Effort with the OMNI Picture System.* Champaign, IL: Human Kinetics, 2004.

Spriet, L. L., and M. J. Gibala. Nutritional strategies to influence adaptations to training. *Journal of Sports Science* 22(1):127–141, 2004.

Warburton, D. E., N. Gledhill, and A. Quinney. Musculoskeletal fitness and health. *Canadian Journal of Applied Physiology* 26(2):217–237, 2001.

Chapter 4

American College of Sports Medicine. Quantity and quality of exercise for developing and maintaining cardiorespiratory, musculoskeletal, and neuromotor fitness in apparently healthy adults: Guidance for prescribing exercise. *Medicine and Science in Sports and Exercise* 43(7):1334–1359, 2011.

Baechle, T. R., and R. Earle. *Essentials of Strength Training and Conditioning*, 3rd ed. Champaign, IL: Human Kinetics, 2008.

Bishop P. A., E. Jones, and A. K. Woods. Recovery from training: A brief review. *Journal of Strength and Conditioning Research* 22(3):1015–1024, 2008.

Folland, J. P., and A. G. Williams. The adaptations to strength training: Morphological and neurological contributions to increased strength. *Sports Medicine* 37(2):145–168, 2007.

Hoffman, J. (Ed.). *National Strength and Conditioning Association's Guide to Program Design*. Champaign, IL: Human Kinetics, 2012.

Hurley, B., E. D. Hanson, and A. K. Sheaff. Strength training as a countermeasure to aging muscle and chronic disease. *Sports Medicine* 41(4):289–306, 2011.

Knuttgen, H. G. Strength training and aerobic exercise: Comparison and contrast. *Journal of Strength and Conditioning Research* 21(3):973–978, 2007.

Krieger, J. W. Single vs. multiple sets of resistance exercise for muscle hypertrophy: A meta-analysis. *Journal of Strength and Conditioning Research* 24(4):1150–1159, 2010.

Martel, G. F., S. M. Roth, F. M. Ivey, J. T. Lemmer, B. L. Tracy, D. E. Hurlbut, E. J. Metter, B. F. Hurley, and M. A. Rogers. Age and sex affect human muscle fiber adaptations to heavy-resistance strength training. *Experimental Physiology* 91(2):457–464, 2006.

Phillips, S. M. The science of muscle hypertrophy: Making dietary protein count. *Proceedings of the Nutrition Society* 70(1):100–103, 2011.

Phillips, S. M., and R. A. Winett. Uncomplicated resistance training and health-related outcomes: Evidence for a public health mandate. *Current Sports Medicine Report* 9(4):208–213, 2010.

Zatsiorsky, V. M., and W. J. Kraemer. *Science and Practice of Strength Training*, 2nd ed. Champaign, IL: Human Kinetics, 2006.

Chapter 5

American College of Sports Medicine. American College of Sports Medicine position stand: Quantity and quality of exercise for developing and maintaining cardiorespiratory, musculoskeletal, and neuromotor fitness in apparently healthy adults: Guidance for prescribing exercise. *Medicine and Science in Sports and Exercise* 43(7):1334–1359, 2011.

Behm, D. G., and A. Chaouachi. A review of the acute effects of static and dynamic stretching on performance. *European Journal of Applied Physiology* 111(11): 2633–26351, 2011.

Cruz-Ferreira, A., J. Fernandes, L. Laranjo, L. M. Bernardo, and A. Silva. A systematic review of the effects of Pilates method of exercise in healthy people. *Archives of Physical Medicine and Rehabilitation* 92(12):2071–2081, 2011.

da Costa, B. R., and E. R. Vieira. Stretching to reduce work-related musculoskeletal disorders: A systematic review. *Journal of Rehabilitation Medicine* 40(5):321–328, 2008.

Herbert, R. D., M. de Noronha, and S. J. Kamper. Stretching to prevent or reduce muscle soreness after exercise. *Cochrane Database of Systematic Reviews* 6(7):CD004577, 2011.

Herman, S. L., and D. T. Smith. Four-week dynamic stretching warm-up intervention elicits longer-term performance benefits. *Journal of Strength and Conditioning Research* 22(4):1286–1297, 2008.

Jenkins, J., and J. Beazell. Flexibility for runners. *Clinics in Sports Medicine* 29(3):365–377, 2010.

Rubini, E. C., A. L. L. Costa, and P. S. C. Gomes. The effects of stretching on strength performance. *Sports Medicine* 37(3):213–224, 2007.

Small, K., L. McNaughton, and M. Matthews. A systematic review into the efficacy of static stretching as part of a warm-up for the prevention of exercise-related injury. *Research in Sports Medicine* 16(3):213–231, 2008.

Chapter 6

Bouchard, C., S. Blair, and W. Haskell (Eds.). *Physical Activity and Health*. Champaign, IL: Human Kinetics, 2012.

Bouchard, C., and P. Katzmarzyk (Eds.). *Physical Activity and Obesity*. Champaign, IL: Human Kinetics, 2010.

Church, T., and S. N. Blair. Does physical activity ameliorate the health hazards of obesity? *British Journal of Sports Medicine* 43:80–81, 2009.

Donnelly, J., S. Blair, J. Jakicic, M. Manore, J. Rankin, and B. Smith. American College of Sports Medicine position stand: Appropriate physical activity intervention strategies for weight loss and prevention of weight gain for adults. *Medicine and Science in Sports and Exercise* 41:459–471, 2009.

Heshmat, S. *Eating Behavior and Obesity.* New York: Springer, 2011.

Howley, E., and D. Thompson. *Fitness Professional's Handbook.* Champaign, IL: Human Kinetics, 2012.

Kumanvika, S., R. Brownson, and D. Satcher. *Handbook of Obesity Prevention.* New York: Springer. 2010.

Lee, R., K. McAlexander, and J. Banda. *Reversing the Obesogenic Environment.* Champaign, IL: Human Kinetics, 2011.

Powers, S., and E. Howley. *Exercise Physiology: Theory and Application to Fitness and Performance*, 8th ed. New York: McGraw-Hill, 2012.

Waisted: Abdominal obesity and your health. *Harvard Men's Health Watch* 13:1–6, 2009.

Chapter 7

Baechle T., and R. Earle. *Essentials of Strength Training and Conditioning.* Champaign, IL: Human Kinetics, 2008.

Byrd, N. What gets measured is more likely to get done. *ACSM's Health and Fitness Journal* 15:26–29, 2011.

Donatelle, R. J. *My Health: An Outcomes Approach.* San Francisco: Benjamin Cummings, 2013.

Fieger, H. *Behavior Change.* New York: Morgan James, 2009.

Howley, E., and D. Thompson. *Fitness Professional's Handbook.* Champaign, IL: Human Kinetics, 2012.

Pate, R. Overcoming barriers to physical activity: Helping youth be more active. *ACSM's Health and Fitness Journal* 15:7–12, 2011.

Powers, S., and E. Howley. *Exercise Physiology: Theory and Application to Fitness and Performance*, 8th ed. New York: McGraw Hill, 2012.

Shumaker, S. A., J. K. Ockene, and K. A. Riekert. *The Handbook of Health Behavior Change*, 3rd ed. New York: Springer, 2008.

Turner, S. L., A. M. Thomas, and P. J. Wagner. A collaborative approach to wellness: Diet, exercise, and education to impact behavior change *Journal of the American Academy of Nurse Practitioners* 20(6):339–344, 2008.

Volpe, S. L. Can dogs help with maintaining motivation? *ACSM's Health and Fitness Journal* 15:36–37, 2011.

Chapter 8

Block, G. Junk foods account for 30% of caloric intake. *Journal of Food Composition and Analysis* 17: 439–447, 2004.

Heber, D. Vegetables, fruits and phytoestrogens in the prevention of diseases. *Journal of Postgraduate Medicine* 50(2):145–149, 2004.

Kant, A. K. Dietary patterns and health outcomes. *Journal of the American Dietetic Association* 104(4): 615–635, 2004.

Maughan, R. J., D. S. King, and T. Lea. Dietary supplements. *Journal of Sports Sciences* 22(1):95–113, 2004.

Position of the American Dietetic Association, Dietitians of Canada, and the American College of Sports Medicine: Nutrition and athletic performance. *Journal of the American Dietetic Association* 109(3):509–527, 2009.

Spriet, L. L., and M. J. Gibala. Nutritional strategies to influence adaptations to training. *Journal of Sports Sciences.* 22(1):127–141, 2004.

Srinath, R. K., and M. B. Katan. Diet, nutrition and the prevention of hypertension and cardiovascular diseases. *Public Health and Nutrition* 7(1A):167–186, 2004.

Thompson, J., and M. Manore. *Nutrition: An Applied Approach, MyPlate edition*, 3rd ed. San Francisco: Benjamin Cummings, 2012.

Wood, O. B., and C. M. Bruhn. Position of American Dietetic Association: Food irradiation. *Journal of the American Dietetic Association* 100(2):246–253, 2000.

Chapter 9

Centers for Disease Control. Obesity at a Glance. 2011.

Donnelly, J., S. Blair, J. Jakicic, M. Manore, J. Rankin, and B. Smith. ACSM position stand: Appropriate physical activity intervention strategies for weight loss and prevention of weight regain for adults. *Medicine and Science in Sports and Exercise* 41:459–471, 2009.

Gaesser, G., and K. Kratina. *It's the Calories Not the Carbs.* New York: Trafford Publishing, 2006.

Martins, C., L. Morgan, and H. Truby. A review of the effects of exercise on appetite regulation: An obesity perspective. *International Journal of Obesity* 32: 1337–1347, 2008.

Powers, S., and E. Howley. *Exercise Physiology: Theory and Application to Fitness and Performance*, 8th ed. New York: McGraw-Hill, 2012.

Sherer, E., and J. Sherer. Examining the most popular weight loss diets: How effective are they? *Journal of the American Academy of Physician Assistants* 21:31–34, 2008.

Stensel, D. Exercise, appetite, and appetite-regulating hormones: Implications for food intake and weight control. *Annals of Nutrition and Metabolism* 57:36–42, 2010.

Wolff, E., and M. Dansinger. Soft drinks and weight gain: How strong is the Link? *Medscape Journal of Medicine* 10:89–97, 2008.

Chapter 10

American Heart Association. Heart disease and stroke statistics—2012 update. *Circulation* 125:e2–e220, 2012.

Franklin, B., and C. Lavie. Triggers of acute cardiovascular events and potential strategies: Prophylactic role of regular exercise. *Physician and Sports Medicine* 39:11–21, 2011.

Franklin, B., J. Trivax, and T. Vanhecke. New insights in preventive cardiology and cardiac rehabilitation. *Current Opinion in Cardiology* 23:477–486, 2008.

Löllgen, H., A. Böckenhoff, and G. Knapp. Physical activity and all-cause mortality: An updated meta-analysis with different intensity categories. *International Journal of Sports Medicine* 30:213–224, 2009.

Powers, S., and E. Howley. *Exercise Physiology: Theory and Application to Fitness and Performance*, 8th ed. New York: McGraw-Hill, 2012.

Trogdon, P., O. Khavjou, J. Butler, K. Dracup, M. Ezekowitz, et al. Forecasting the future of cardiovascular disease in the United States: A policy statement from the American Heart Association. *Circulation* 123:933–944, 2011.

Waisted: Abdominal obesity and your health. *Harvard Men's Health Watch* 13:1–6, 2009.

Chapter 11

Atkinson, D. *Live Right! Beating Stress in College and Beyond*. San Francisco: Benjamin Cummings, 2008.

Barrett, S., W. London, R. S. Baratz, and M. Kroeger. *Consumer Health: A Guide to Intelligent Decisions*, 8th ed. New York: McGraw-Hill, 2006.

Benson, H. *The Relaxation Response*. New York: Avon, Wholecare, 2000.

Daniel, E. (Ed.). *Annual Editions: Health*, 25th ed. Guilford, CT: McGraw-Hill, 2004.

Donatelle, R. *Health: The Basics*, 10th ed. San Francisco: Pearson Education, 2013.

Greenberg, J. *Comprehensive Stress Management*, 10th ed. Dubuque, IA: McGraw-Hill, 2006.

References

Chapter 1

1. Margen, S., et al. (Eds.). *The Wellness Encyclopedia*. Boston: Houghton Mifflin, 1995.

2. National Institute of Mental Health. *The Numbers Count: Mental Disorders in America*. Fact Sheet. http://www.nimh.nih.gov/publicat/numbers.cfm#MajorDepressive.

3. Koeing, H. G. Religion, spirituality and medicine: Research findings and implications for clinical practice. *Southern Medical Journal* 97:1194–1200, 2004.

4. Katon, W., E. H. B. Lin, and K. Kroenke. The association of depression and anxiety with medical symptom burden in patients with chronic medical illness. *General Hospital Psychiatry* 29:147–155, 2007.

5. Weaver, A. J., and K. J. Flannelly. The role of religion/spirituality for cancer patients and their caregivers. *Southern Medical Journal* 97:1210–1214, 2004.

6. Caspersen, C. J., K. E. Powell, and G. M. Christenson. Physical activity and exercise: Definitions and distinctions for health related-fitness research. *Public Health Reports* 100:126–130, 1985.

7. Paffenbarger, R., J. Kampert, I. Lee, R. Hyde, R. Leung, and A. Wing. Changes in physical activity and other lifeway patterns influencing longevity. *Medicine and Science in Sports and Exercise* 26:857–865, 1994.

8. Paffenbarger, R., R. Hyde, A. Wing, and C. Hsieh. Physical activity, all-cause mortality, longevity of college alumni. *New England Journal of Medicine* 314:605–613, 1986.

9. Helmrich, S., D. Ragland, and R. Paffenbarger. Prevention of non-insulin-dependent diabetes mellitus with physical activity. *Medicine and Science in Sports and Exercise* 26:824–830, 1994.

10. Wood, P. Physical activity, diet, and health: Independent and interactive effects. *Medicine and Science in Sports and Exercise* 26:838–843, 1994.

11. Morris, J. Exercise in the prevention of coronary heart disease: Today's best buy in public health. *Medicine and Science in Sports and Exercise* 26:807–814, 1994.

12. Blair, S. N., M. LaMonte, and M. Nichaman. The evolution of physical activity recommendations: How much is enough? *American Journal of Clinical Nutrition* 79:913S–920S, 2004.

13. Thompson, P., et al. Exercise and physical activity in the prevention and treatment of atherosclerotic cardiovascular disease. *Circulation* 107:3109–3116, 2003.

14. Brooks, G. A., N. Butte, W. Rand, J. Flatt, and B. Caballero. Chronicle of the Institute of Medicine physical activity recommendation: How a physical activity recommendation came to be among dietary recommendations. *American Journal of Clinical Nutrition* 79:921S–930S, 2004.

15. Brown, D., D. Brown, G. Heath, L. Balluz, W. Giles, E. Ward, and A. Mokdad. Associations between physical activity dose and health-related quality of life. *Medicine and Science in Sports and Exercise* 36:890–896, 2004.

16. U.S. Department of Health and Human Services. *Physical Activity and Health: A Report of the Surgeon General*. Atlanta, GA: U.S. Department of Health and Human Services, Centers for Disease Control and Prevention, National Center for Chronic Disease Prevention and Health Promotion, 1996.

17. Rogers, V. L. et al. Heart disease and stroke statistics—2012 update. *Circulation* 125:e12–e230, 2012.

18. Barrow, M. *Heart Talk: Understanding Cardiovascular Diseases*. Gainesville, FL: Cor-Ed Publishing, 1992.

19. Williams, P. T. Relationship between distance run per week to coronary heart disease risk factors in 8283 male runners: The National Runners Health Study. *Archives of Internal Medicine* 157:191–198, 1997.

20. Fagard, R. Physical activity in the prevention and treatment of hypertension in the obese. *Medicine and Science in Sports and Exercise* 31:S624–S630, 1999.

21. Williams, P. Physical fitness and activity as separate heart disease risk factors: A meta-analysis. *Medicine and Science in Sports and Exercise* 33:754–761, 2001.

22. Lennon, S., J. Quindry, K. Hamilton, J. French, J. Staib, J. Mehta, and S. K. Powers. Loss of cardioprotection after cessation of exercise. *Journal of Applied Physiology* 96: 299–1305, 2004.

23. Powers, S., M. Locke, and H. Demirel. Exercise, heat shock proteins, and myocardial protection from I-R injury. *Medicine and Science in Sports and Exercise* 33:386–392, 2001.

24. Hamilton, K., J. Staib, T. Phillips, A. Hess, S. Lennon, and S. Powers. Exercise, antioxidants, and HSP72: Protection against myocardial ischemia-reperfusion. *Free Radicals in Biology and Medicine* 34:800–809, 2003.

25. Lee, I., and R. Paffenbarger. Associations of light, moderate, and vigorous intensity physical activity with longevity: The Harvard Alumni Health Study. *American Journal of Epidemiology* 151:293–299, 2000.

26. Powell, K., and S. Blair. The public health burdens of sedentary living habits: Theoretical but realistic estimates. *Medicine and Science in Sports and Exercise* 26:851–856, 1994.

27. Rodnick, K., J. Holloszy, C. Mondon, and D. James. Effects of exercise training on insulin-regulatable glucose-transporter protein levels in rat skeletal muscle. *Diabetes* 39:1425–1429, 1990.

28. Pan, X. R., et al. Effects of diet and exercise in preventing NIDDM in people with impaired glucose tolerance. *Diabetes Care* 20:537–544, 1997.

29. Rankin, J. Diet, exercise, and osteoporosis. *Certified News* (American College of Sports Medicine) 3:1–4, 1993.

30. Wheeler, D., J. Graves, G. Miller, R. Vander Griend, T. Wronski, S. K. Powers, and H. Park. Effects of running on the torsional strength, morphometry, and bone mass on the rat skeleton. *Medicine and Science in Sports and Exercise* 27:520–529, 1995.

31. Taaffe, D., T. Robinson, C. Snow, and R. Marcus. High impact exercise promotes bone gain in well-trained female athletes. *Journal of Bone and Mineral Research* 12:255–260, 1997.

32. Hagberg, J. Effect of training in the decline of VO2max with aging. *Federation Proceedings* 46:1830–1833, 1987.

33. Fleg, J., and E. Lakatta. Role of muscle loss in the age-associated reduction in VO2max. *Journal of Applied Physiology* 65:1147–1151, 1988.

34. Nakamura, E., T. Moritani, and A. Kanetaka. Effects of habitual physical exercise on physiological age in men and women aged 20–85 years as estimated using principal component analysis. *European Journal of Applied Physiology* 73:410–418, 1996.

35. Hammeren, J., S. Powers, J. Lawler, D. Criswell, D. Martin, D. Lowenthal, and M. Pollock. Exercise training–induced alterations in skeletal muscle oxidative and antioxidant enzyme activity in senescent rats. *International Journal of Sports Medicine* 13:412–416, 1992.

36. Powers, S., J. Lawler, D. Criswell, Fu-Kong Lieu, and D. Martin. Aging and respiratory muscle metabolic plasticity: Effects of endurance training. *Journal of Applied Physiology* 72:1068–1073, 1992.

37. Holloszy, J. Exercise increases average longevity of female rats despite increased food intake and no growth retardation. *Journal of Gerontology* 48:B97–B100, 1993.

38. Lee, I., R. Paffenbarger, and C. Hennekens. Physical activity, physical fitness, and longevity. *Aging* (Milano) 9:2–11, 1997.

39. Franklin, B. Improved fitness = increased longevity. *ACSM's Health and Fitness Journal* 5:32–33, 2001.

40. Blair, S. N., and M. Wei. Sedentary habits, health, and function in older men and women. *American Journal of Health Promotion* 15:1–8, 2000.

41. Blair, S. N., H. W. Kohl, R. Paffenbarger, D. Clark, K. Cooper, and L. Gibbons. Physical fitness and all-cause mortality: A prospective study of healthy men and women. *Journal of the American Medical Association* 262:2395–2401, 1989.

42. Penedo, F. J., and J. R. Dahn. Exercise and well-being: A review of mental and physical health benefits associated with physical activity. *Current Opinion in Psychiatry* 18:198–193, 2005.

43. Jones, M. A., G. Stratton, T. Reilly, and V. B. Unnithan. Biological risk indicators for recurrent non-specific low back pain in adolescents. *British Journal of Sports Medicine* 39:137–140, 2005.

44. Mikkelson, L. O., H. Nupponen, J. Kaprio, H. Kautiainen, and U. M. Kujala. Adolescent flexibility, endurance strength, and physical activity as predictors of adult tension neck, low back pain and knee injury: A 25 year follow up. *British Journal of Sports Medicine* 40:107–113, 2006.

Chapter 2

1. Howley, E., and D. Thompson. *Fitness Professional's Handbook.* Champaign, IL: Human Kinetics, 2012.

2. Powers, S., and E. Howley. *Exercise Physiology: Theory and Application to Fitness and Performance,* 8th ed. New York: McGraw-Hill, 2012.

3. Stone, M., S. Plisk, and D. Collins. Training principles: Evaluation of modes and methods of resistance training—A coaching perspective. *Sports Biomechanics* 1:79–103, 2002.

4. Abernethy, P., J. Jurimae, P. Logan, A. Taylor, and R. Thayer. Acute and chronic response of skeletal muscle to resistance exercise. *Sports Medicine* 17:22–28, 1994.

5. Powers, S., D. Criswell, J. Lawler, L. Ji, D. Martin, R. Herb, and G. Dudley. Influence of exercise and fiber type on antioxidant enzyme activity in rat skeletal muscle. *American Journal of Physiology* 266:R375–R380, 1994.

6. Coyle, E., W. Martin, D. Sinacore, M. Joyner, J. Hagberg, and J. Holloszy. Time course of loss of adaptations after stopping prolonged intense endurance training. *Journal of Applied Physiology* 57:1857–1864, 1984.

7. Costill, D., and A. Richardson. *Handbook of Sports Medicine: Swimming.* London: Blackwell Publishing, 1993.

8. Bushman, B. (Ed). *ACSM's Complete Guide to Fitness and Health.* Champaign, IL: Human Kinetics, 2011.

9. Bouchard, C., R. Shephard, T. Stephens, J. Sutton, and B. McPherson (Eds.). *Exercise, Fitness, and Health: A Consensus of Current Knowledge.* Champaign, IL: Human Kinetics, 1990.

10. Bonow, R., D. Mann, D. Zipes, and P. Libby. *Braunwald's Heart Disease. A Textbook of Cardiovascular Medicine.* Philadelphia, Saunders, 2011.

11. Morris, J. Exercise in the prevention of coronary heart disease: Today's best buy in public health. *Medicine and Science in Sports and Exercise* 26:807–814, 1994.

12. Warburton, D., C. Nicol, and S. Bredin. Prescribing exercise as preventative therapy. *Canadian Medical Association Journal* 28:961–974, 2006.

13. Walsh, N., M. Gleeson, D. Pyne, D. Nieman, Dhabhar, R. Shephard, S. Oliver, S. Bermon, and A. Kajeniene. Position statement. Part two: Maintaining immune health. *Exercise Immunology Review.* 17:64–103, 2011.

14. Paffenbarger, R., J. Kampert, I. Lee, R. Hyde, R. Leung, and A. Wing. Changes in physical activity and other lifeway patterns influencing longevity. *Medicine and Science in Sports and Exercise* 26:857–865, 1994.

15. Williams, P. Physical fitness and activity as separate heart disease risk factors: A meta-analysis. *Medicine and Science in Sports and Exercise* 33:754–761, 2001.

16. Garber, C. B. Blissmer, M. Deschenes, B. Franklin, M. Lamonte, I. Lee, D. Nieman, D. Swain. American College of Sports Medicine position stand. Quality and quantity of exercise for developing and maintaining cardiorespiratory, musculoskeletal, and neuromotor fitness in apparently healthy adults: Guidance for prescribing exercise. *Medicine and Science in Sports and Exercise.* 43:1334–1359, 2011.

17. Howley, E. T. You asked for it: Is rigorous exercise better than moderate activity in achieving health-related goals? *ACSM's Health and Fitness Journal* 4(2):6, 2000.

18. Thompson, P., et al. Exercise and physical activity in the prevention and treatment of atherosclerotic cardiovascular disease. *Circulation* 107:3109–3116, 2003.

19. Blair, S., M. LaMonte, and M. Nichman. The evolution of physical activity recommendations: How much exercise is enough? *American Journal of Clinical Nutrition* 79: 913S–920S, 2004.

20. Brooks, G., N. Butte, W. Rand, J. P. Flatt, and B. Caballero. Chronicle of the institute of medicine physical activity recommendation: How a physical activity recommendation came to be among dietary recommendations. *American Journal of Clinical Nutrition* 79:921S–930S, 2004.

21. Brown, D., D. Brown, G. Heath, L. Balluz, W. Giles, E. Ford, and A. Mokdad. Associations between physical activity dose and health-related quality of life. *Medicine and Science in Sports and Exercise* 36:890–896, 2004.

22. Swain, D. Moderate or vigorous intensity exercise: What should we prescribe? *ACSM's Health and Fitness Journal* 10:21–27, 2006.

23. Ishikawa-Takata, K., T. Ohta, and H. Tanaka. How much exercise is required to reduce blood pressure in essential hypertensive: A dose-response study. *American Journal of Hypertension* 16:629–633, 2003.

24. U.S. Department of Health and Human Services. *2008 Physical Activity Guidelines for Americans.* 2008. http://www.health.gov/paguidelines.

25. Blair, S. N. Physical inactivity: The biggest public health problem of the 21st century. *British Journal of Sports Medicine* 43:1–2, 2009.

26. Powell, K. A. Paluch, and S. Blair. Physical activity for health: What kind? How much? How intense? On top of what? *Annual Review of Public Health.* 32:349–395, 2011.

27. Lee, D., E. Artero, X. Sui, and S. Blair. Mortality trends in the general population: The importance of cardiorespiratory fitness. *Journal of Psychopharmacology.* 24:27–35, 2010.

28. Gleeson, M., N. Bishop, D. Stensel, M. Lindley, S. Mastana, and M. Nimmo. The anti-inflammatory effects of exercise: Mechanisms and implications for the prevention and treatment of disease. *Nature Review Immunology.* 11:607–615, 2011.

Chapter 3

1. Ross, R., and I. Janssen. Physical activity, total and regional obesity: Dose-response considerations. *Medicine and Science in Sports and Exercise* 33(6):S345–S641, 2001.

2. Kohl, H. W. Physical activity and cardiovascular disease: Evidence for a dose response. *Medicine and Science in Sports and Exercise* 33(6):S472–S483, 2001.

3. Powers, S., and E. Howley. *Exercise Physiology: Theory and Application to Fitness and Performance,* 8th ed. New York: McGraw-Hill, 2012.

4. Laursen, P. B., and D. G. Jenkins. The scientific basis for high-intensity interval training: Optimising training programmes and maximising performance in highly trained endurance athletes. *Sports Medicine* 32(1):53–73, 2002.

5. Kesaniemi, Y. A., E. Danforth, M. D. Jensen, P. G. Kopelman, P. Lefebvre, and B. A. Reeder. Dose-response issues concerning physical activity and health: An evidence-based symposium. *Medicine and Science in Sports and Exercise* 33(6):S351–S358, 2001.

6. Dunn, A. L., M. H. Trivedi, and H. A. O'Neal. Physical activity dose-response effects on outcomes of depression and anxiety. *Medicine and Science in Sports and Exercise* 33(6):S587–S597, 2001.

7. Gambelunghe, C., R. Rossi, G. Mariucci, M. Tantucci, and M. V. Ambrosini. Effects of light physical exercise on sleep regulation in rats. *Medicine and Science in Sports and Exercise* 33(1):57–60, 2001.

8. American College of Sports Medicine. *ACSM's Guidelines for Exercise Testing and Prescription,* 7th ed. Philadelphia: Lippincott Williams, & Wilkins, 2006.

9. Cooper, K. *The Aerobics Program for Total Well-Being.* New York: M. Evans, 1982.

10. Cooper, K. *The Aerobics Way.* New York: Bantam Books, 1977.

11. Fox, E. A simple technique for predicting maximal aerobic power. *Journal of Applied Physiology* 35:914–916, 1973.

12. Rippe, J., A. Ward., J. Porcari, and P. Freedson. Walking for fitness and health. *Journal of the American Medical Association* 259:2720–2724, 1988.

13. Rippe, J. Walking for fitness: A roundtable. *Physician and Sports Medicine* 14:144–159, 1986.

14. Ward, A., and J. Rippe. *Walking for Health and Fitness.* Philadelphia: J. B. Lippincott, 1988.

15. Lox, C. L., K. A. Martin Ginis, and S. J. Petruzzello. *The Psychology of Exercise Integrating Theory and Practice,* 3rd ed. Scottsdale, AZ: Holcomb Hathaway Publishers, 2010.

16. Mullineaux, D. R., C. A. Barnes, and E. F. Barnes. Factors affecting the likelihood to engage in adequate physical activity to promote health. *Journal of Sports Sciences* 19(4):279–288, 2001.

17. Borg, G. *Borg's Perceived Exertion and Pain Scales.* Champaign, IL: Human Kinetics, 1998.

18. Storms, W. W. Review of exercise-induced asthma. *Medicine and Science in Sports and Exercise* 35 (9):1464–1470, 2003.

Chapter 4

1. Kell, R. T., and G. J. Asmundson. A comparison of two forms of periodized exercise rehabilitation programs in the management of chronic nonspecific low-back pain. *Journal of Strength and Conditioning Research* 23(2):513–523, 2009.

2. Olson, T. J., C. Chebny, J. D. Willson, T. W. Kernozek, and J. S. Straker. Comparison of 2D and 3D kinematic changes during a single leg step down following neuromuscular training. *Physical Therapy and Sport* 12(2):93–99, 2010.

3. Sundell, J. Resistance training is an effective tool against metabolic and frailty syndromes. *Advances in Preventive Medicine* 2011:984683.

4. Hopps, E., and G. Caimi. Exercise in obesity management. *Journal of Sports Medicine and Physical Fitness* 51(2):275–282, 2011.

5. Powers, S., and E. Howley. *Exercise Physiology: Theory and Application to Fitness and Performance,* 8th ed. New York: McGraw-Hill, 2012.

6. Oberbach A., Y. Bossenz, S. Lehmann, J. Niebauer, V. Adams, R. Paschke, M. R. Schön, M. Blüher, and K. Punkt. Altered fiber distribution and fiber-specific glycolytic and oxidative enzyme activity in skeletal muscle of patients with type 2 diabetes. *Diabetes Care* 29(4):895–900, 2006.

7. Karjalainen, J., H. Tikkanen, M. Hernelahti, and U. Kujala. Muscle fiber-type distribution predicts weight gain and unfavorable left ventricular geometry: A 19 year follow-up study. *BMC Cardiovascular Disorders* 10(6):1–8, 2006.

8. Ehrenborg, E., and A. Krook. Regulation of skeletal muscle physiology and metabolism by peroxisome proliferator-activated receptor delta. *Pharmacological Reviews* 61(3):373–393, 2009.

9. Monteiro, W. D., R. Simão, M. D. Polito, C. A. Santana, R. B. Chaves, E. Bezerra, and S. J. Fleck. Influence of strength training on adult women's flexibility. *Journal of Strength and Conditioning Research* 22(3):672–677, 2008.

10. American College of Sports Medicine. American College of Sports Medicine position stand: Progression models in resistance training for healthy adults. *Medicine and Science in Sports and Exercise* 41(3):687–708, 2009.

11. Folland, J. P., and A. G. Williams. The adaptations to strength training: Morphological and neurological contributions to increased strength. *Sports Medicine* 37(2):145–168, 2007.

12. Knuttgen, H. G. Strength training and aerobic exercise: Comparison and contrast. *Journal of Strength and Conditioning Research* 21(3):973–978, 2007.

13. American College of Sports Medicine. Quantity and quality of exercise for developing and maintaining cardiorespiratory, musculoskeletal, and neuromotor fitness in apparently healthy adults: Guidance for prescribing exercise. *Medicine and Science in Sports and Exercise* 43(7):1334–1359, 2011.

14. Hubal, M. J., S. R. Rubinstein, and P. M. Clarkson. Muscle function in men and women during maximal eccentric exercise. *Journal of Strength and Conditioning Research* 22(4):1332–1338, 2008.

15. Tillin, N. A., M. T. G. Pain, and J. P. Folland. Short-term training for explosive strength causes neural and mechanical adaptations. *Experimental Physiology* 23(8):817–824, 2012.

16. Rønnestad, B. R., B. S. Nymark, and T. Raastad. Effects of in-season strength maintenance training frequency in professional soccer players. *Journal of Strength and Conditioning Research* 25(10): 2653–2660, 2011.

Chapter 5

1. Ylinen, J., T. Kankainen, H. Kautiainen, A. Rezasoltani, T. Kuukkanen, and A. Häkkinen. Effect of stretching on hamstring muscle compliance. *Journal of Rehabilitation Medicine* 41(1):80–84, 2009.

2. Esposito, F., E. Limonta, and E. E. Cè. Passive stretching effects on electromechanical delay and time course of recovery in human skeletal muscle: new insights from an electromyographic and mechanomyographic combined approach. *European Journal of Applied Physiology* 111(3):485–495, 2011.

3. Ryan, E. E., M. Rossi, and R. Lopez. The effects of the contract-relax-antagonist-contract form of proprioceptive neuromuscular facilitation stretching on postural stability. *Journal of Strength and Conditioning Research* 24(7):1888–1894, 2010.

4. American College of Sports Medicine position stand: Quantity and quality of exercise for developing and maintaining cardiorespiratory, musculoskeletal, and neuromotor fitness in apparently healthy adults: Guidance for prescribing exercise. *Medicine and Science in Sports and Exercise* 43(7):1334–1359, 2011.

5. Small, K., L. McNaughton, and M. Matthews. A systematic review into the efficacy of static stretching as part of a warm-up for the prevention of exercise-related injury. *Research in Sports Medicine* 16(3):213–231, 2008.

6. Rubin, D. I. Epidemiology and risk factors for spine pain. *Neurologic Clinics* 25(2):353–371, 2007.

7. Brackley, H. M., J. M. Stevenson, and J. C. Selinger. Effect of backpack load placement on posture and spinal curvature in prepubescent children. *Work* 32(3):351–360, 2009.

8. O'Hora, J., A. Cartwright, C. D. Wade, A. D. Hough, and G. L. K. Shum. Efficacy of static stretching and proprioceptive neuromuscular facilitation stretch on hamstrings length after a single session. *Journal of Strength and Conditioning Research* 25(6):1586–1591, 2011

9. Fasen, J. M., A. M. O'Connor, S. L. Schwartz, J. O. Watson, C. T. Plastaras, C. W. Garvan, C. Bulcao, S. C. Johnson, and V. Akuthota. A randomized controlled trial of hamstring stretching: Comparison of four techniques. *Journal of Strength and Conditioning Research* 23(2):660–667, 2009.

Chapter 6

1. Thompson, W. (Ed.). *ACSM'S Resource Manual for Guidelines for Exercise Testing and Prescription.* Philadelphia: Lippincott, Williams and Wilkins, 2009.

2. Kumanyika, S., and R. Brownson (Ed.). *Handbook of Obesity Prevention: A Resource for Health Professionals.* New York: Springer, 2010.

3. Rosen, L., and E. Rossen. *Obesity 101.* New York: Springer, 2011.

4. Cook, C., and D. Schoeller. Physical activity and weight control. *Current Opinion in Clinical Nutrition and Metabolic Care* 14:419–424, 2011.

5. Hu, F. *Obesity Epidemiology.* New York: Oxford Press, 2008.

6. Dubnov-Raz, G., and E. Berry. The dietary treatment of obesity. *Medical Clinics of North America* 95:939–952, 2011.

7. Bouchard, C., S. Blair, and W. Haskell (Eds.). *Physical Activity and Health.* Champaign, IL: Human Kinetics, 2012.

8. Center for Disease Control. Statistics on obesity and overweight. 2012. http://www.cdc.gov/obesity/data/index.html.

9. Van Itallie, T. Health implications of overweight and obesity in the United States. *Annals of Internal Medicine* 103:983–988, 1985.

10. Frieden, T. Centers for Disease Control Annual Report, 2010.

11. Weight Control Information Network, National Institute of Diabetes and Digestive and Kidney Diseases, National Institutes of Health. http://win.niddk.nih.gov/statistics.

12. Stein, C., and G. Colditz. The epidemic of obesity. *Journal of Clinical Endocrinology and Metabolism* 89:2522–2525, 2004.

13. Hedley, A., C. Ogden, C. Johnson, M. Carroll, L. Curtin, and K. Flegal. Prevalence of overweight and obesity among US children, adolescents, and adults, 1999–2002. *Journal of the American Medical Association* 16:2847–2850, 2004.

14. Bouchard, C., A. Tremblay, J. Despres, et al. The response to long-term overfeeding in identical twins. *New England Journal of Medicine* 322:1477–1482, 1990.

15. Stunkard, A., T. Sorensen, C. Hanis, et al. An adoption study of human obesity. *New England Journal of Medicine* 314:193–198, 1986.

16. Kohl, H., and T. Murray. *Foundations of Physical Activity and Public Health.* Champaign, IL: Human Kinetics, 2012.

17. Health implications of obesity: National Institutes of Health consensus development conference. *Annals of Internal Medicine* 103:977–1077, 1985.

18. Diabetes Prevention Research Group. Impact of intensive lifestyle and Metformin therapy on cardiovascular disease risk factors in the diabetes prevention program. *Diabetes Care* 28:888–894, 2005.

19. Wing, R. R., E. Venditti, J. M. Jakicic, B. A. Polley, and W. Lang. Lifestyle intervention in overweight individuals with a family history of diabetes. *Diabetes Care* 21:350–359, 1998.

20. Cohen, T., and M. Esther. Depressed mood and concern with weight and shape in normal women. *International Journal of Eating Disorders* 14:223–227, 1993.

21. Kirkcaldy, B. D., M. Eysenck, A. F. Furnham, and G. Siefen. Gender, anxiety, and self-image. *Personality and Individual Differences* 24:677–684, 1998.

22. Mokdad, A. H., M. K. Serdula, W. H. Dietz, B. A. Bowman, J. S. Marks, and J. P. Koplan. Prevalence of obesity, diabetes, and obesity-related health risk factors, 2001. *Journal of the American Medical Association* 289:76–79, 2003.

23. McGinnis, J. M., and W. H. Foege. Actual cases of death in the United States. *Journal of the American Medical Association* 270:2207–2212, 1993.

24. Howley E., and Thompson D. *Fitness Professional's handbook.* Champaign, IL: Human Kinetics, 2012.

25. DiGirolamo, M. Body composition—roundtable. *Physician and Sports Medicine* 14:144–162, 1986.

26. Van Itallie, T. Topography of body fat: Relationship to risk of cardiovascular and other diseases. In *Anthropometric Standardization Reference Manual,* T. Lohman et al. (Eds.). Champaign, IL: Human Kinetics, 1988.

27. Powers, S., and E. Howley. *Exercise Physiology: Theory and Application to Fitness and Performance,* 8th ed. New York: McGraw-Hill, 2012.

28. Jackson, A., and M. Pollock. Practical assessment of body composition. *Physician and Sports Medicine* 13:76–90, 1985.

29. Stunkard, A., and T. Wadden, eds. *Obesity: Theory and Therapy.* New York: Raven Press, 1993.

30. Lee, S., and D. Gallagher. Assessment methods in body composition. *Current Opinion in Clinical Nutrition and Metabolic Care* 11:566–572, 2008.

31. Dehghan, M., and A. Merchant. Is bioelectrical impedance accurate for use in large epidemiological studies? *Nutrition Journal* 7:26–35, 2008.

32. Rankinen, T., T. Rice, M. Teran-Garcia, D. Rao, and C. Brouchard. FTO genotype is associated with exercise training-induced changes in body composition. *Obesity* 18:322–326, 2010.

Chapter 7

1. Byrd, N. What gets measured is more likely to get done. *ACSM's Health and Fitness Journal* 15:26–29, 2011.

2. Fieger, H. *Behavior Change.* New York: Morgan James, 2009.

3. Howley, E., and D. Thompson. *Fitness Professional's Handbook.* Champaign, IL: Human Kinetics, 2012.

4. Baechle, T., and R. Earle. *Essentials of Strength Training and Conditioning.* Champaign, IL: Human Kinetics, 2008.

5. Powers, S., and E. Howley. *Exercise Physiology: Theory and Application to Fitness and Performance,* 8th ed. New York: McGraw Hill, 2012.

6. Earle, R., and T. Baechle. *NSCA's Essentials of Personal Training.* Champaign, IL: Human Kinetics, 2003.

7. Volpe, S. L. Can dogs help with maintaining motivation? *ACSM's Health and Fitness Journal* 15:36–37, 2011.

8. Pate, R. Overcoming barriers to physical activity: helping youth be more active. *ACSM's Health and Fitness Journal* 15:7–12, 2011.

9. Chaput, J. P., L. Klingenberg, and A. Sjodin. Do all sedentary activities lead to weight gain: sleep does not. *Current Opinion in Clinical Nutrition and Metabolic Care* 13:601–607, 2010.

10. Walsh, N. P., M. Gleeson, D. B. Pyne, D. C. Nieman, F. S. Dhabhar, R. J. Shephard, S. J. Oliver, S. Bermon, and A. Kajeniene. Position statement. Part 2: Maintaining immune health. *Exercise Immunology Review* 17:64–103, 2011.

11. Bonnet, M. H., and D. L. Arand. Clinical effects of sleep fragmentation versus sleep deprivation. *Sleep Medicine Reviews* 7:297–310, 2003.

12. Bonnet, M. H., and D. L. Arand. We are chronically sleep deprived. *Sleep* 18:908–911, 1995.

13. Kokkinos, P., H. Sheriff, and R. Kheirbek. Physical inactivity and mortality risk. *Cardiology Research and Practice* 2011:1–10, 2011.

14. Warburton, D. E., C. W. Nicol, and S. S. Bredin. Health benefits of physical activity: The evidence. *Canadian Medical Association Journal* 174:801–809, 2006.

15. Edwards, R. ABC of smoking cessation: The problem of smoking. *British Medical Journal* 328:217–219, 2004.

16. Doran, C. M., L. Valenti, M. Robinson, H. Britt, and R. P. Mattick. Smoking status of Australian general practice patients and their attempts to quit. *Addictive Behaviors* 31:758–766, 2005.

Chapter 8

1. Nutrition Business Journal. *NBJ's Supplement Business Report 2010*. http://newhope360.com/2010-supplement-business-report-0.

2. Mokdad, A. H., J. S. Marks, D. F. Stroup, and J. L. Gerberding. Actual causes of death in the United States, 2000. *Journal of the American Medical Association* 291(10):1238–1245, 2004.

3. Byrd-Bredbenner, C., G. L. Moe, D. Beshagetoor, and J. R. Berning. *Wardlaw's Perspectives in Nutrition*, 7th ed. Columbus, OH; McGraw-Hill, 2009.

4. Jenkins, D., C. Kendall, and V. Vuksan. Viscous fibers, health claims, and strategies to reduce cardiovascular disease risk. *American Journal of Clinical Nutrition* 71(2):401–402, 2000.

5. Tucker, K. L. Dietary intake and coronary heart disease: A variety of nutrients and phytochemicals are important. *Current Treatment Options in Cardiovascular Medicine* 6(4):291–302, 2004.

6. Dragsted, L. O., A. Pedersen, A. Hermetter, S. Basu, M. Hansen, G. R. Haren, M. Kall, V. Breinholt, J. J. Castenmiller, J. Stagsted, J. Jakobsen, L. Skibsted, S. E. Rasmussen, S. Loft, and B. Sandstrom. The 6-a-day study: Effects of fruit and vegetables on markers of oxidative stress and antioxidant defense in healthy nonsmokers. *American Journal of Clinical Nutrition* 79(6):1060–1072, 2004.

7. Powers, S., and E. Howley. *Exercise Physiology: Theory and Application to Fitness and Performance*, 8th ed. New York: McGraw-Hill, 2012.

8. Karppanen, H., and E. Mervaala. Sodium intake and hypertension. *Progress in Cardiovascular Disease* 49(2):59–75, 2006.

9. Food and Nutrition Information Center, U.S. Department of Agriculture. *Dietary Reference Intakes (DRI) and Recommended Dietary Allowances (RDA)*. http://www.nal.usda.gov/fnic.

10. Keen, R. Osteoporosis: Strategies for prevention and management. *Best Practice and Research Clinical Rheumatology* 21(1):109–122, 2007.

11. Jones, N. L., and K. J. Killian. Exercise limitation in health and disease. *New England Journal of Medicine* 343(9):632–641, 2000.

12. Tipton, K. D., and R. R. Wolfe. Exercise, protein metabolism, and muscle growth. *International Journal of Sport Nutrition and Exercise Metabolism* 11(1):109–132, 2001.

13. Lemon. P. W., J. M. Berardi, and E. E. Noreen. The role of protein and amino acid supplements in the athlete's diet: Does type or timing of ingestion matter? *Current Sports Medicine Reports* 1(4):214–221, 2002.

14. Lukaski, H. C. Vitamin and mineral status: Effects on physical performance. *Nutrition* 20(7–8):632–644, 2004.

15. Young, I. S., and J. V. Woodside. Antioxidants in health and disease. *Journal of Clinical Pathology* 54(3):176–186, 2001.

16. Powers, S. K., K. C. DeRuisseau, J. Quindry, and K. L. Hamilton. Dietary antioxidants and exercise. *Journal of Sports Sciences* 22(1):81–94, 2004.

17. Food Safety Policy, Science, and Risk Assessment: Strengthening the Connection: Workshop Proceedings (2001), Institute of Medicine. Washington, DC: National Academy Press, 2001.

Chapter 9

1. Centers for Disease Control. Obesity at a Glance, 2011. http://www.cdc.gov/chronicdisease/resources/publications/AAG/obesity.htm.

2. Hu, F. *Obesity Epidemiology*. New York: Oxford University Press, 2008.

3. American Society for Metabolic and Bariatric Surgery. News release: Bariatric Surgical Society Takes on New Name, New Mission and New Surgery. August 22, 2007. http://www.asbs.org/Newsite07/resources/press_release_8202007.pdf.

4. Thompson, W. (Ed.). *ACSM'S Resource Manual for Guidelines for Exercise Testing and Prescription*. Philadelphia: Lippincott, Williams and Wilkins, 2009.

5. Raloff, J. Still hungry? Fattening revelations—and new mysteries—about the hunger hormone. *Science News Online* 167: April 2, 2005.

6. Morton, G., D. Cummings, D. Baskin, G. Barsh, and W. Schwartz. Central nervous system control of food intake and body weight. *Nature* 443:289–295, 2006.

7. Trayhurn, P., and C. Bing. Appetite and energy balance signals from adipocytes. *Philosophical Transactions of the Royal Society* 361:1237–1249, 2006.

8. deKloet, A., and S. Woods. Molecular neuroendocrine targets for obesity therapy. *Current Opinion in Endocrinology, Diabetes, and Obesity* 17:441–445, 2010.

9. Fry, M., and A. Ferguson. Ghrelin: Central nervous system sites of action in regulation of energy balance. *International Journal of Peptides* 616757:1–8, 2010.

10. Kraemer, R. R., and V. D. Castracane. Exercise and humoral mediators of peripheral energy balance: Ghrelin and adiponectin. *Experimental Biology and Medicine* 232:184–194, 2007.

11. Stensel, D. Exercise, appetite, and appetite-regulating hormones: Implications for food intake and weight control. *Annals of Nutrition and Metabolism* 57:36–42, 2010.

12. Cummings, D. E., D. S. Weigle, R. S. Frayo, P. A. Breen, M. K., Ma, E. P. Dellinger, and J. Q. Purnell. Plasma ghrelin levels after diet-induced weight loss or gastric bypass surgery. *New England Journal of Medicine* 346:1623–1630, 2002.

13. Powers, S., and E. Howley. *Exercise Physiology: Theory and Application to Fitness and Performance*, 8th ed. New York: McGraw-Hill, 2012.

14. Thorogood, A., S. Mottillo., A. Shimony, K. Fillion, L. Joseph, J. Genest, L. Pilote, P. Poirier, E. Schiffrin, and M. Eisenberg. Isolated aerobic exercise and weight loss: A systematic review and meta-analysis of randomized controlled studies. *American Journal of Medicine* 124:747–755, 2011.

15. Ismail, L., S. Keating, M. Baker, and N. Johnson. A systematic review and meta-analysis of the effect of aerobic vs. resistance exercise training on visceral fat. *Obesity Reviews* 13:68–91, 2012.

16. Power, M., and J. Schulkin. *The Evolution of Obesity*. Baltimore, MD: John Hopkins University Press. 2009.

17. Melanson, E., P. MacLean, and J. Hill. Exercise improves fat metabolism in muscle but does not increase 24-h fat oxidation. *Exercise and Sport Science Reviews* 37:93–101, 2009.

18. Steelman, G. and E. Westman (Eds.). Obesity: Evaluation and treatment essentials. *Informa Healthcare*, 2010.

19. Sharkey, B., and S. Gaskill. *Fitness and Health*. Champaign, IL: Human Kinetics, 2006.

20. Ross, R., J. Freeman, and I. Janssen. Exercise alone is an effective strategy for reducing obesity and related comorbidities. *Exercise and Sport Sciences Reviews* 28(4):165–170, 2000.

21. Jakicic, J., et al. ACSM position stand: Appropriate intervention strategies for weight loss and prevention of weight regain for adults. *Medicine and Science in Sports and Exercise* 33:2145–2156, 2001.

22. Broeder, C., K. Burrhus, L. Svanevik, and J. Wilmore. The effects of either high intensity resistance or endurance training on resting metabolic rate. *American Journal of Clinical Nutrition* 55:802–810, 1992.

23. Romijn, J., E. Coyle, L. Sidossis, et al. Regulation of endogenous fat and carbohydrate metabolism in relation to exercise and duration. *American Journal of Physiology* 265:E380–E391, 1993.

24. Yeomans, M. Alcohol, appetite, and energy balance: Is alcohol intake a risk for obesity? *Physiology of Behavior* 100:82–89, 2010.

25. Stallknecht, B., F. Dela, and J. Helge. Are blood flow and lipolysis in subcutaneous adipose tissue influenced by contractions in adjacent muscles in humans? *American Journal of Physiology* 292:394–399, 2007.

26. Weight-Control Information Network. *Gastrointestinal Surgery for Severe Obesity*. NIH Publication No. 04-4006. December 2004. http://win.niddk.nih.gov/publications/gastric.htm.

27. American Psychiatric Association. APA Expert Opinion: Pauline S. Powers, MD. http://healthyminds.org. Accessed July 2007.

28. Office on Women's Health, U.S. Department of Health and Human Services. Eating Disorders. February 2000. http://www.womenshealth.gov/body-image/eating-disorders.

29. Johnson, R., M. Segal, Y. Sautin, T. Nakagawa, D. Feig, D. Kang, M. Gersh, S. Benner, and L. Sanchez-Lozada. Potential role of sugar (fructose) in the epidemic of hypertension, obesity and the metabolic syndrome, diabetes, kidney disease, and cardiovascular disease. *American Journal of Clinical Nutrition* 86:899–906, 2007.

30. Samuel, V. Fructose induced lipogenesis: From sugar to fat to insulin resistance. *Trends in Endocrinology and Metabolism* 22:60–65, 2011.

31. Stanhope, K. Role of fructose-containing sugars in the epidemics of obesity and metabolic syndrome. *Annual Review of Medicine* 63:19.1–19.15, 2012.

32. Wolff, E., and M. Dansinger. Soft drinks and weight gain: How strong is the Link? *Medscape Journal of Medicine* 10:89–97, 2008.

33. Johnson, R. J., and R. Murray. Fructose, exercise, and health. *Current Sports Medicine Reports* 9:253–258, 2010.

34. Onakpoya, I., R. Perry, J. Zhang, and E. Ernst. Efficacy of calcium supplementation for management of overweight and obesity: Systematic review of randomized clinical trials. *Nutrition Reviews* 69:335–343, 2011.

35. Manore, M. Dietary supplements for improving body composition and reducing body weight: Where is the evidence? *International Journal of Sport Nutrition and Exercise Metabolism* 22:139–154, 2012.

36. Jeukendrup, A., and R. Randell. Fat burners: Nutrition supplements that increase fat metabolism. *Obesity Reviews* 12:841–851, 2011.

37. Sherer, E., and J. Sherer. Examining the most popular weight loss diets: How effective are they? *Journal of the American Academy of Physician Assistants* 21:31–34, 2008.

38. Dansinger, M., J. Gleason, and J. Griffith, H. Selker, and E. Schaefer. Comparison of the Atkins, Ornish, Weight Watchers, and Zone diets for weight loss and heart disease risk reduction. *Journal of American Medical Association* 293:43–53, 2005.

39. Gardner, C., A. Kizzand, S. Alhassan, S. Kim, R. Stafford, R. Balise, H. Kraemer, and A. King. Comparison of the Atkins, Zone, Ornish, and LEARN diets for change in weight and related risk factors among overweight premenopausal women. *Journal of American Medical Association* 297:969–977, 2007.

40. Shai, I., D. Schwarzfuchs, et al. Weight loss with a low carbohydrate, Mediterranean, or low-fat diet. *New England Journal of Medicine* 359:229–241, 2008.

41. Sachs, F., G. Bray, et al. Comparison of weight-loss diets with different compositions of fat, protein, and carbohydrates. *New England Journal of Medicine* 360:859–873, 2009.

Chapter 10

1. American Heart Association. Heart disease and stroke statistics—2012 update. *Circulation* 125:e2–e220, 2012.

2. Trogdon, P., O. Khavjou, J. Butler, K. Dracup, M. Ezekowitz, et al. Forecasting the future of cardiovascular disease in the United States: A policy statement from the American Heart Association. *Circulation* 123:933–944, 2011.

3. Centers for Disease Control and Prevention. Heart Disease and Stroke Prevention: At a Glance, 2011. http://www.cdc.gov/chronicdisease/resources/publications/AAG/dhdsp.htm.

4. Powers, S., and E. Howley. *Exercise Physiology: Theory and Application to Fitness and Performance*, 8th ed. New York: McGraw-Hill, 2012.

5. Powers, S., Z. Murlasits, M. Wu, and A. Kavazis. Ischemia-reperfusion-induced cardiac injury: A brief review. *Medicine and Science in Sports and Exercise* 39:1529–1536, 2007.

6. American Cancer Society. *Fifty Most Often Asked Questions about Smoking and Health and the Answers*. New York: American Cancer Society, 1990.

7. Pollack, M., and D. Schmidt. *Heart Disease and Rehabilitation*. Champaign, IL: Human Kinetics, 1995.

8. Durstine, J. L., and R. Thompson. Exercise modulates blood lipids and exercise plan. *ACSM's Health and Fitness Journal* 4(4):44–46, 2000.

9. Third report of the National Cholesterol Education Program Expert Panel on Detection, Evaluation, and Treatment of High Blood Cholesterol in Adults. *Journal of the American Medical Association* 285(19): 1–19, 2001.

10. Thomas, T., and T. LaFontaine. Exercise, nutritional strategies, and lipoproteins. In *ACSM's Resource Manual for Guidelines for Exercise Testing and Prescription*, 4th ed., J. Roitman (Ed.). Philadelphia: Lippincott Williams & Wilkins, 2001.

11. Morris, J., J. Heady, P. Raffle, C. Roberts, and J. Parks. Coronary heart disease and physical activity of work. *Lancet* 2:1053–1057, 1953.

12. Blair, S. N., H. W. Kohl, R. S. Paffenbarger, D. G. Clark, K. H. Cooper, and L. W. Gibbons. Physical fitness and all-cause mortality: A prospective study of healthy men and women. *Journal of the American Medical Association* 262:2395–2401, 1989.

13. American Heart Association. Risk Factors and Coronary Heart Disease, 2012. http://www.americanheart.org.

14. Paffenbarger, R. S., R. T. Hyde, A. L. Wing, and C. C. Hsieh. Physical activity, all-cause mortality of college alumni. *New England Journal of Medicine* 314:605–613, 1986.

15. Kohl, H. Physical activity and cardiovascular disease: Evidence for a dose-response. *Medicine and Science in Sports and Exercise* 33(Suppl.): S472–S483, 2001.

16. Powers, S., J. Quindry, and A. Kavazis. Exercise-induced cardioprotection against myocardial ischemia-reperfusion injury. *Free Radical Biology and Medicine* 44:193–201, 2008.

17. Wood, P. Physical activity, diet, and health: Independent and interactive effects. *Medicine and Science in Sports and Exercise* 26:838–843, 1994.

18. Durstine, J., and W. Haskell. Effects of training on plasma lipids and lipoproteins. *Exercise Reviews* 22:477–521, 1994.

19. Batty, G., and I. Lee. Physical activity and coronary heart disease. *British Medical Journal* 328:1089–1090, 2004.

20. Zalesin, K., B. Franklin, W. Miller, E. Peterson, and P. McCullough. Impact of obesity on cardiovascular disease. *Medical Clinics of North America* 95:919–937, 2011.

21. Asplund, K., J. Karvanen, S. Giampaoli, P. Jousilahti, et al. Relative risks for stroke by age, sex, and population based on a follow-up of 18 European populations in the Morgam projection. *Stroke* 40: 2319–2326, 2009.

22. Lee, I., C. Hsieh, and R. Paffenbarger. Exercise intensity and longevity in men: The Harvard Alumni Health Study. *Journal of American Medical Association* 273:1179–1184, 1995.

23. Lee, Y., K. Min, E. Talbert, A. Kavazis, A. Smuder, W. Willis, and S. K. Powers. Exercise protects cardiac mitochondria against ischemia-reperfusion injury. *Medicine and Science in Sports and Exercise* 44:397–405, 2012.

24. Quindry, J., K. Hamilton, J. French, Y. Lee, Z. Murlasits, N. Tumer, and S. Powers. Exercise-induced HSP-72 elevation and cardioprotection against infarct and apoptosis. *Journal of Applied Physiology* 103:1056–1062, 2007.

25. Powers, S., J. Quindry, and A. Kavazis. Exercise-induced cardioprotection against myocardial ischemia-reperfusion injury. *Free Radical Biology and Medicine* 44:193–201, 2008.

26. Gotto, A. Statins: Powerful drugs for lowering cholesterol. *Circulation* 105:1514–1516, 2002.

27. Bybee, K., J. Lee, and J. O'Keefe. Cumulative clinical trial data on atorvastatin for reducing cardiovascular events: The clinical impact of atorvastatin. *Current Medical Research Opinion* 24:1217–1229, 2008.

28. Franklin, B. Aspirin for the primary prevention of cardiovascular events: Considerations regarding the risk/benefit. *Physician and Sports Medicine* 38:158–161, 2010.

29. Thompson, P. D., et al. Exercise and acute cardiovascular events placing the risks into perspective: A scientific statement from the American Heart Association Council on Nutrition, Physical Activity, and Metabolism and Council on Clinical Cardiology. *Circulation* 115:2358–2368. 2007.

Chapter 11

1. Canon, W. *The Wisdom of the Body*. New York: Norton Publishing, 1963.

2. Selye, H. *The Stress of Life*, rev. ed. New York: McGraw-Hill, 1978.

3. Friedman, M., and R. H. Rosenman. Type A behavior pattern: Its association with coronary heart disease. *Annals of Clinical Research* 3(6):300–312, 1971.

4. Knox, S. S., G. Wiedner, A. Adelman, S. M. Stoney, and R. C. Ellison. Hostility and physiological risk in the National Heart, Lung, and Blood Institute Family Heart Study. *Archives of Internal Medicine* 164(22): 2442–2448, 2004.

5. DeFruyt, F., and J. Denollet. Type D personality: A five factor model perspective. *Psychology and Health* 17(5): 671–683, 2002.

6. Albus, C., J. Jordan, and C. Herrmann-Lingen. Screening for psychosocial risk factors in patients with coronary heart disease: Recommendations for clinical practice. *European Journal of Cardiovascular Rehabilitation* 11(1):75–79, 2004.

7. Kessler, R. C., W. T. Chui, O. Demler, K. R. Merikangas, and E. E. Walters. Prevalence, severity, and comorbidity of 12-month DSM-IV disorders in the National Comorbidity Survey Replication Study. *Archives of General Psychiatry* 62:590–592, 2005.

8. American Psychological Association Help Center. May 2007. How Does Stress Affect Us? http://www.apahelpcenter.org.

9. Weil, A. Stress and Relaxation: An Introduction. June 2007. http://www.drweil.com/drw/u/id/ART00534.

10. Margen, S., et al. (Eds.). *The Wellness Encyclopedia*. Boston: Houghton Mifflin, 1992.

11. Lovallo, W. R. *Stress and Health: Biological and Psychological Interactions*. Thousand Oaks, CA: Sage Publications, 1997.

12. McEwen, B. S. Allostasis and allostatic load: Implications for neuropsychopharmacology. *Neuropsychopharmacology* 22:108–124, 2000.

13. Abercrombie, H., et. al. Flattened cortisol rhythms in metastatic breast cancer patients. *Psychoneuroendocrinology* 29(8):1082–1092, 2004.

14. Holroyd, K. A., et al. Management of chronic tension-type headache with tricyclic antidepressant medication, stress management therapy, and their combination: A randomized trial. *Journal of the American Medical Association* 285(17):2208–2215, 2001.

15. Howley, E., and B. D. Franks. *The Fitness Professional's Handbook*, 5th ed. Champaign, IL: Human Kinetics, 2007.

16. Petruzzello, S. J., D. M. Landers, B. D. Hatfield, K. A. Kubitz, and W. Salazar. Meta-analysis on the anxiety-reducing effects of acute and chronic exercise: Outcomes and mechanisms. *Sports Medicine* 11:143–182, 1991.

17. Tsai, J. C., et al. The beneficial effects of tai chi chuan on blood pressure and lipid profile and anxiety status in a randomized controlled trial. *Journal of Alternative Complementary Medicine* 9(5):747–754, 2003.

18. Rocha, K. K., A. M. Ribeiro, K. C., Rocha, F. S. Albuquerque, S. Ribeiro, and R. H. Silva. Improvement in physiological and psychological parameters after 6 months of yoga practice. *Consciousness and Cognition*. [Epub ahead of print] 2012. http://www.ncbi.nlm.nih.gov/pubmed/22342535.

19. Oliver, S., and D. Alfermann. Effects of physical exercise on resources evaluation, body self-concept and well-being among older adults. *Anxiety, Stress, and Coping* 15(3):311–320, 2002.

20. Breus, M. J., and P. J. O'Connor. Exercise-induced anxiolysis: A test of the "time out" hypothesis in high anxious females. *Medicine and Science in Sports and Exercise* 30(7):1107–1112, 1998.

21. Dishman, R. K. and P. J. O'Connor. Lessons in exercise neurobiology: the The case of endorphins. *Mental Health and Physical Activity* 2:4–9, 2009.

Photo Credits

Glossary

A

adaptations Semipermanent changes that occur over time with regular exercise. Adaptations can be reversed when a regular exercise program is stopped for an extended period of time.

adenosine triphosphate (ATP) A high-energy compound that is synthesized and stored in small quantities in muscle and other cells. The breakdown of ATP results in a release of energy that can be used to fuel muscular contraction.

adipose tissue Tissue where fat is stored in the body.

aerobic "With oxygen"; in cells, pertains to biochemical pathways that use oxygen to produce energy.

aerobic exercise A common term to describe all forms of exercises that primarily use the aerobic energy system and that are designed to improve cardiorespiratory fitness.

air displacement A technique used to assess body composition by estimating body volume based on air displaced when a person sits in a chamber.

allostasis The ability to maintain homeostasis through change.

allostatic load The inability to respond appropriately to stress; leads to compromised health.

alveoli Tiny air sacs in the lungs that receive carbon dioxide and other wastes from oxygen-depleted blood.

amino acids The building blocks of protein. There are 20 different amino acids that can be linked in various combinations to create different proteins.

anaerobic "Without oxygen"; in cells, pertains to biochemical pathways that do not require oxygen to produce energy.

android pattern A pattern of fat distribution characterized by fat stored in the abdominal region; more common in men.

anemia Deficiency of red blood cells and/or hemoglobin that results in decreased oxygen-carrying capacity of the blood.

anorexia nervosa An eating disorder in which a person severely restricts caloric intake because of an intense fear of gaining weight.

antagonist The muscle on the opposite side of a joint.

antioxidants Molecules that neutralize free radicals, thereby preventing them from causing damage to cells.

arrhythmia An irregular heartbeat.

arteries The blood vessels that carry blood away from the heart.

arteriosclerosis A group of diseases characterized by a narrowing, or "hardening," of the arteries.

atherosclerosis A special type of arteriosclerosis that results in arterial blockage due to buildup of a fatty deposit (called *atherosclerotic plaque*) inside the blood vessel.

autonomic nervous system The branch of the nervous system that controls basic bodily functions that do not require conscious thought; includes the parasympathetic and sympathetic branches.

B

ballistic stretching A type of stretch that involves sudden and forceful bouncing to stretch the muscles.

binge eating disorder The compulsive need to gorge on food without purging.

bioelectrical impedance analysis (BIA) A method of assessing body composition by running a low-level electrical current through the body.

body composition The relative amounts of fat and fat-free mass in the body.

body composition The relative amounts of fat and fat-free tissue (muscle, organs, bone) found in the body.

body mass index (BMI) A ratio of body weight (kg) divided by height squared (m^2) used to determine whether a person is at a healthy body weight; BMI is related to the percentage of body fat.

Borg Rating of Perceived Exertion (RPE) A subjective way of estimating exercise intensity based on a numerical scale of 6 to 20.

bulimia nervosa An eating disorder that involves overeating (called *binge eating*) followed by vomiting (called *purging*).

burnout The loss of physical, emotional, and mental energy, which, if ignored, can lead to emotional exhaustion and withdrawal.

C

capillaries Thin-walled vessels that permit the exchange of gases (oxygen and carbon dioxide) and nutrients between the blood and tissues.

carbohydrate A macronutrient that is a key energy source for muscular contraction.

cardiac output The amount of blood the heart pumps per minute.

cardiorespiratory endurance A measure of the heart's ability to pump oxygen-rich blood to the working muscles during exercise and of the muscles' ability to take up and use the oxygen.

cardiovascular disease (CVD) Any disease of the heart and blood vessels.

cartilage A tough connective tissue that forms a pad on the end of long bones such as the femur, tibia, and humerus. Cartilage acts as a shock absorber to cushion the weight of one bone on another and to provide protection from the friction due to joint movement.

cholesterol A type of lipid that is necessary for cell and hormone synthesis. Found naturally in animal foods, but made in adequate amounts in the body.

complete proteins Proteins containing all the essential amino acids; found only in soy and animal foods (meats and dairy products).

complex carbohydrates Long chains of sugar units linked together to form starch or fiber.

concentric muscle action Action in which the muscle develops tension as it shortens against resistance and/or gravity. Also called *positive work*.

cool-down A 5- to 15-minute period of low-intensity exercise that immediately follows the primary conditioning period; sometimes called a *warm-down*.

coronary heart disease (CHD) Also called *coronary artery disease;* the result of atherosclerotic plaque blocking one or more coronary arteries (the blood vessels that supply the heart).

cortisol A hormone secreted by the outer layer (cortex) of the adrenal gland.

creeping obesity A slow increase in body weight and percentage of body fat over several years.

cross training The use of a variety of activities for training the cardiorespiratory system.

curl-up test A test to evaluate abdominal muscle endurance.

cycle ergometer A stationary exercise cycle that provides pedaling resistance so the amount of work can be measured.

D

Daily Values Standard values for nutrient needs, used as a reference on food labels. The Daily Values may not exactly reflect the true nutrient needs for all people.

diabetes A metabolic disorder characterized by high blood glucose levels that is associated with increased risk for heart disease, kidney disease, nerve dysfunction, and eye damage.

diabetes A metabolic disorder characterized by high blood glucose levels. Chronic elevation of blood glucose is associated with increased incidence of heart disease, kidney disease, nerve dysfunction, and eye damage.

distress Negative stress that is harmful to performance.

dual energy X-ray absorptiometry (DXA) A technique for assessing body composition using a low-radiation X-ray; it is typically used in research or clinical settings and is considered a gold-standard measure.

duration of exercise The amount of time invested in performing the primary workout.

dynamic stretching Stretching that involves moving the joints through the full range of motion to mimic a movement used in a sport or exercise.

E

eccentric muscle action Action in which the muscle develops tension as it lengthens while controlling the movement with gravity. Also called *negative work*.

endocrine system A series of glands and tissues in the body that secrete hormones to regulate bodily processes.

endorphins A group of hormones (endogenous opioids, or "painkillers") released during the stress response.

energy balance The state of consuming a number of calories that is equal to the number expended. Over the long term, energy balance results in maintenance of a constant body weight.

epinephrine A hormone secreted by the inner core (medulla) of the adrenal gland; also called *adrenaline*.

essential amino acids The nine amino acids that cannot be manufactured by the body and must therefore be consumed in the diet.

essential fat Body fat that is necessary for physiological functioning.

eustress A stress level that results in improved performance; also called *positive stress*.

exercise metabolic rate (EMR) The amount of energy expended during any form of exercise.

exercise prescription The individualized amount of exercise that will effectively promote physical fitness for a given person.

exercise Planned, structured, and repetitive bodily movement done to improve or maintain one or more components of fitness.

F

fascia A thin layer of connective tissue that surrounds the muscle.

fast-twitch fibers White muscle fibers that contract rapidly but fatigue quickly. These fibers have a low aerobic capacity and produce ATP anaerobically.

fats (triglycerides) The form of lipid that is broken down in the body and used to produce energy to power muscle contractions during exercise.

fatty acids The basic structural unit of triglycerides; they are important nutritionally not only because of their energy content, but also because they play a role in cardiovascular disease.

fiber A stringy, nondigestible complex carbohydrate found in whole grains, vegetables, and fruits.

fiber recruitment The process of involving more muscle fibers to increase muscular force.

fight-or-flight response A series of physiological reactions by the body to prepare to combat a real or perceived threat.

flexibility The ability to move joints freely through their full range of motion.

free radicals Oxygen molecules that can potentially damage cells.

frequency of exercise The number of times per week that one exercises.

G

general adaptation syndrome A pattern of responses to stress that consists of an alarm stage, a resistance stage, and an exhaustion stage.

ghrelin A hormone that contributes to feelings of hunger.

glucose A simple carbohydrate (sugar) that can be used/directly by the body. All other carbohydrates must be converted to glucose before being used for fuel.

glycemic index A ranking system for carbohydrates based on a food's effect on blood glucose levels.

glycogen The storage form of glucose in the liver and skeletal muscles.

glycolysis A process during which carbohydrates are broken down in cells. Much of the anaerobic ATP production in muscle cells occurs during glycolysis.

Golgi tendon organs The type of proprioceptor found within tendons.

gynoid pattern A pattern of fat distribution characterized by fat stored in the hips and thighs; more common in women

H

heart attack Stoppage of blood flow to the heart resulting in the death of heart cells; also called *myocardial infarction*.

heart rate reserve (HRR) The difference between your maximal heart rate and resting heart rate.

high-density lipoproteins (HDL) A combination of protein, fat, and cholesterol in the blood, composed of relatively large amounts of protein. Protects against the fatty plaque accumulation in the coronary arteries that leads to heart disease; also called "good" cholesterol.

hydrostatic weighing A method of determining body composition that involves weighing an individual on land and in a tank of water.

hyperplasia An increase in the number of muscle fibers.

hypertension High blood pressure.

hypertrophy An increase in muscle fiber size.

hypokinetic disease Disease associated with a lack of exercise.

I

incomplete proteins Proteins that are missing one or more of the essential amino acids; found in plant sources such as nuts and legumes.

insoluble fiber Type of fiber found in whole wheat and vegetables.

intensity of exercise The amount of physiological stress or overload placed on the body during exercise.

intermediate fibers Muscle fibers with a combination of the characteristics of fast- and slow-twitch fibers. They contract rapidly and are fatigue resistant because they have a well-developed aerobic capacity.

interval training Type of training that includes repeated sessions or intervals of relatively intense exercise alternated with lower-intensity periods to rest or recover.

irradiation The use of radiation (high-energy waves or particles, including radioactivity and X-rays) to kill microorganisms that grow on or in food.

isokinetic A type of exercise that can include concentric or eccentric muscle actions performed at a constant speed using a specialized machine.

isometric A type of exercise in which muscular tension is developed but the body part does not move. Also called *static* exercise.

isotonic A type of exercise in which there is movement of a body part. Most exercise or sports skills are isotonic exercise. Also called *dynamic* exercise.

K

kilocalorie The unit of measure used to quantify food energy or the energy expended by the body. Technically, a kilocalorie is the amount of energy necessary to raise the temperature of 1 gram of water 1°C. The terms *kilocalorie* and *calorie* are often used interchangeably.

L

lactic acid A by-product of glucose metabolism, produced primarily during intense exercise (i.e., greater than 50%-60% of maximal aerobic capacity).

leptin A hormone that appears to depress appetite.

ligaments Connective tissues within the joint capsule that hold bones together.

lipids A group of insoluble compounds that include fats and cholesterol.

lipoproteins Combinations of protein, triglycerides, and cholesterol in the blood that are important because of their role in influencing the risk of heart disease.

low-density lipoproteins (LDL) A combination of protein, fat, and cholesterol in the blood, composed of relatively large amounts of cholesterol. LDLs promote the fatty plaque accumulation in the coronary arteries that leads to heart disease; also called "bad" cholesterol.

M

macronutrients Carbohydrates, fats, and proteins, which are necessary for building and maintaining body tissues and providing energy for daily activities.

maintenance phase The third phase of an exercise program. The goal of this phase is to maintain the increase in strength obtained during the first two phases.

maintenance program Exercising to sustain a desired level of physical fitness.

meditation A method of relaxation that involves sitting quietly, focusing on a word or image, and breathing slowly.

micronutrients Vitamins and minerals. Micronutrients are involved in many body processes, including regulating cell function.

minerals Chemical elements (e.g., sodium and calcium) that are required by the body in small amounts for normal functioning.

mode of exercise The specific type of exercise to be performed.

motor unit A motor nerve and all of the muscle fibers it controls.

muscle action The shortening of a skeletal muscle (causing movement) or the lengthening of a skeletal muscle (resisting movement)

muscle spindles The type of proprioceptor found within muscle.

muscular endurance The ability of a muscle to generate a submaximal force over and over again.

muscular strength The maximal ability of a muscle to generate force.

N

nonessential amino acids Eleven amino acids that the body can make and are therefore not necessary in the diet.

norepinephrine A hormone secreted by the inner core (medulla) of the adrenal gland.

nutrients Substances in food that are necessary for good health.

nutrition The study of food and the way the body uses it to produce energy and build or repair body tissues.

O

obese An excessive amount of fat in the body, typically above 25% for men and 35% for women.

omega-3 fatty acid A type of unsaturated fatty acid that lowers both blood cholesterol and triglycerides and is found abundantly in some fish.

1.5-mile run test One of the simplest and most accurate assessments of cardiorespiratory fitness.

one-repetition maximum (1 RM) test Measurement of the maximum amount of weight that can be lifted one time.

organic Plant or animal foods that are grown without the use of pesticides, chemical fertilizers, antibiotics, or hormones.

osteoporosis A condition that results from the loss of bone mass and strength.

osteoporosis Bone disease in which the mineral content of bone is reduced and the bone is weakened and at increased risk of fracture.

overload principle A basic principle of physical conditioning that states that in order to improve physical fitness, the body or specific muscles must be stressed.

overtraining The result of failure to get enough rest between exercise training sessions.

overweight A weight above the recommended level for health.

P

parasympathetic branch The division of the autonomic nervous system that is dominant at rest and controls the energy conservation and restoration processes.

phospholipid A type of lipid that contains phosphorus and is an important component of cell membranes.

physical activity Any movement of the body produced by a skeletal muscle that results in energy expenditure, especially through movement of large muscle groups.

principle of progression A principle of training that states that overload should be increased gradually.

principle of recuperation The body requires recovery periods between exercise training sessions to adapt to the exercise stress. Therefore, a period of rest is essential for achieving maximal benefit from exercise.

principle of reversibility The loss of fitness due to inactivity.

principle of specificity The effect of exercise training is specific to those muscles involved in the activity.

progressive resistance exercise (PRE) Application of the overload principle to strength and endurance exercise programs.

proprioceptive neuromuscular facilitation (PNF) A series of movements combining stretching with alternating contraction and relaxation of muscles.

proprioceptor Specialized receptor in muscle or tendon that provides feedback to the brain about the position of body parts.

pulmonary circuit The vascular system that circulates blood from the right side of the heart, through the lungs, and back to the left side of the heart.

push-up test A fitness test designed to evaluate endurance of shoulder and arm muscles.

R

range of motion The amount of movement possible at a joint.

responses The changes that occur during exercise to help you meet the demands of the exercise session. These changes return to normal levels shortly after the exercise session.

resting energy expenditure The amount of energy expended during all sedentary activities. Also called *resting metabolic rate.*

S

saturated fatty acid A type of fatty acid that comes primarily from animal sources and is solid at room temperature.

set The number of repetitions performed consecutively without resting.

shaping Breaking a behavior or task into small steps to accomplish the larger goal.

shoulder flexibility test A fitness test that measures the ability of the shoulder muscles to move through their full range of motion.

sit-and-reach test A fitness test that measures the ability to flex the trunk.

sit-up test A test to evaluate abdominal and hip muscle endurance.

skinfold test A field test used to estimate body composition; representative samples of subcutaneous fat are measured using calipers to estimate the overall level of body fat.

slow progression phase The second phase of an exercise program. The goal of this phase is to increase muscle strength beyond the starter phase.

slow-twitch fibers Red muscle fibers that contract slowly and are highly resistant to fatigue. These fibers have the capacity to produce large quantities of ATP aerobically.

soluble fiber Viscous fiber found in oats, barley, peas, and citrus fruits.

specificity of training The concept that the development of muscular strength and endurance, as well as cardiorespiratory endurance, is specific to both the muscle group exercised and the training intensity.

Stages of Change Model A framework for understanding how individuals move toward adopting and maintaining health behavior changes.

starches Long chains of glucose units; commonly found in foods such as corn, grains, and potatoes.

starter phase The beginning phase of an exercise program. The goal of this phase is to build a base for further physical conditioning.

static stretching Stretching that slowly lengthens a muscle to a point where further movement is limited.

sterol A type of lipid that does not contain fatty acids; cholesterol is the most commonly known sterol.

storage fat Excess fat reserves stored in the body's adipose tissue.

stress A state of physical and mental tension in response to a situation that is perceived as a threat or challenge.

stress response The physiological and behavioral changes that take place when a person is presented with a stressor.

stressor A factor that produces stress.

stretch reflex Involuntary contraction of a muscle due to rapid stretching of that muscle.

stroke Brain damage that occurs when the blood supply to the brain is reduced for a prolonged period of time.

stroke volume The amount of blood pumped per heartbeat (generally expressed in milliliters).

subcutaneous fat Fat stored just beneath the skin.

sympathetic branch The division of the autonomic nervous system that is in control when we need to react or respond to challenges; the excitatory branch.

systemic circuit The vascular system that circulates blood from the left side of the heart, throughout the body, and back to the right side of the heart.

T

target heart rate (THR) The range of heart rates that corresponds to an exercise intensity of approximately 50%–85% $\dot{V}O_2$max. This is the range of training heart rates that results in improvements in aerobic capacity.

ten percent rule The training intensity or duration of exercise should not be increased by more than 10% per week.

tendons A fibrous connective tissue that attaches muscle to bone.

threshold for health benefits The minimum level of physical activity required to achieve some of the health benefits of exercise.

training threshold The training intensity above which there is an improvement in cardiorespiratory fitness. This intensity is approximately 50% of $\dot{V}O_2$max.

trans fatty acid A type of fatty acid that increases cholesterol in the blood and is a major contributor to heart disease.

U

unsaturated fatty acid A type of fatty acid that comes primarily from plant sources and is liquid at room temperature.

V

Valsalva maneuver Breath holding during an intense muscle contraction; can reduce blood flow to the brain and cause dizziness and fainting.

veins The blood vessels that transport blood toward the heart.

visceral fat Fat stored in the abdomen and around the organs.

visualization A relaxation technique that uses appealing mental images to promote relaxation and reduce stress; also called *imagery*.

vitamins Micronutrients that play a key role in many body functions, including the regulation of growth and metabolism. They are classified according to whether they are soluble in water or fat.

$\dot{V}O_2$ max The maximum amount of oxygen the body can take in and use during exercise.

W

waist-to-hip ratio A ratio of the waist and hip circumferences used to determine the risk for disease associated with the android pattern of obesity.

warm-up A brief (5- to 15-minute) period of exercise that precedes a workout.

wellness The state of healthy living achieved by the practice of a healthy lifestyle, which includes regular physical activity, proper nutrition, eliminating unhealthy behaviors, and maintaining good emotional and spiritual health.

Index

('b' indicates boxed material; 'f' indicates a figure;
't' indicates a table)